THE NEW
LIVING
HEART

THE NEW LIVING HEART

Michael E. DeBakey, MD
Antonio M. Gotto, Jr., MD, DPhil

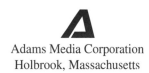

Adams Media Corporation
Holbrook, Massachusetts

Published by Adams Media Corporation
260 Center Street, Holbrook, MA 02343

ISBN: 1-55850-722-1

Printed in the United States of America.

J   I   H   G   F   E   D   C   B

Library of Congress Cataloging-in-Publication Data
DeBakey, Michael E. (Michael Ellis),
The new living heart / Michael E. Debakey, Antonio M. Gotto.
p.   cm.
ISBN 1-55850-722-1 (pb)
1. Cardiovascular system—Diseases—Popular works. 2. Heart—Diseases—Popular works. I. Gotto, Antonio M. II. Title.
RC672.D413   1997
616.1—dc21   97–365
CIP

This publication is designed to provide accurate and authoritative information with regard to the subject matter covered. It is sold with the understanding that the publisher is not engaged in rendering professional medical advice. If assistance is required, the services of a competent professional person should be sought.

This book is available at quantity discounts for bulk purchases.
For information, call 1-800-872-5627 (in Massachusetts, 617-767-8100).

Visit our home page at http://www.adamsmedia.com

Contents

Foreword

Heart disease before the age of 80 is not God's will, but due to our own faults.
Paul Dudley White

Therapeutics is of two types: that which promotes strength in the healthy, and that which alleviates disorders.
Charaka Samhita (1000 B.C.)

Heart diseases have been the leading cause of death in the United States for many decades. Although considerable progress has been made in the battle against these diseases, and although public concern about them has been eclipsed by the fear of other conditions such as AIDS and some cancers, they remain by far the main avenue to the grave in our country. One American dies from a heart disease approximately every 30 seconds, and one from a heart attack every minute.

Because of their greater longevity, more women than men die from heart diseases. Nevertheless, many, many American men and women die prematurely from them.

Years of successful research supported by a strong commitment from the public and from political leaders have yielded very significant progress. The death rate from all cardiovascular diseases today is only 45 percent of what it was in 1963; the cerebrovascular disease death rate decreased 65 percent while that from heart attack decreased 58 percent during that period of time. In fact, the increased life expectancy of the American population is largely due to the reduction in death rates from cardiovascular diseases.

In examining the reasons for this magnificent success—which is the envy of many other countries—it became clear that the improvements are largely due to better therapeutic modalities, which have increased the survival of heart disease patients. At the same time, the emergence of a "prevention culture" in the United

States has resulted in a slight decrease in the incidence of some heart diseases, especially heart attacks, and often delayed their occurrence and minimized their morbidity.

We would be remiss, however, if we allowed these successes to overshadow the problems that remain with us and the new problems that are emerging.

Clearly, our vigilance must not diminish; in fact, it must increase because we have in hand opportunities and approaches to confront the problems and to successfully reduce their burden. That is what this book is all about.

Throughout its chapters, the book gives the reader the most recent information about the heart and how it functions in health and disease. It discusses the cause and characteristics of the most common heart diseases and explains their therapeutic options.

Woven through this information is the thread that will lead to future success. Today, we have the tools and the ideas to keep the heart healthy and to fight diseases, if and when they occur. However, the battle cannot be waged only by physicians; it also requires the understanding and the willingness of the patients. Fortunately, today's public—both healthy and ill—is eager to know and to learn about health issues and to establish a partnership with the physicians. This volume is presented and written to help achieve that goal. In a way its title, *The New Living Heart,* symbolizes the

prospects before us—the public, the patients, and the physicians.

Scientific pursuits are extraordinarily productive and in most instances almost immediately applicable, that is, they directly benefit the patients. The field of cardiovascular disease is full of excitement and promise that have captured the enthusiasm of researchers and clinicians working in this area. The book's descriptions of the new developments in cardiovascular knowledge and therapeutic options convey this excitement powerfully. The readers, be they health care professionals or laypersons, will see that we are on the threshold of new and significant developments ranging from gene therapy or genetic substitution to total heart replacement.

However, this new and promising knowledge cannot be fully exploited without patient-physician partnership. This was implied by Paul Dudley White, the father of modern cardiology, when he said, "Heart disease before the age of 80 is not God's will, but due to our own faults." What this really says is that if we, the public, the persons who may become heart disease patients, know about these diseases, know about the therapeutic options, and know about the trade-offs that are necessary, we can curtail or forestall, if not eliminate, some of the consequences of these diseases. If the public, the patient, appreciates the power and potential of partnership with physicians, this will result in a stronger collaboration and, more importantly, in a better outcome.

Although this concept of patient-physician partnership is not new, the message here takes on a renewed, if not unique, strength because of the stature of those who deliver it.

Doctors Michael F. DeBakey and Antonio M. Gotto, Jr. are international figures in medicine. They bring into this book years of worldwide recognized successes in medical care, in biomedical research, and in medical education. In addition, both have been leaders in prevention; their practice has been to "promote strength in the healthy and [to] alleviate disorders."

Michael DeBakey is unquestionably the father of cardiovascular surgery as we know it today. During the last 50 years, no revolutionary new surgical procedure in this field has emerged with which his name is not associated, either as a developer or as a perfecter! Nearly all the world's cardiovascular surgeons have either been trained or influenced by him. Yet, his vision of medicine and the impact he has had on it are best established by the fact that his love for surgery has never obscured his greater love for prevention and good health, as well as his compassion for patients. And so, no voice could be stronger in talking about *The New Living Heart.*

Antonio Gotto, Jr. is another force that has driven the effort to overcome heart diseases in the most significant and successful manner. His early research led him to discover risk factors for heart diseases and to apply this knowledge to the prevention and treatment of some of these disorders. Medical communities throughout the world recognize his approach, and this led him to become our medical ambassador. Dr. Gotto is a true pioneer in his own right who has had, and continues to have, a remarkable impact on the cardiovascular health of this nation.

Surely, it was no accident that Drs. DeBakey and Gotto decided to combine their interests and talents. This is clearly an association that is much, much stronger than the sum of its components, and the public and the patients are the beneficiaries of this association. This book presents a new opportunity for people to help themselves if their cardiovascular health begins to fail. As one who has had the opportunity to witness the changing state of cardiovascular disease in this country and elsewhere for many years, I applaud this effort. I believe that *The New Living Heart* will bring better cardiovascular health to all.

Claude Lenfant, MD
Director
National Heart, Lung, and Blood Institute
Bethesda, Maryland

Preface

Heart Disease in the United States, as well as in Europe, Russia, and China, is by far the most common cause of death. Indeed, it accounts for more deaths than all other diseases combined. Well over one million people die annually, or more than 2,500 daily, from cardiovascular disease in the United States. About 60 million Americans have one or more forms of cardiovascular disease, and about 5 million Americans alive today have coronary artery disease. One in four people suffer from some form of heart disease, and the economic drain, in cost of treatment and loss of productivity, approaches 50 billion dollars. These facts and figures emphasize the magnitude and gravity of this disease and underscore the need for concerted efforts to effectuate its control. Toward that goal much can be done by individual persons along with members of their families, if they would apply available knowledge to reduce and even eliminate some of the risk factors that contribute to this disease. It is the purpose of this book to provide the lay reader with this knowledge and with a better understanding of the various specific conditions comprising cardiovascular disease and their current therapeutic modalities.

During the past half century, truly momentous progress has been made—greater than in all previously recorded history—in our understanding of mechanisms (biochemical, physiologic, molecular biologic, and genetic processes) involved in disease of the heart and blood vessels. Similar progress has been made in the medical and surgical treatment, as well as in prevention, of these disorders. This has ensued from the intensification and expansion of medical research, largely supported by the National Institutes of Health beginning in the late 1940s and early 1950s. Much credit for this truly humanitarian endeavor belongs to imaginative leadership in Congress and the Administrations that recognized, along with the public, that medical research was essential for the control and elimination of disease.

The term heart disease often strikes terror in the patient and the family, but this is unnecessarily alarming in a substantial proportion of cases. Because the term is imprecise and all-encompassing, it can often be misleading. For this reason, it is important to understand, and indeed to learn, that there are a number of different types of diseases of the heart and blood vessels. In actual fact, about three-fourths of all diseases under the term cardiovascular or heart disease, are diseases of the arteries. The term heart attack, for example, is caused by occlusive disease of the coronary arteries that supply blood to the heart and is usually due to arteriosclerosis or atherosclerosis. A similar type of atherosclerotic blockage of the arteries supplying blood to the brain is a common cause of stroke. This same type of disease affecting the arteries supplying blood to the legs can result in walking disability and even gangrene. In addition, arteriosclerosis may cause weakening of the wall of the aorta and major arteries, resulting in a ballooning out (aneurysmal formation) that can lead to rupture and fatal hemorrhage. There are, of course, certain specific diseases of the heart itself, such as heart muscle weakness (termed cardiomyopathy), diseases of the valves of the heart, and congenital anomalies, all of which can lead to heart failure. In this book, we have endeavored to provide the reader with a more specific definition and description of the various forms of diseases of the heart and blood vessels, along with current knowledge about their management, which has greatly improved in recent years.

Arteriosclerosis or atherosclerosis, commonly referred to as "hardening of the arteries," is the most common underlying pathologic process in cardiovascular disease. Although the terms arteriosclerosis and atherosclerosis are of relatively recent origin, the former having been coined by Jean-Frederic-Martin Lobstein, Professor of Pathological Anatomy in Strasbourg (1829–33), and the latter by Felix Marchaud of Leipzig in 1904, the disease was prevalent in ancient times, as demonstrated by studies of arterial specimens of Egyptian mummies (1580 B.C. to A.D. 525) reported in 1911 by Marc Armand Ruffler. Whereas extensive studies have been made on the pathologic features of the disease during the past several hundred years, only during the past half century, and indeed during the past few decades, has there evolved a much better understanding of the initiation and progressive development of the disease. This has led to a growing recognition of factors contributing to its development, such as abnormally high cholesterol in the blood, high blood pressure, and smoking, whose control or elimination can reduce the risk of the disease. These factors are discussed in great detail in the text dealing with this disease.

It has also been demonstrated that the disease tends to assume distinctive patterns, with the occlusive lesions being well localized in certain segments of the arterial bed, with relatively normal patent portions of the artery above and below the diseased segment. This constitutes the basis for effective surgical treatment, consisting in restoration of normal circulation by one of several surgical technical procedures.

Still another important observation concerning the disease is that its rate of development or progression varies considerably from patient to patient. In some, for example, the disease tends to progress slowly over long periods, as much as 10 to 20 years, whereas in others it may progress rapidly, causing serious consequences within a few years. In most patients, however, it tends to progress moderately over a period of 5 to 7 years. There are now some reasons to believe that the rate of progression can be modified or can even be made to regress by specific regimen, as described in the text.

Significant progress has also been made in the development of diagnostic procedures that are not only precise, but are also relatively simple and noninvasive, such as Doppler ultrasonography and echocardiography, both based on the principle of ultrasound. Also now available are radionuclide scintigraphy and computed tomography (CT). These highly sophisticated diagnostic imaging technologic developments make it possible virtually to see through the body and observe the actual function of the heart and blood vessels and to obtain precise measurements that readily demonstrate any abnormality.

The diagnosis of heart disease should no longer be an alarming report. In most patients, considerable improvement, and even cure, can be anticipated. The steady decline in the mortality rate for stroke and coronary artery disease, about 50 and 40 percent, respectively, during the past three decades, is a reflection of this encouraging news. Whereas there still remain some forms of heart disease for which little or nothing can be done at present, in most cases today highly effective medical and surgical treatment can enable patients to resume a normal life and begin preventive regimens that can help sustain it.

Almost 20 years ago, we published a book called *The Living Heart* to provide the layman with a better understanding of heart disease. The book was prompted by inquiries from our patients and members of their families who wanted more information about their condition in a readily available and convenient form. The response to that book was highly gratifying. Since then, substantially greater advances have been made in this field, and the present book incorporates these new developments. It thus provides the layman with a still better understanding of heart disease, with special emphasis on the many different diseases of the heart and blood vessels and the therapeutic procedures for each of them, including a preventive regimen that can help maintain better health.

There is no intent to present a comprehensive treatise or textbook on cardiovascular disease; such texts are readily available to the medical community. This book is intended to provide the lay reader, in a succinct but compendious form, current knowledge about the more common forms of the disease, and particularly those for which the most can be done in treatment and prevention. The selection of historical material is based on relevance of the material to an understanding of current concepts of cardiovascular problems. It is our hope that this book will supplement the physician's judgment and recommendations by providing the patient and other interested people with a better understanding of the problem. We are convinced that an informed public is more capable of addressing and resolving problems, and we therefore hope that this book will provide such enlightenment about heart disease.

Acknowledgments
Michael E. DeBakey, MD

I wish to express my grateful appreciation to Selma DeBakey, Professor of Scientific Communication at Baylor College of Medicine, for her invaluable editorial counsel. I am also grateful to Dr. James Young for the preparation of the chapters on Controlling Arrhythmias and on Advanced Heart Failure and to Dr. John Winikates for the preparation of the chapter on Medical Aspects of Stroke. My thanks, also, to Bronwyn Wallace for her diligent preparation of the manuscript and her attention to grammatical and mechanical aspects of the text. Finally, I should like to express grateful appreciation to Mr. Herbert R. Smith, Jr. for the lucid illustrations, which not only supplement the text, but also provide the reader with a much better understanding of it.

Michael E. DeBakey, MD
Chancellor Emeritus
Olga Keith Wiess and Distinguished Service Professor of Surgery
Director, DeBakey Heart Center
Baylor College of Medicine, Houston, Texas 77030

Acknowledgments
Antonio M. Gotto, Jr., MD, DPhil

I wish to express my deep appreciation to Lynne W. Scott, M.A., R.D., for her guidance and counsel, to Beth W. Allen, M.A., for her editorial support, and to Suzanne Simpson, B.A., for her excellent medical editing. Carol V. Bryce, B.S., and Marianne Doran, M.A., helped guide the project to completion. Jesse Y. Jou, B.A., served as a valuable editorial assistant, and Daphna Gregg helped in the early stages.

Many colleagues provided invaluable insight and comments, in particular John Farmer, M.D., and also James K. Alexander, M.D., Christie M. Ballantyne, M.D., Chu-Huang Chen, M.D., Ph.D., G. Kenneth Goodrick, Ph.D., Bassem El-Masri, M.D., Ryan Neal, M.D., David P. Via, Ph.D., Dennis W. Zhu, M.D., Georgia White, R.N., Bobby Griffin, and Joan Seidel, R.N., C.N.S., C.C.R.N.

Jan Redden, M.S., Sharon D. Carmichael, M.S., Carl G. Clingman, M.A., Carol Pienta Larson, C.M.I., and Bharat Parikh of the Department of Medical Illustration and Audiovisual Education at Baylor College of Medicine worked to help produce drawings and photographs for the text. Barbara Hatton efficiently managed typing and other technical tasks.

All these professionals brought their individual gifts to this project, contributing talent, time, and energy beyond what was required. For this, I acknowledge my debt and gratitude and applaud their performance.

Antonio M. Gotto, Jr., MD, DPhil
Provost for Medical Affairs
Stephen and Suzanne Weiss Dean
Cornell University Medical College
New York, New York

CHAPTER ONE

Introduction: Early Knowledge of the Heart

The organs of the body might be likened to a series of working engines. For example, the heart, which is linked to all of them, is a two-stage stroke pump. The liver and the intestines refine the fuels used by the body's engines. The kidneys, lungs, intestines, and liver are sanitation units, disposing of potential pollutants, wastes, or the refuse left after fuel is consumed. From the air, the lungs mine oxygen, a vital component required by any internal combustion engine. The central nervous system serves as a computer, programming the work demanded by the body's engines and monitoring the level of performances.

The human body is not a self-contained apparatus—outside supplies of food, oxygen, and water must be brought into the body to stoke the machinery. An ecologic efficiency, however, characterizes bodily functions. Blood cells, for example, nourish the tissues, which in turn help produce new blood cells. The heart keeps the digestive organs alive, and these, in turn, reciprocate. Worn-out cells are broken

down, and some elements are salvaged and recycled back into the system. For this reason, too, in any consideration of heart disease, it is important to realize that the heart itself is but a link in a complex machine known as the cardiovascular system (Figure 1.1) and is itself a part of the infinitely more complex microcosm constituting the whole individual.

To the ancients, this chain of organs beneath the skin posed as much of a mystery as the world that lay beyond, a few days' journey from their homeland. One of the first scholars to begin to clarify knowledge about the structure of the heart and other organs was the Alexandrian physician Erasistratus, who recorded his observations of dissected animals and human beings 2,300 years ago. To be sure, the cave paintings made by our ancestors some 20,000 years ago depicted the heart in its proper position on the outlines of the bison and elephant they hunted; its shape was much like the stylized heart we see today on St. Valentine's Day. Undoubtedly,

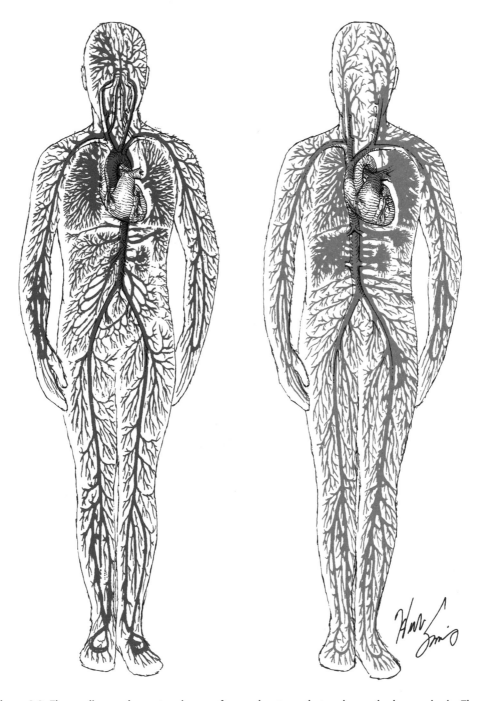

Figure 1.1. The cardiovascular system is one of several systems that make up the human body. The arteries carry bright red oxygenated blood from the heart to the various tissues of the body. Veins then carry the bluish blood back to the heart, which then pumps it through the lungs for a fresh supply of oxygen.

they had an idea of its vital nature. It was not, however, until the time of the Greeks that their more enlightened religious and philosophical outlook permitted anatomic studies to be undertaken on man himself.

Before the time of the Greeks, disease was attributed more often to supernatural than to natural causes. Indeed, during the early years of Greek history, medical care was often provided by the priest, who specialized as a healer. Much earlier than this, treatment of "disease" became separated because an understanding of the supernatural was not needed to explain the occurrence of a simple wound. This distinction between surgeons and physicians continued for many hundreds of years, and we find the barber-surgeon active during the Middle Ages and the Renaissance. Hippocrates, the great Greek physician, had a keen eye for physical diagnosis and compiled the first descriptions of many ailments that we know today. He recognized that diseases run a course, ascribing sickness to imbalance in the "humours" or juices of the body. Even today we talk of a "good humored" or a "bilious" person.

Probably because the Egyptians had earlier practiced the art of embalming and had removed some of the body's organs, Erasistratus was able to study some of the organs rather thoroughly. He discovered three pathways—*veins, arteries,* and *nerves** extending through the body. He also described the appearance of the heart and its valves fairly accurately. But, unable to grasp the notion of muscular tissue, Erasistratus decided the heart itself consisted of a conjunction of veins, arteries, and nerves. Obedient to the dogma of his predecessors, he accepted the theory that the arteries contained an air or spirit or soul, called "pneuma," which was replenished by breathing. The pneuma was supposed to enter the body through the nose, throat, and lungs. According to Erasistratus and other physicians of the time, the veins contained blood, which flowed along these pathways to feed the rest of the body. To Erasistratus, blood was found in arteries only after the surgeon cut the vessel open; as the pneuma rushed out, the blood poured into the empty space.

Erasistratus also pointed out specific changes in the organs of the dead that could be related to the cause of death. Four centuries later, the insights of Erasistratus were vastly reinforced by the power of Galen, the great physician of the Roman Empire, who was born a Greek in A.D. 130. Practicing in the Roman city of Perzmos in Asia Minor, Galen dissected the great apes and lesser animals brought to the gladiatorial ring by the roving Roman legions. He expanded anatomic knowledge enormously with his recognition of muscle as one of

---

* Definitions and/or explanations of the italicized words that appear throughout the text can be found either in the surrounding copy or in the glossary at the back of the book.

the substances that make up the human heart. He demonstrated that the arteries hold blood, not air, as Erasistratus had insisted. Galen even spoke of the movement of blood, although he asserted that the fluid in the arteries ebbed and flowed with the heart's pulsation. He viewed the liver as being the center of the circulation, rather than the heart.

Relying heavily on the correlation of experimental findings and careful clinical observations, Galen began to correlate function and structure. Like Erasistratus, he too proposed hypotheses about the way organs of the body work, based on what he had learned from his experiments. One hypothesis concerned the relation of the right and left ventricles, the two largest chambers of the heart. Galen hypothesized that tiny pores in the wall that separates these chambers permit blood to pass from the right side to the left, from whence it enters the arteries and passes throughout the body. Although he was in error, Galen was on the right track in his suggestion that blood moved from one side of the heart to the other. He was so highly regarded as a physician that his sugges-

tions were accepted as dogma until the time of William Harvey, who was not born until 1578, which was 1,448 years after Galen's birth. Galen is quoted as saying that ". . . if anyone desires to become famous, all that is necessary is to accept what I have established . . ." and ". . . never yet have I gone astray."

Between the era of Galen and the Renaissance was a period of dangerous decline in medical knowledge, particularly in the search for new knowledge. Although in Europe there were a few men who respected knowledge, they no longer searched for new information because they were convinced that everything had been revealed. Advancement of scientific and medical knowledge came to a halt. In Europe, Galen's theories, codified and made rigid, stood as the limits of information in medicine. Superstition and religion prohibited autopsies of the dead. Not until the thirteenth century at Bologna is there any record of dissection of the human body.

Fortunately, medical scholarship did not die out. A Christian sect, the Nestorians,[1] were proscribed as heretics and forced to flee eastward, carrying with

---

[1] Nestorians were named after Nestorius, appointed the Patriarch of Constantinople by Emperor Theodosius in 428. Nestorius outraged the Catholic world by opposing the use of the title Mother of God for the Virgin on the grounds that while the Father begot Jesus as God, Mary bore him as a man. This view was contradicted by Cyril, Patriarch of Alexandria, and both sides appealed to Pope Celestine I. In 431, the Council of Ephesus was convened to settle the matter, and the decision was made to excommunicate Nestorius and his followers. Nestorius was then deposed and exiled by Theodosius, who ordered the consecration of a new Patriarch of Constantinople.

them the whole of the Greek culture, that of medicine included. Reestablished in Persia, the cult flourished; a great medical school was established; and the works of Hippocrates, Galen, and many more were translated into Persian. As Persia was conquered by the Moslems, the whole of this culture was incorporated into the new Islamic culture. Great physicians founded hospitals; medical schools were established; new medical works began to appear; and new diseases were described. Physicians were respected as never before, regardless of their religion. When Europe was again prepared to receive its medical culture, it was ready and waiting, preserved by cultures in the East.

The Renaissance brought a new thirst for exploration. Along with daring voyages on the seas came a new breed of scientists peering into the mysteries of life. They soon found that the learning of the past was overly dogmatic; it had lost the very spirit of medical inquiry that brought greatness to Hippocrates and Galen, and fruitless theories had been exaggerated beyond all reason. One who dared to challenge the static dogma of Galen was the itinerant Swiss physician Paracelsus, the son of a physician. Success with notables brought his appointment as town physician at Basel, with the right to lecture at the university. Like so many of his predecessors, Paracelsus tried to create a philosophy that might explain birth, growth, and

death. Out of the depths of his own experiences, he rejected the theories of Hippocrates and Galen. To scholars at the university, Paracelsus thundered,

> We shall free it [medicine] from its worst errors, not by following that which those of old taught, but by our own observation of nature, confirmed by extensive practice and long experience. Who does not know that most doctors make terrible mistakes, greatly to the harm of their patients? Who does not know that this is because they cling too anxiously to the teachings of Hippocrates, Galen . . . .

To demonstrate his own independence, Paracelsus made a public bonfire of his personal collection of the teachings of Galen.

In an era when the Protestant Reformation had begun to dispute the dogma and works of the Roman Catholic Church, Paracelsus decided against the rebellion and remained in the Church. Nevertheless, because of his outspoken views, town authorities usually encouraged him to move on before he stayed very long, condemning him to a peripatetic existence much like the old Greek physicians. The life suited Paracelsus, however, and each town gave him something new to study and time to work on a new book, perhaps, before he moved on. In one town, Paracelsus saw miner's disease and described an occupational disease for the first time. In another he studied the mineral springs known for their health-giving qualities and wrote, again as a first, a book on balneotherapy. He introduced mercury for the treatment of syphilis, the only successful therapy for nearly 400 years, until Ehrlich introduced the arsenicals at the beginning of the twentieth century. He also had modern ideas about the natural care of wounds. So Paracelsus's legacy was to open the door to scientific study a crack wider; eventually most of his findings were published with their cryptic statements and self-coined words, full of hidden meanings for us to puzzle over.

In their pursuit of knowledge, Renaissance thinkers wandered from one discipline to another, their curiosity boosting them over the barriers that normally separate one field of thought from another. To the Renaissance scholar, botany, astronomy, physiology, mathematics, painting, poetry, and theology were all interrelated. If this led to the well-rounded man that we praise as the shining achievement of the Renaissance, it also posed a distinct threat to his survival, for the intertwining of empirical scientific knowledge with the dogma of theology can result in serious problems.

The Spaniard Michael Servetus (1511–1553), who was the first to describe the pulmonary circulation, provided a perfect illustration of the danger of combining scientific endeavor with theologic proclamation. Geographer, mathematician, astronomer, and part-time investigator of human anatomy, Servetus also showed an intense interest in religion. As a traveling scholar in Europe, he proclaimed that the God-sent spirit, so grandly infused by Galen into the veins and arteries of man, happened to be only air. Furthermore, in contradiction to Galen, Servetus wrote,

> The communication between right and left ventricle does not, as generally believed, take place through the mid-wall of the heart, but in a wonderful way the subtle blood is conducted through a long passage from the right ventricle to the lungs where it is rendered light, becomes bright red in color and passes from the vein-like artery (arteria venosa) into the artery-like vein (vena arteriosa), whence it is finally carried . . . into the left ventricle.

Servetus had offered an accurate description of the process by which blood becomes saturated with oxygen.

Servetus's revelations were, unfortunately, part of a book that attacked a variety of prevailing theologic dogmas. John Calvin, the Protestant reformer, proved he could be as fiery in zeal as the Roman Catholic Inquisitors, who had Servetus on their proscribed list. By order of Calvin, Servetus went to the stake along with his books. Although the scholar perished, he had succeeded in shedding an additional ray of light on the workings of the circulatory system.

The quest for knowledge, however, continued. The Flemish anatomist, Andreas Vesalius, born in Brussels in 1514 into a family of physicians, compiled a mammoth amount of anatomic information, based on his own dissections and the discoveries of others. As a boy, he dissected all the animals he could find. He went to Paris at age 18 to study anatomy, a field which was hampered by an edict of Pope Boniface VIII, in the 1300s, forbidding the cutting or dismemberment of dead bodies. The original intent of the edict had been to curb the practice during the Crusades of cutting off parts of the body, boiling the parts, and preserving them until they could be taken home and buried. An unintended consequence of the edict was to impair the study of anatomy. But in Paris the Renaissance was in full swing, and two great teachers, Winter of Andernach and Sylvius, became his special mentors; he performed many of the dissections for their classes.

He then went to Padua, where he obtained the degree of Doctor of Medicine "with highest distinction." On the following day, at the age of 23 years, he was appointed Professor of Anatomy and Surgery. His duties in this position included the teaching of anatomy and holding of public dissections. He pursued his subject with an enthusiasm that to a non-medical person might seem to border on the morbid. One day he noticed the intact skeleton of a man hanging from the gallows. Carrion eaters had picked the body clean of flesh. Vesalius immediately secured the "perfect" specimen. In his enthusiasm, Vesalius courted the local magistrates to obtain a convenient time for the execution and the right to perform dissections on the condemned. He did not hesitate at grave robbery, spiriting away the corpse of a monk's concubine and skinning it before the bereaved could search and recognize his deceased lover.

During the next five years, he worked on the monumental task of preparing an entirely new book of the complete anatomy of the human body based on his personal dissections. He was able to enlist an excellent artist, Jan Stefan van Calcar, also a native of Flanders and Titian's favorite pupil. Entitled *De Humani Corporis Fabrica,* a masterpiece of anatomic scholarship, the seven books were published in Basel in 1543, when the author was 28 years old (Figure 1.2).

This work constituted a major contribution to science and medicine because the knowledge of the anatomy of the human body is indispensable to any understanding of normal physiology or disease processes. Vesalius discovered and exposed more than 200 errors of Galen; this is easily understood today. Galen had written presumptuously about the anatomy of the monkey, and he himself made this clear, but in time, this fact was forgotten and Galen's anatomy was accepted as that of man. Vesalius's demonstration of so many errors of Galen's anatomy undermined the traditional authority vested in Galen's theories.

Lectures by Vesalius were like mob scenes with violent shouting and cheering, and along with his book, they made him a controversial figure. Attacks from pro-Galenic forces, including Vesalius's former teacher Sylvius, eventually caused him to become embittered and disillusioned. Vesalius retired from further academic pursuits and began practicing surgery, serving in several military campaigns. In the preface of his book addressed to "The Divine Charles V," the Emperor of Spain, whose physician he became after resigning his chair at Padua, he expressed his resentment and obvious bitterness against the physicians' attitude toward surgeons as follows:

> There in course of time the art of healing has been so wretchedly rent asunder that certain doctors, advertising themselves under the name of physicians, have arrogated to themselves alone the prescriptions of drugs and diet for obscure diseases, and have relegated the rest of medicine to those they call surgeons and scarcely regard as slaves, disgracefully banishing from themselves the chief and most ancient branch of the medieval art, and that which principally (if indeed there be any other) bases itself upon the investigation of nature.

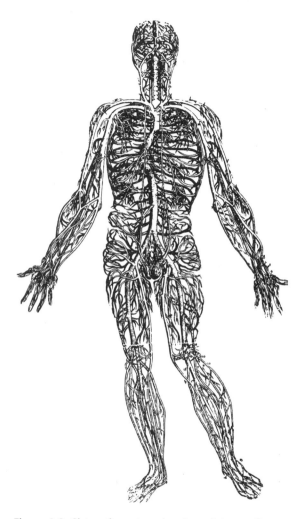

Figure 1.2. Sixteenth-century drawing of the cardio-vascular system from the book *De Humani Corporis Fabrica* by Andreas Vesalius (courtesy of the Bettmann Archive).

Vesalius's remarkable contribution to human anatomy, considered among the greatest of medical texts, revolutionized medicine and stimulated the development of pathology and physiology.

Surgical treatment of disease during the Middle Ages and Renaissance was limited by the lack of adequate information about human anatomy, and by the inability to control the loss of blood. Surgery was limited to very few procedures, such as pouring boiling metal or oil on wounds, excising skin tumors, and removing bladder stones. The work of barber-surgeons was supervised by a physician, who did not himself practice surgery but who had a degree.

An immediate result of the spread of the new knowledge of anatomy was a great forward step for surgery. The man person-ally associated with this advance was Ambroise Paré, a contemporary of Vesalius. Paré, born in 1510, had a great influence on the adoption of an humani-tarian approach to the surgical treatment of battlefield wounds and the control of bleeding. He arrived at the Hôtel Dieu near Notre Dame in Paris to become a surgeon. The Hôtel Dieu was used as a hospital, though it was actually an ancient hotel dating back to 660. The stench of dying and decaying flesh and the cries of the ill and near dead were overwhelming when Paré arrived. After working in this hospital for three years, he left to travel as personal surgeon to various aristocratic army offi-cers and eventually to the King of France.

One of the battle surgeon's greatest challenges was the treatment of gunshot wounds. On one occasion the casualty list was so long that Paré ran out of boiling oil and had recourse only to soothing salves.

Anxiously visiting the wounded the next day and expecting to find these patients either dead or dying, he was surprised to see that they were in better condition and in less pain than those treated with the boiling oil. Soon he abandoned the use of oil cautery entirely and used only salves, a number of which he concocted. One employed rose oil and egg yolk, and another contained 2 new-born puppies boiled alive, 1 pound of earthworms drowned in white wine, 2 pounds of oil of lilies, 16 ounces of Venetian turpentine, and 1 ounce of aqua vitae. Whereas these recipes might not have promoted healing, the results they yielded convinced Paré that the wounds healed better if they were not cauterized with burning oil, a treat-ment that not only was extremely painful but actually inflicted much additional damage to the tissues of the poor soldiers. Paré used humanitarian arguments in support of his new treatment with salves.

Another major surgical contribution of Paré was the reintroduction of the control of bleeding by tying off the damaged blood vessel. Paré used forceps to pick up the vessel and then secured it with a liga-ture. This relatively simple procedure was a giant advance in the application of surgical technique. Incidentally, ligatures to tie off blood vessels were used and clearly described approximately 1,500 years earlier and were subsequently abandoned, to be revived by Paré. The procedure was precisely described both by Aulus Aurelius Cornelius Celsus in his *De Re Medica Libra Octo* (*Eight Books on Medicine*) published in A.D. 30 and by Galen (A.D. 130–199), who even told where to obtain the "Celtic linen thread" that he used for this purpose—at a shop between "the Temple of Rome and the Forum."

As a better knowledge of human anatomy led to surgical advances, it gave rise to one of the most significant discoveries in the history of medicine. As a student of medicine at Padua some 50 years after Vesalius made his mark there, William Harvey, appropriately enough,

studied under Hieronymus Fabricius, then at the height of his power and fame as Professor of Anatomy.

Although Fabricius accepted the entire Galenic system, he provided a key to the discovery of the circulation of the blood with his study on the valves of the veins, showing that they permitted only one-way flow to the heart. A famous sketch by Harvey shows the effect of the finger pressure upon a vein in the arm (Figure 1.3). When pressure is applied, the vein collapses on the side of the pressure point closer to the heart, an action that demonstrates that the blood in the veins flows toward the heart.

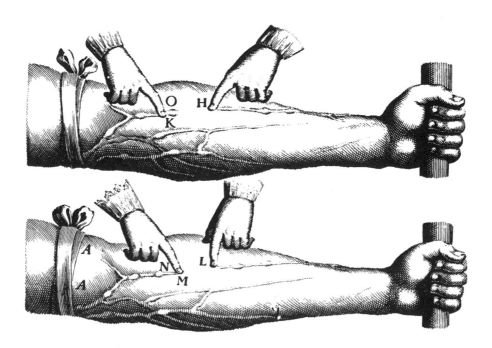

Figure 1.3. Classic drawing by William Harvey showing that the valves of the veins permit only one-way flow toward the heart (courtesy of the Bettmann Archive).

Harvey returned from Padua to London to practice medicine, but actually spent most of his time studying the circulation of the blood. He was small in stature and independent in character, working virtually in isolation. The prevailing theory of the circulation at that time was that there are two kinds of blood that ebb back and forth between the arteries and the veins like a tide.

Harvey's younger contemporary, the chemist and philosopher Robert Boyle, who promulgated the laws regarding gases, once asked Harvey what inspired him to concentrate upon the heart and the circulatory system. Boyle said of the reply:

> He answer'd me that when he took notice that the Valves in the Veins of so many several Parts of the Body, were so plac'd that they gave free passage to the Blood Towards the Heart, but oppos'd the passage of the Venal blood the Contrary way: He was invited to imagine that so Provident a Cause as Nature had not so Plac'd so many Valves without design: and no Design seem'd more probable, than that, since the Blood could not well, because of the interposing Valves, be sent by the Veins to the limbs, it should be sent through the Arteries, and return through the Veins, whose Valves did not oppose its course that way.

Harvey studied cold-blooded animals because their circulatory systems seemed to work considerably slower than those of warm-blooded ones. He observed that the transparent body walls of small shrimp, taken from the sea and the Thames River, permitted him to see heart action while the subject lived. He also watched the earliest development of a chick heart in a hen's egg, where the tiny drop of blood actually disappears during the *systolic phase* of heart action (contraction of the heart), only to reappear slightly larger, visible to the naked eye, during the *diastolic phase* (relaxation of the heart). Harvey discovered that the function of the heart is the same in all animals, that is, to pump blood, but that the anatomic structures of the heart and circulatory system differ in various species.

In one of his more conclusive studies, Harvey tied off the *aorta*, the main channel of blood from the heart, of a fish. He watched the aorta become bloated above the ligature as the dammed blood expanded the walls of the vessel. He then tied off the *inferior vena cava*, the main channel bringing blood back to the heart, and saw the lower half of the vessel swell with the accumulation of blood. In the aorta and its branching arteries, the blood flows from the heart to the distant parts of the body; in the veins, it flows back to the heart.

A simple exercise in logic made his point about the circularity of the cardiovascular system. Harvey calculated that each beat of the heart expels about two fluid ounces of blood, or 8,400 ounces per hour. Since this much blood adds up to three times the weight of an average person, the only explanation for this volume of blood was that the same six quarts of fluid were constantly circulating within the same closed system in the body.

Harvey conclusively demonstrated that blood alone travels through the arteries and veins. He demolished the Galenic notion that the heartbeat and respiration were identical twins and that the air seeped into the body by means of the pores.

> For, if pulsation and respiration serve the same purposes, and if [as is commonly stated] in diastole the arteries take air into their cavities and in systole expel sooty vapours through the same pores of flesh and skin; further, if between systole and diastole they contain air, and at any given time air or spirits or sooty vapours, what answer can those holding such views make to Galen, who wrote in his book that the arteries normally contain blood and nothing but blood, certainly no spirits or air, as one can readily ascertain from his experiments, and from his arguments in that book? . . . as all arteries, deep as well as cutaneous, are distended simultaneously and at equal speed, how will air be able to pass so freely and rapidly through skin, flesh and body fabric into the depths as it will through the skin alone?

Harvey's major achievement was not his destruction of the dogma of the ancients, but his conception of the heart

and blood as elements within a closed, circulating system. He described the path of blood into the right side of the heart, then to the lungs and the rest of the body. He concluded that the force driving the blood through the arteries comes from the pumping action of the heart, which alternately contracts and relaxes. The arteries contain no "air or spirits or sooty vapours" but just blood, which is returned to the heart in its rest phase through the veins. This cycle is then repeated time and time again throughout a lifetime. A few years later, it remained for successors Marcello Malpighi and Antonius van Leeuwenhoek, with the aid of a new tool, the microscope, to describe the tiniest blood vessels, *capillaries* and *venules,* and to report the final link in the system.

Harvey was able to carry out his research while he was physician-in-chief to St. Bartholomew's Hospital in London. He treated patients and consulted with other physicians at the hospital one day a week. Most of the remainder of the time he devoted to his research. Harvey's discoveries, published in *De Motu Cordis* (*The Motion of the Heart*), brought him no immediate acclaim. Instead, people began to doubt his clinical ability. A contemporary reported that Harvey suffered an immediate decline in the number of patients he treated as a result of the "strange theories" he proposed. Another physician ridiculed, "Anatomy is no further necessary to the surgeon than the knowledge of the nature of wood to a carpenter or of stone to a stone cutter." Perhaps the best indication of the times is exemplified by an assignment Harvey performed six years after he described the circulation of blood. Along with 6 other surgeons, 10 midwives, and a lecturer on anatomy, Harvey served on a panel that examined 4 women accused of witchcraft. Stubbornly adhering to the science of empirical anatomy, Harvey found none of the extra organs or accessories with which folklore endowed witches. The women were spared the stake.

Eventually, the world did honor Harvey. He was elected President of the College of Physicians, but declined the honor. Harvey's genius explained more than the route followed by the blood stream. He conceived of the heart, lungs, and blood vessels as an interdependent system. What Harvey recognized then holds true today—that which is labelled heart disease may not lie in the actual heart but in other areas of the anatomy, and especially in the arterial system. And even if the problem happens to be within the heart itself, it is of little value to be described simply as heart disease, for the cure and care depend upon a more precise diagnosis. Treatment demands knowledge of exactly what segment of the heart is injured and what the threat is to the entire cardiovascular system.

With Harvey's discovery of the circulatory system, the study of anatomy was once again undertaken with a new perspective. Such studies, conducted by the great surgeon and anatomist John Hunter (1728–1793), gave rise to the field of surgical pathology, which opened doors to new knowledge about changes in the body's tissues when diseased. Here, at last, was a study of disease or pathologic processes as they affect the body's organs and tissues.

There are many other milestones in medical knowledge after Harvey that are relevant to the treatment of heart disease. Among these, three are particularly important because of their great significance in surgery. The first is the development and use of anesthetics during surgery; the second is the introduction of the concept of antisepsis and asepsis to control and prevent wound infection; and the third is the advance of the knowledge of blood groups, which led to the successful introduction of blood transfusion.

An anesthetic was first used by Crawford Williamson Long of Jefferson, Georgia, who had witnessed "ether frolics" at the University of Pennsylvania. On March 30, 1842, he removed a tumor from the neck of a patient with use of ether anesthesia, but he did not report it until 1846. The method, however, gained general acceptance and worldwide adoption after its successful demonstration by W. T. G. Morton, a Boston dentist, on a patient with a vascular tumor of the neck that was removed by John Collins Warren at Massachusetts General Hospital on October 17, 1846.

The second important contribution, namely, the concept of antisepsis and asepsis, was made by Joseph Lister, who, as a young Glasgow surgeon, recognized the significance of the earlier discovery by Louis Pasteur in 1862—the existence of bacteria. Lister reasoned that it was these minute organisms suspended in the atmosphere that were responsible for wound infection. He stated, ". . . it occurred to me that decomposition of the injured part might be avoided without excluding the air, by applying as a dressing some material capable of destroying life of the floating particles." Lister then used carbolic acid as a carbolized dressing and as a spray to prevent infection, with considerable success. His first publication on this antiseptic method appeared in 1876, but these early reports were met with indifference and even violent opposition—mostly by his British colleagues, interestingly enough. During the next 20 years, Lister continued to work at perfecting the method, accumulating impressive evidence of its validity. Eventually, it gained worldwide acceptance, and thus greatly expanded the horizons of surgery.

A third major advance was the transfusion of whole blood to replace loss of blood during surgery or after trauma or burns. Early on, man had learned the danger of severe blood loss, or hemorrhage. It is a curious thing that the removal of blood from a vein, called bloodletting or venesection, gained acceptance by physicians more than 4,000 years ago as a therapeutic method for many forms of disease. Both Hippocrates and Galen strangely subscribed to this mode of therapy. Galen prescribed the removal of one-half to one and one-half pints of blood. In some parts of the world, bloodletting was used until relatively recent times. Blood transfusions, on the other hand, were not successfully used until the twentieth century.

To be sure, historical references to blood transfusion may be found as early as the fifteenth century, particularly after the discovery of circulation by William Harvey in 1628.[2] Experiments were performed on animals and, in a few cases, lambs' blood was transfused into humans. Although some success was recorded, the fatalities that occurred created much opposition and led to legal prohibition of the procedure throughout most of Europe. Not until the nineteenth century was there a revival of interest in blood transfusion. Various investigations, mostly of a tech-

[2] Robert A. Kilduffe and Michael E. DeBakey: *The Blood Bank and the Technique and Therapeutics of Transfusions.* (St. Louis: C.V. Mosby Co., 1942).

nical nature, were carried out, and a few actual transfusions were performed on humans with some success, but the major obstacles of serious and even fatal complications resulting from incompatible blood, hindered its adoption and widespread use.

This problem was solved by the monumental, pioneering work of K. Landsteiner, a German scientist, in 1900. In brief, Landsteiner discovered that humans can be divided into different *blood groups*, which are determined by the presence of certain factors on the red blood cells and in the individual's serum. Some blood groups are compatible with each other for purposes of transfusion, whereas others are not. It was not until the problems of incompatibility of blood were solved that blood transfusions could be used therapeutically.

Subsequent significant developments in this field include the use of sodium citrate to facilitate blood storage by preventing clotting, advances in blood preservation, and the establishment of blood banks for matching and storing blood and its components.

It is important to be aware of the fact that many patients with cardiovascular disease before the twentieth century were doomed with no hope for any kind of treatment. Before World War II, no effective treatment was known for vascular disease, such as aneurysms and occlusive disease, and prior to the era of open heart surgery (1953), no effective treatment was available for many forms of congenital and acquired cardiac disease. There were no antibiotics for treating or preventing *bacterial endocarditis, rheumatic fever, streptococcal infections,* and *cardiovascular syphilis.* Effective drug treatment for control of high blood pressure has become available only in recent times.

Today the most prevalent form of cardiovascular disease that the physician encounters is that affecting the coronary arteries (the affliction that probably killed John Hunter during a fit of anger). There has been considerable disagreement as to whether the frequency of coronary artery disease has actually increased in the twentieth century. We suspect that it has. *Angina pectoris,* or chest pain, which is a symptom of coronary artery disease, was clearly described by William Heberden in an article entitled, "Some Account of a Disorder of the Breast," published in the *Medical Transactions of the Royal College of Physicians of London* in 1772. Heberden, however, did not realize that angina pectoris was associated with disease of the coronary arteries; this was discovered later by William Jenner. In 1812, John Warren wrote about angina pectoris in the first issue of the new publication, *The New England Journal of Medicine.* Some patients with angina pectoris were noted to die suddenly during an attack. The cause was usually given as acute indigestion. One of the most important papers ever written on this subject, "Clinical Features of Sudden Obstructions of the Coronary Arteries," was published by James Herrick in the *Journal of the American Medical Association* in 1912. Though the paper was largely ignored for several years, it clearly related obstruction of the coronary arteries to chest pain, and in some instances, sudden death. Another important treatise relating angina pectoris to coronary artery disease is that of C. S. Keefer and W. H. Resnik in the *Archives of Internal Medicine* (1928) entitled, "Angina Pectoris: A Syndrome Caused by Anoxemia of the Myocardium."

To return to the question of whether heart disease is becoming more frequent or whether it is being more accurately diagnosed, we refer to the experience in New York of Austin Flint, who wrote in 1866 that he observed only 7 cases of angina pectoris in more than 150 patients with organic heart disease. It is unlikely that a physician as astute a clinician as Flint would have failed to diagnose angina pectoris had it been as common as it is today. Other causes of disease and deaths from disease, including various forms of severe infection, were far more common prior to the era of antimicrobial therapy. This is reflected, along with other causes of early death, in the survival expectancy. Thus, the survival expectancy in 1900 was 47 years, and now it is 76 years. Since arteriosclerosis is more common in the elderly, and since the proportion of the elderly in our population is increasing, it follows that arterial occlusive disease is actually increasing.

CHAPTER TWO

The Healthy Heart and How It Works

Look at your fist and you'll see an approximation of the size of your heart. In appearance, the heart more closely resembles a thick cone than the conventional valentine representation. A normal adult heart weighs about 11 ounces, although in a highly trained athlete it may be as much as a pound. This center of the cardiovascular system sits between the lungs, with its top tilted toward the right side of the body (Figure 2.1). Most of the heart consists of muscle, known in medical terms as the *myocardium.* Actually, this muscle is sandwiched between two thin protective layers: the *epicardium* (the outer layer) and the *endocardium* (the inner layer). The interior of the heart harbors two pairs of hollow chambers. We refer to these chambers as the right and left sides of the heart, but in fact the right side is located almost in front of the left side if one looks at the heart head on. Each pair contains a small antechamber—an *atrium,* or *auricle*—and a larger section called a *ventricle.*

Let us follow the circulation cycle, beginning in the right atrium (Figure 2.2). Blood that has completed its mission of delivering oxygen and nutrition to the rest of the body empties into the right atrium from two large veins, the *inferior vena cava* and the *superior vena cava.* The former collects its cargo from the area of the body below the heart, the latter from above the heart.

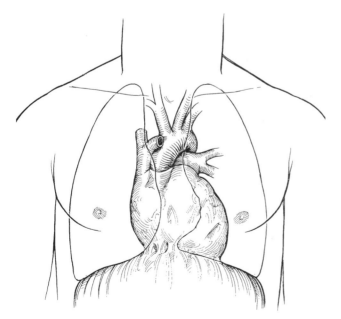

Figure 2.1. Relative position of the heart in the pericardial sac in the chest.

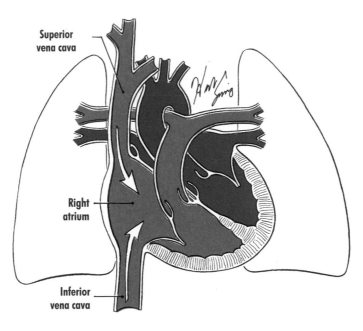

Figure 2.2. Deoxygenated blood from the veins of the body enters the right atrium through the superior and inferior venae cavae.

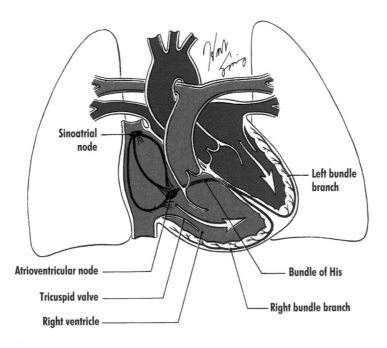

Figure 2.3. Normal pacemaker and conduction system.

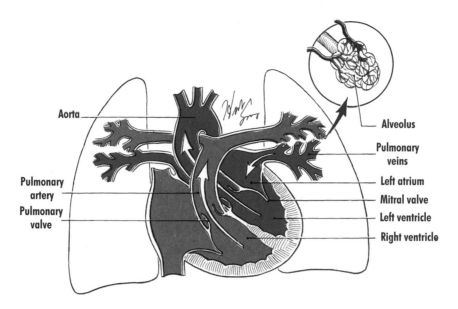

Figure 2.4. From the right ventricle blood is pumped through the pulmonary artery into the lungs, where it is oxygenated in the alveoli. The blood returns from the lungs through the pulmonary veins into the left atrium. After passing through the mitral valve, the blood is then pumped out of the left ventricle into the aorta and the arteries of the body.

Inside the top of the right atrium sits a small bundle of muscle fibers and nerves. This is the *sinoatrial node,* or *pacemaker* (Figure 2.3), and at regular intervals an electrical impulse shoots out from the sinoatrial node. That charge causes the muscles of the right atrium to contract in a wavelike motion from top to bottom. The squeeze of muscle fibers exerts pressure on the blood in the atrium, and the fluid seeks an outlet. Between the atrium and a much larger chamber, the right ventricle, lies the outlet, the *tricuspid valve,* a one-way opening named for the three leaves of tissue that form it. Pressure forces the valve open, and blood pours into the right ventricle.

Just as the right ventricle fills with blood, an electrical impulse fired by the sinoatrial node reaches the *atrioventricular node* (Figure 2.3). This is another bundle of muscle and nerves, located in the wall, or septum, between the two ventricles. The atrioventricular node, triggered by the charge from the sinoatrial node, passes the shock wave along two routes, quickly stimulating the rest of the heart's muscle.

The muscles of the right ventricle contract, but as the blood seeks to return to the opening from which it came, the tricuspid valve shuts when pressure in the right ventricle exceeds that in the right atrium. Since the tricuspid valve opens only one way, there can be no return of blood from the right ventricle to the right atrium. Within the right ventricle, mounting pressure forces the trapped blood to find an escape route. As the pressure in the right ventricle becomes greater than that in the *pulmonary artery,* the *pulmonary valve* is pushed open to expose a hoselike tube that divides into left and right branches leading to the two lungs (Figure 2.4). Passing through the branches of the pulmonary artery, the blood eventually comes in contact with the alveoli, which hold oxygen inhaled through the mouth and nose.

The freshly oxygenated blood, bright crimson as a result of the infusion of oxygen, drains into a pair of pulmonary veins that lead out of each lung. These veins, like the inferior and superior venae cavae, empty into another chamber of the heart, the left atrium, which is slightly larger than its colleague on the right (Figure 2.4).

The electrical impulse that initiated the squeezing of the muscles of the right side of the heart almost simultaneously energizes the left side, beginning with the left atrium. The contraction forces the blood in the left atrium to seek an outlet, but the route from the veins is again one-way. Pressure forces open a two-leaved valve, called the *mitral valve,* and oxygenated blood enters the largest chamber of the heart, the left ventricle. Now the rolling wave of muscular contraction begins to compress the left ventricle. The mitral valve shuts to prevent blood from returning to the atrium. The only escape is through a valve that leads to the aorta, the

main artery, or pathway, of the cardiovascular system. Oxygenated blood is now on its journey to the farthest reaches of the body, bearing life-supporting supplies for the cells.

Actually, the entire process of blood's filling and emptying the heart lasts less than a second. The contraction phase is called *systole,* while the relaxation period, when blood fills the atria and the ventricles, is known as *diastole* (Figure 2.5). Said the observant William Harvey, "Those two movements, one of the auricles and the other of the ventricles, occur successively, but so harmoniously and rhythmically that both [appear to] happen together and only one movement can be seen,

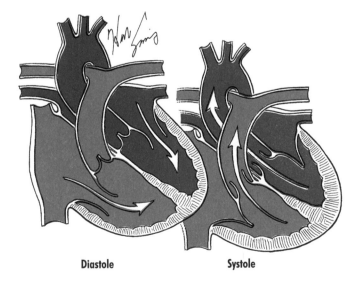

Diastole   **Systole**

Figure 2.5. During diastole, the heart relaxes and blood fills the atria and ventricles. During systole, the ventricles contract and drive the blood from the right ventricle into the lungs, and from the left ventricle into the aorta and its branching arteries throughout the body.

The Medical Arts: Listening to the Heart

The history of physicians' listening to their patients' hearts is long. Even the school of Hippocrates described a cacophony of noises within the chests of patients: "It bubbles like boiling vinegar," or "It creaks like a new leather strap." In the eighteenth century, physician Leopold Auenbrugger (1722–1809), the son of an Austrian innkeeper, drew his inspiration from the practice of tradesmen like his father, who tapped wine vats to determine the level of the contents. Auenbrugger began tapping humans, starting with himself, testing all parts of his body, and then experimenting on corpses. Auenbrugger managed to distinguish between the sounds due to fluid in the chest, enlargement of the heart, or thickening of the lungs. In 1761 he published these results. He observed, for example, that upon striking the thorax, or chest, "The sound thus elicited from the healthy chest resembles the stifled sound of a drum covered with a thick woolen cloth or other envelope." He also cataloged the many dismal sounds of chest ailments.

Auenbrugger became so discouraged by the scorn heaped upon him that he shifted his public interest to music but quietly pursued further study of chest percussion. Some 40 years later, French physician Jean Nicolas Corvisart (1755–1821) took command of Napoleon's medical corps and adopted the technique of percussion. When Napoleon's renowned chief doctor advised tapping, all of France's healers listened. Doctors even began to take the use of sound as a means of diagnosis a step further: they listened to the heart with an ear on the chest.

Prudery, fashion, and anatomy all conspired against this form of study. Modest female patients did not dare undress before a doctor. Coarse fabrics and thick layers of undergarments muffled any sounds that might reach the ear of a discreet physician. Obesity, a common ailment among the well-to-do, the class most likely to obtain the services of a doctor, made listening difficult as well. Poor hygiene also contributed to the unpleasantness of auscultation.

All of these obstacles to diagnosis through listening faced youthful French doctor René Laënnec (1781–1826) in 1816. As a doctor at Paris's Necker Hospital, he started to walk home one day while pondering what to do in the case of a plump, 17-year-old patient. When he passed through a restoration project in the Louvre, he noticed some children playing among the building materials. In a happy accident of discovery, he saw one boy put his ear to the end of a piece of lumber while another youngster thumped the opposite end. Immediately, Laënnec recalled the well-known acoustic phenomenon and walked back to the hospital. He seized the nearest magazine, and rolled it into a cylinder for the first use of what we know today as a *stethoscope*, whose roots mean to observe the chest (Greek *stēthos*). Laënnec later refined the instrument from a paper cylinder to a wooden tube.

Laënnec embarked on an intensive research project on auscultation. At first, publication of his results brought either indifference or opposition; gradually, however, the technique gained adherents. In Austria–Hungary, Laënnec's text fascinated medical student Josef Skoda (1805–1881), who became such an ardent convert to the stethoscope that he took an unpaid job as an underdoctor in the Vienna General Hospital, in the hope that he might be allowed to listen to the chests of patients. His incessant application of auscultation caused patients to complain. Hospital officials transferred Skoda to the mental patients' ward. But even these unfortunates wearied of Skoda's obsession with listening to their chests. He accepted a post as a physician to paupers, since they could not afford to complain about their

doctors. Vindication came when Skoda published a textbook, and he returned to the Vienna General Hospital in a higher capacity. Tapping and listening finally became an accepted technique of medicine with nineteenth-century physicians, who even stowed the stethoscope in their top hats.

especially in warmer animals in rapid movement."

The action of the heart produces sounds, and long before the perfection of electrocardiography, doctors examined patients by means of techniques that came under the headings of *percussion* (tapping) and *auscultation* (listening). The stethoscope carries two distinct sounds to the ear of the doctor. When the heart begins a contraction, the tricuspid and mitral valves (which lead from the right and left atria to their respective ventricles) slam shut. The pulmonary and aortic valves (which are gates to the pulmonary artery and the aorta) open, and the leaves of these two valves vibrate from the pressure of the blood forcing them to expand. This tremor adds to the noise of the tricuspid and mitral valves' closing, and a sound describable as a *lub* can be heard (Figure 2.6).

Just as the *lub* fades away, the pressure within the ventricles falls low enough for the aortic and pulmonary valves to swing shut, and a fraction of a second later the tricuspid and mitral valves open. This

creates a vibrating noise that supplements the sound of the closing valves. To the ear at the end of the stethoscope comes a *dub*. Then there is perceivable silence, since diastole ordinarily lasts longer than

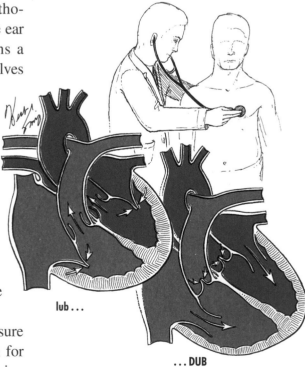

lub ...

... DUB

Figure 2.6. The sounds a physician hears through the stethoscope are caused by the opening and closing of the various valves of the heart.

systole. The normal sequence heard is *lub-DUB*, silence, *lub-DUB*, silence.

Occasionally, vibrations of the ventricular cavity can be heard as it fills with blood pouring from the atrium, and a physician will hear a third sound. Through the stethoscope a doctor can hear if valves fail to close properly, or if some blood backs up into a ventricle instead of being pumped out. The normal heart rate of 70 beats per minute pumps little more than $2^1/_2$ fluid ounces per stroke, which adds up to 6 quarts of output per minute. But when necessary, the heart can boost its performance to as much as 30 to 35 quarts per minute.

Heart rate seems to bear some relation to the size of the species, varying from 1,000 beats per minute in a canary, to about 25 beats per minute in an elephant. In humans, an infant's heart beats about 120 times per minute, while an adult's heart beats 65 to 75 times per minute. This rate in an adult adds up to approximately 100,000 beats per day, or 2.5 billion in a lifetime. Pulse rate sharply increases with physical exertion, from a mild increase of 20 to 30 beats per minute upon walking, to more than twice as fast during sexual intercourse.

The cardiovascular system has a computerlike ability to direct a heavier flow of blood to areas that require it and to order a detour around organs not needing it. This enhances circulatory efficiency. For example, gastric organs need an added amount of oxygenated blood during the digestion of food. But when no food is in the stomach, a series of shunts blocks off the flow of blood to these organs, and the extra supply is then available to the legs and arms for physical work. This mechanism explains why athletes forgo a meal just before engaging in competition.

The pump itself can contribute greatly to an increased supply of blood to tissues in need. The duration, and even the intensity, of cardiac systole (contraction) alter when the heart receives a demand for more oxygenated blood. To push the blood along faster, the time of diastole (relaxation) shortens. At rest, for example, systole lasts about one-third of a second and diastole about one-half of a second. During exercise the heart sustains the pressure stroke for perhaps one-fifth of a second and cuts its filling time to one-quarter of its normal time. The quantity of blood that is able to enter the heart drops, and the output of oxygenated blood per stroke falls, although the total output per minute is, of course, much higher than normal.

Dr. Roger Bannister, the first person to run a mile in under four minutes, thinks that the enormous reduction in distance-running times is due to an increased blood oxygen efficiency that can result from training. In fact, Dr. Bannister has predicted a 3.5-minute mile because of new methods to boost oxygen usage.

Let us consider the responses of the cardiovascular system to exercise. Picture for a moment the kickoff returner on a professional football team awaiting the kickoff near his goal line. His athletically trained heart may be beating about 60 times per minute at rest. However, in anticipation of the demands about to be placed upon his body, the player's sympathetic nervous system has already boosted his heart rate. In addition to the action of the nervous system, the adrenal glands have been stimulated to release adrenaline and noradrenaline, which initiate a series of reactions to prepare the player for "fight or flight." The player catches the ball and begins to run. Depending on the degree of his exertion and the rate at which he is being pursued, his pulse rate may reach nearly 200 beats per minute, and his cardiac output may become as high as 36 quarts of blood per minute. This will almost certainly occur if he succeeds in running the full length of the field for a touchdown.

Ordinarily, a healthy, trained athlete is unable to sustain exertion to the point that his or her heart muscle (myocardium) will suffer damage. Long before the myocardium reaches the danger point in terms of oxygen deficiency, other muscles in the body will suffer fatigue. It is indeed extraordinary to think that the heart must operate for 70 years without ever being permitted to rest or shut down for extensive repairs. It staggers the imagination to think of the wear and tear that the heart valves, those critically important parts of the cardiovascular machinery, must sustain in opening and shutting with considerable hydraulic pressure 2.5 billion times in a

lifetime. The magnitude of these forces is apparent to a surgeon when replacing a defective heart valve with a prosthetic device consisting of a silicone ball in a steel cage. Some of these hard silicone balls become pitted, rutted, and battered out of shape after only three or four years of being pounded by the blood. Because of this constant hammering, materials that are even stronger and more resilient than silicone are now being used. Yet in a normal, healthy heart, the delicate flesh of the valves stands up for 70 years or more.

Changes in cardiac output reflect biochemical and physiologic adaptations of the muscle cells of the myocardium. There are two types of muscle cells in the body: striated and smooth. The skeletal or voluntary muscles that we call on to do physical work are made up of many individual striated cells, or fibrils (Figure 2.7). The muscle tissue of the heart is also composed of striated muscle cells, although it is not, of course, under voluntary control. Altogether, muscle accounts for approximately 40 to 50 percent of a person's weight. The individual muscle cell is a highly specialized structure whose function is to produce chemical energy that can be converted into mechanical work. Sustained contraction of muscles demands consumption of oxygen to burn fuels that provide the necessary energy.

Both striated and smooth muscle cells contain myofibrils, which are the basic

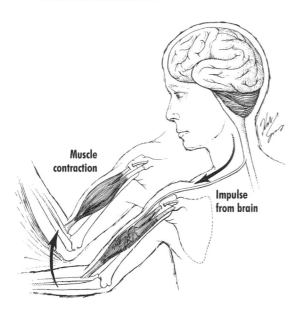

Muscle
contraction

Impulse
from brain

Figure 2.7. The skeletal muscles of the body perform their mechanical function by contracting and relaxing in accordance with physical labor when electrical impulses are received from the brain through the nerves.

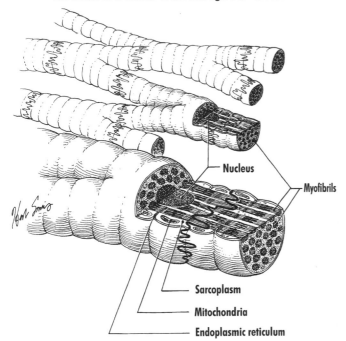

Nucleus

Myofibrils

Sarcoplasm

Mitochondria

Endoplasmic reticulum

Figure 2.8. The structure of the striated muscle of the heart. The substance surrounding the nucleus of the muscle cell is called the *sarcoplasm*. The sarcoplasm contains mitochondria and endoplasmic reticulum, similar to all cells.

structural units of the muscle (Figure 2.8). In the striated muscle, the myofibril contains multiple striations, or crossbands, while in the smooth muscle, no such striations are present. The sequence of events thought to culminate in muscle contraction begins with an electrical impulse from the nervous system that results in the electrical depolarization of the membrane of the cell (Figure 2.7).

The length of the muscle fiber prior to contraction is very important in determining the force developed during contraction. This is the basic principle behind the Frank–Starling law of the heart. This law describes the functioning of the heart and states that the work done by the heart varies with the diastolic volume of the ventricle, which determines the length of the myocardial muscle fibers. Thus, when venous return to the heart is increased, there is an increased filling pressure of the heart, a rise in the diastolic volume, and a greater stretching of the myocardial muscle fibers of the ventricle. This results in a higher stroke volume. When the heart is failing, the stroke volume produced by the left ventricle decreases. In the failing heart, the contraction is inadequate for biologic reasons that are still not clearly understood. One possibility is that there is a dysfunction between the coupling of the chemical energy and the mechanical work to be done by the heart. When the heart fails, there is insufficient mechanical energy to adequately pump blood to meet the needs of the body's tissues. The drug digitalis tends to increase the contractile force of the failing heart.

When the body is subjected to physical exertion, the tissues use more oxygen. In order to provide enough oxygen, the body responds by increasing the output of the heart, largely through a faster pulse rate, a more rapid respiration rate, and an increase in oxygen extracted from the bloodstream by organs and tissues. Cardiac output also is increased through a decrease in the resistance to blood flow near the extremities of the cardiovascular system. In another of nature's ingenious engineering triumphs, a sensing mechanism reduces resistance to the flow of blood by widening the blood vessels that supply the working muscle tissue.

If an individual is in good physical health, his or her oxygen will be supplied at a slower pulse rate than it is in a person in poor condition. While both individuals can reach the same maximal pulse rate for their age, the subject in good condition is able to achieve a higher level of work owing to the greater amount of oxygen that can be carried to and extracted by the tissues. This maximum oxygen uptake reached by an individual during exercise is sometimes referred to as *aerobic capacity*. This capacity declines as people get older and can be decreased further by cardiovascular disease or other forms of illness.

The conversion of chemical energy into mechanical work by muscle can be achieved only by shortening of the fibers or by an increase in their tension. A number of years ago, the great physiologist A. V. Hill described the fundamental relation between these two parameters; in simple terms, the rate of shortening of the muscle fiber varies inversely with the degree of tension achieved. Thus, if tension is great, as when a heavy object is lifted, the shortening of the muscle will occur at a relatively slow velocity. On the other hand, if a light object is to be raised, requiring only a small degree of tension, the rate of shortening will be much faster. Changes in the contractile state of the heart muscle may be altered by varying the resting length of the muscle fiber or by changing the contractility of the fiber. Practical ways to accomplish this are by giving agents such as noradrenaline or digitalis, both of which increase the force and velocity of contraction that the heart can achieve.

Maintenance of the normal contractility of the heart depends upon innervation by sympathetic nerve endings that release noradrenaline. This sympathetic control tends to speed up the heart, increase the rate at which the muscle fibers contract, and augment the pace at which the left ventricle ejects the blood.

During exercise, ventricular filling pressure rises because of an increase in the venous return to the heart. At the same time, the sympathetic nerve fibers and the circulating adrenaline and noradrenaline speed up the rate of the heart and increase venous return to the heart. The sympathetic nerve fibers and the circulating adrenaline and noradrenaline also increase the contractility of the myocardium. All of these forces tend to increase the diastolic volume and the length of the heart fibers, greatly augmenting cardiac output.

These changes occur to a lesser degree or not at all in the failing heart. In heart failure, the pumping action of the heart is inadequate to meet the metabolic demands of the tissues. It is important to emphasize that the exact biochemical basis for ordinary heart failure is not known. There appears to be a decrease in the amount of noradrenaline stored and released. Whatever the cause, there is simply a diminished output of the heart in relation to tissue demands. The most common causes of this type of heart failure are atherosclerotic coronary artery disease, hypertension, and valvular disease. Energy production by the heart appears to be normal, but its capacity to produce useful mechanical work is impaired. Heart failure may also be caused by pulmonary embolism, by an infection of the heart valves known as bacterial endocarditis, by severe systemic infection, or by other heart abnormalities.

Clinical manifestations of heart failure include fluid accumulation in the peripheral tissues (particularly the legs), the liver, and the lungs. Pulmonary congestion and eventually a highly dangerous condition known as *pulmonary edema* may result. The old term *dropsy* was used to describe congestive heart failure. This condition is characterized by a shortness of breath upon exertion and an abnormal degree of fatigue and weakness. It is a rarity when heart failure is a "high-output" rather than a "low-output" type. High-output heart failure may result from thiamine deficiency in beriberi, or from hyperthyroidism, severe anemia, or arteriovenous fistula.

Digitalis and noradrenaline administered to a patient may improve the contractility of a failing heart. Such drugs as barbiturates and such conditions as *myocardial infarction,* severe *hypoxia,* or *acidosis* may depress myocardial contractility. When heart failure cannot be corrected by medical measures, surgical placement of a cardiac assist device may sometimes be employed.

Muscular efforts are one type of request for additional work by the heart, but there are others. In everyday life we become aware of changes in heartbeat caused by some sensory or intellectual perception. Getting ready to make a speech or witnessing an emergency situation, for example, can turn the heartbeat from a stately march to a quick step. This is caused by a signal from the brain, which receives information from the eye and combines it with certain stored impressions to produce an increased heartbeat. Two separate nerve lines link heart and brain: the sympathetic, or accelerator, nerves, which liberate noradrenaline, and the vagus system, which tends to inhibit, or slow, the heart action (Figure 2.9).

The vagus system is a major influence in depressing the frequency of impulses from the pacemaker sinoatrial node of the heart. Sometimes surgical repair of the heart cuts the vagal connection and, inevitably, the patient's heartbeat, even while the patient is at rest, exceeds the accepted norm. The accelerator system reaches beyond the heart's pacemaker nodes and can be traced into the heart muscle itself. In extreme surgery, such as heart transplantation, in which accelerator and vagus lines into the heart have been severed, the nervous system can no longer affect the heart rate. But the heart still retains a regular rhythm through its own pacemaker, the sinoatrial node, and its relay to the atrioventricular node. While the heart is capable of generating its own rhythm, in a healthy body its tempo and electrical activity are, in fact, modulated by impulses from the brain.

A major advance in the study of the physiology of the heart was the discovery that the electrical discharge from the two cardiac nodes provides an excellent way to measure heart action by means of electrocardiography. As early as 1856, two German scientists reported that the heartbeat of a frog was accompanied by an elec-

trical impulse. Researchers experimented with measurement of this current in animals. But not until London physiologist Augustus Waller (1816–1870) learned how to record this electrical impulse without opening the patient's chest was it deemed possible to work with humans. Waller gave the technology a name, *electrocardiography*, but not even he thought it more than just an interesting toy. The problem was that Waller's machine lacked stability and the capacity to follow precisely the rapid

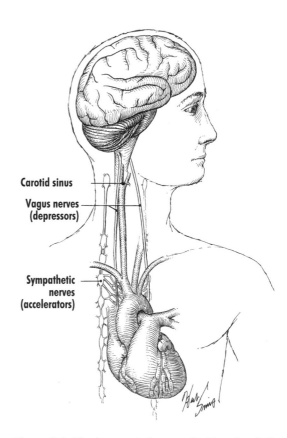

Carotid sinus

Vagus nerves (depressors)

Sympathetic nerves (accelerators)

Figure 2.9. The heart rate is controlled by electrical impulses from the brain through the vagus and sympathetic nerves.

changes in the minute variations of current associated with the heartbeat.

The need for an instrument adequate to register electrical current in the heart attracted the attention of a physiology professor named Willem Einthoven (1860–1927) at the University of Utrecht. Starting in 1893, he worked for seven years on the problem of designing a more satisfactory machine. The result was what Einthoven called the *string galvanometer*. The electrical current flowed from electrodes in the body's surface through a quartz thread. The thread was suspended in the force field of an electromagnet, and the thread vibrated as the current flowing through it interacted with the force field. An optical system focused the shadow cast by the quartz thread upon a light-sensitive surface, which recorded its deflections. This Rube Goldberg–like machine weighed 600 pounds and, to operate properly, needed five technicians. But the electrocardiograms provided such superior records of heart activity that Einthoven subsequently earned the Nobel Prize.

The invention of vacuum tubes did away with the cumbersome string galvanometers. The weight of a modern electrocardiography unit amounts to perhaps 30 pounds, with only one person needed to run it. In operating rooms and intensive care units, cathode ray oscilloscope versions monitor cardiac performance, and electrical impulses of the heart send beams of electrons dancing across a screen for an immediately visible record of heart function. To chart the passage of the electrical impulse, a technician places electrodes, or receivers of current, on the chest, arms, and legs. The machine then records the passage of electrical energy from the heart on a graph. The voltage of these impulses is only a matter of millivolts, yet these tiny impulses are enough to excite heart muscle. On a normal electrocardiogram, each vertical line on the graph-paper background represents one-fifth of a second in time, and each horizontal line indicates one-half of a millivolt (Figure 2.10).

The measurement begins with the P wave, which indicates the discharge of electrical energy by the sinoatrial node, which swiftly fans out over the right and left atria. This electrical phenomenon is called *depolarization*. The P wave thus reflects the activation of the atria. The QRS segment follows the subsequent depolarization of the atrioventricular node and reflects the electrical current's journey through the conduction system of the heart and into the muscular walls of the right and left ventricles. Portions of the conduction pathway beyond the node are called the bundle of His; the left and right bundle branches supply the left and right ventricles. Measurement of the interval between the P wave and the R wave indicates the length of time between the discharges of the sinoatrial node and the atrioventricular node. The first down-

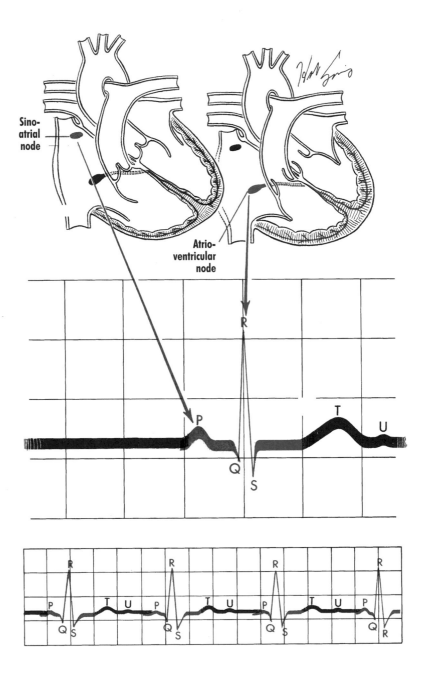

Figure 2.10. The electrocardiogram records the electrical activity of the conduction system of the heart.

ward (negative) deflection of the QRS complex is designated as the Q wave; the initial upward (positive) deflection, the R wave; and the second negative deflection, the S wave. The T wave indicates how long it takes for the recharging (repolarization) of the ventricles. From the distance between the Q and T waves, the physician observes the duration of excitation, ventricular contraction, and repolarization, or recovery, of the heart.

By recording an electrocardiogram over time, a physician can see irregularities in the rhythm of a heart. Sometimes a patient will be asked to run in place so that the cardiogram can show the effect of exercise upon the heart. But whether the body is at

rest or in motion, the heart's rhythm should accelerate and decelerate smoothly. Abnormal rhythms and rates on the electrocardiogram are indications of malfunction. Occasionally, an individual will have an abnormal rhythm that actually works fine for him. If the physician has kept a series of electrocardiograms on this patient over a period of years, the seemingly aberrant heart action will not be disturbing. For this particular heart, the action is normal. On the other hand, a slight variation in the cardiogram of an individual whose previous medical history showed a perfectly normal graph may indicate serious trouble. For this reason, we urge regular electrocardiography as part of everyone's annual physical examination, and exercise cardiograms for adults who are about to undertake a new program of physical exercise.

An abnormality of cardiac rate, or rhythm, is called an *arrhythmia.* The commonest is a slowing of the heart to less than 50 beats per minute, usually due to an excess of vagal inhibition at the sinoatrial node. This condition is called *sinus bradycardia* (Figure 2.11). Athletes may have a slow pulse and sinus bradycardia as their normal rhythm. Emotional excitement may produce the opposite effect, *sinus tachycardia,* in which the pulse rate is greater than 100 beats per minute. An increase in vagal tone slows the heart, and an increase in sympathetic tone speeds the heart. Generally, there is a balance between

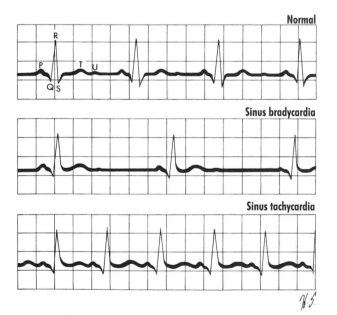

Figure 2.11. The electrocardiogram shows a slower heartbeat during sinus bradycardia, and a faster rhythm during sinus tachycardia.

vagal tone and sympathetic tone. Any removal of vagal input will increase the heart rate, or an increase in sympathetic tone with a constant vagal input will also result in tachycardia. Hyperthyroidism, congestive heart failure, and fever are all causes of sinus tachycardia.

An arrhythmia that arises outside the normal conduction pathway of the heart is called an *ectopic focus.* Such a focus, or site, generally represents an area of irritability within the myocardium that is able to initiate and sustain a pattern of extra heartbeats. An ectopic stimulus arising from the muscle of the atria can produce premature atrial contractions, whereas one coming from the ventricles can cause premature ventricular contractions (Figure 2.12). In order to induce a premature beat, the irritable focus of electrical activity must stimulate the heart muscle at a point in the cardiac cycle when it is susceptible to activation. The heart is vulnerable to reactivation at about the time of the T wave. The particular type of arrhythmia induced depends on the precise timing in the cardiac cycle when the irritable focus discharges, as well as its location within the heart. Premature atrial or ventricular beats may occur with almost any type of heart disease, particularly coronary artery disease. Excessive fatigue, smoking, consumption of coffee and other stimulants, emotional stress, febrile illness, and various metabolic and electrolyte distur-

bances can precipitate premature beats in the normal heart. Premature ventricular beats frequently occur during heart catheterization, after heart surgery, or during a heart attack.

Premature contractions may be perceived by the patient as a skipped beat, although premature ventricular contractions are generally asymptomatic. In the absence of underlying heart disease, premature atrial and occasional premature ventricular beats may be effectively treated by rest, sedatives, and withdrawal of stimulants. If there is underlying heart disease, or if premature ventricular contractions become too frequent, the use of an antiarrhythmic drug may be indicated. For an

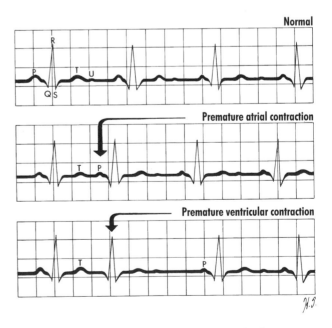

Figure 2.12. Premature contractions can occur in the atria or in the ventricles.

individual patient, the choice of drug depends on the type of arrhythmia and the cardiac and clinical status.

In addition to premature contractions, other frequently encountered atrial arrhythmias include paroxysmal atrial tachycardia, atrial flutter, and atrial fibrillation (Figure 2.13). In paroxysmal atrial tachycardia, an irritable atrial focus takes over from the normal pacemaker, namely, the sinoatrial node, and the pulse rate usually accelerates to about 180 beats per minute. Premature atrial beats usually precede arrhythmia. This cardiac irregularity may occur periodically in otherwise normal

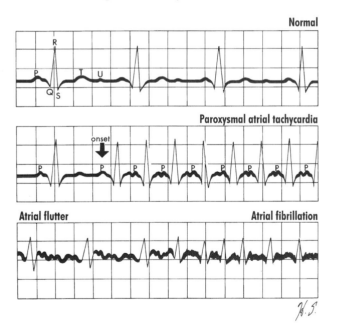

Figure 2.13. When paroxysmal atrial tachycardia occurs, the heart rate increases to about 180 beats per minute. When atrial flutter occurs, the rate increases to over 250 beats per minute. In atrial fibrillation, the atria contract in an irregular and ineffective way.

individuals, or it may be caused by coronary or rheumatic heart disease or by an overactive thyroid. Fatigue, stimulants, or emotional stress may bring on attacks. A patient may learn to terminate an attack by gagging or by external massage of the carotid sinus in the neck, procedures that increase vagal tone.

In atrial flutter, which is thought to be a reentry rhythm, the atrial rate is 250 to 400 beats per minute. The ventricle is unable to respond this rapidly, so the electrical impulses of the sinus node are not all transmitted by the atrioventricular node. The ventricular rate is usually 150 to 200 beats per minute and is regular. This means that not every atrial contraction on the electrocardiogram is followed by a QRS complex, owing to the absence of a 1:1 ventricular response. The P waves are abnormal in atrial flutter, with a "saw-toothed" configuration. Atrial flutter frequently requires electrical cardioversion.

In contrast to atrial flutter, which is not common, atrial fibrillation is very frequently encountered in patients with heart disease of either coronary or rheumatic etiology. In this condition an abnormal atrial focus discharges at a rate greater than 350 beats per minute. As a consequence, the atria do not contract in an effective or organized way. The atrioventricular node and the ventricles respond irregularly. Clinical manifestations depend on the rate of the ventricular response. If this rate is so rapid that the ventricles do not have adequate time to fill, heart failure may ensue. A digitalis preparation is usually given to slow or control the ventricular rate. Patients live many years and carry on their daily functions perfectly well with a properly slowed atrial fibrillation. The pulse is still irregular, however, even when the arrhythmia is well regulated. In some instances after digitalis therapy, it may be possible to convert a patient's atrial fibrillation to a sinus rhythm by administering electrical countershock. A potentially serious complication of atrial fibrillation is that a blood clot, or thrombus, can form within the atria and subsequently dislodge to enter the arterial circulation. A serious stroke, or cerebrovascular accident, may occur if the dislodged thrombus, now called an embolus, is carried to the brain. The electrocardiogram in atrial fibrillation shows normal but irregularly spaced RS complexes and absent P waves.

The arrhythmias ventricular tachycardia, ventricular fibrillation, and ventricular standstill can be deadly (Figure 2.14). Ventricular tachycardia arises from an irritable focus in the myocardium and usually indicates underlying heart disease, especially atherosclerotic coronary disease. This irregularity resembles a series of premature ventricular beats and produces a rate of 140 to 220 beats per minute. Ventricular filling falls off, and heart failure

may follow. The pulse may be absent at the wrist and, if untreated, the patient may go into cardiogenic shock. Intravenous administration of medication or administration of electrical countershock is required and may save the patient's life.

In ventricular fibrillation, the ventricular muscles cannot maintain a coordinated contraction in response to an exceedingly rapid irritable focus. The muscle goes into a kind of rapid twitching and consequently does not effectively pump blood. In ventricular standstill, there is no impulse to stimulate the ventricle, and the muscle, in a sense, stands still. Ventricular

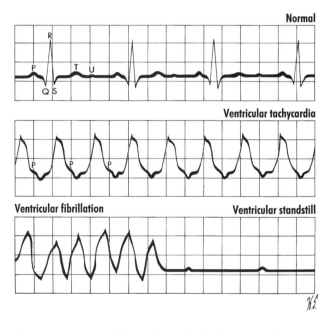

Figure 2.14. In ventricular tachycardia, the heart rate increases to 140 to 220 beats per minute. In ventricular fibrillation, the heart muscle goes into uncoordinated spasmodic contractions and does not effectively pump blood. In ventricular standstill, there is no impulse to stimulate the ventricle.

fibrillation and ventricular standstill produce *cardiac arrest*, in which there is no detectable heartbeat, pulse, or blood pressure. Breathing usually stops. The patient loses consciousness and will suffer irreversible brain damage unless resuscitation or correction of the arrhythmia is carried out within four to six minutes.

In a coronary care unit, the occurrence of a cardiac arrest triggers a number of emergency measures aimed at correcting the condition: The arrhythmia must be corrected by electrical countershock; respiration and the blood pressure must be supported; and acidosis must be reversed. If the arrest occurs outside an area where a defibrillator is available to produce the countershock, cardiopulmonary resuscitation (CPR) must be instituted. As illustrated in Figure 2.15, this procedure involves breathing air into the victim's lungs and

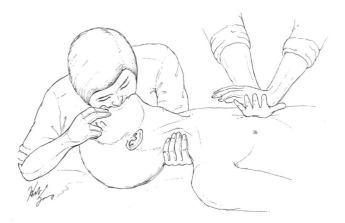

Figure 2.15. Cardiopulmonary resuscitation (CPR) involves breathing air into the victim's lungs and applying external heart massage.

applying external cardiac massage to pump the blood out of the heart. Courses in CPR are available through the American Heart Association and the Red Cross. Being able to carry out CPR may enable you to save someone's life.

There is another group of heart irregularities known collectively as *heart block* (Figure 2.16). The cause of this type of arrhythmia is an interference with the normal conduction system of the heart as the impulses pass through the atrioventricular node. The heart block may be first degree, second degree, or third degree. In first-degree heart block, there is a 1:1 response of atrial and ventricular contractions, but a slowing of conduction through the atrioventricular node, producing an increased P–R interval on the electrocardiogram. In second-degree block, some of the impulses do not pass through the atrioventricular node and the atrial-to-ventricular response is not 1:1 but 2:1, 3:1, or higher. In second-degree heart block, some of the P waves are not followed by a QRS complex. In third-degree heart block, there is no conduction through the atrioventricular node. A slow ventricular rate occurs because a pacemaker within the ventricle itself takes over. In complete heart block, there is no relation between the atrial beats or P waves and the QRS complexes.

If the heart rate slows to the point that the ventricle cannot pump an adequate amount of blood to support the requirements of the body, particularly the brain, heart failure and unconsciousness rapidly occur. The patient with complete heart block may develop cardiac arrest or ventricular fibrillation, both potentially lethal. Loss of consciousness in association with third-degree heart block is called a *Stokes–Adams attack*. Second-degree or third-degree heart block may require treatment if the ventricular rate is not adequate. In some instances it is necessary to insert an artificial pacemaker to control complete heart block.

In concluding this chapter, it may be useful to review some of the awesome statistics concerning the heart and place them in another frame of reference. For example, the 60,000 miles of blood vessels in each adult equals a trip of nearly two and one-half times around the world, or a quarter of the distance from the earth to the moon. A single heart that pumps 6

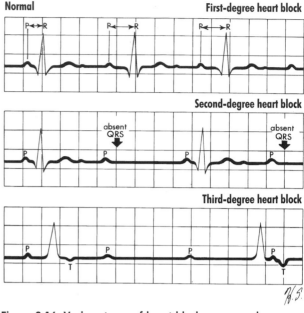

Figure 2.16. Various types of heart block are caused by interference with the normal conduction system of the heart.

quarts of blood per minute (360 quarts per hour) by the end of 70 years will have moved more than 220 million quarts. It's a pretty remarkable piece of machinery.

CHAPTER THREE

Blood Vessels:
The Vascular System

The heart, as we have said, is the center of the cardiovascular system. The body's requirement for oxygen and food is met by a network of blood vessels known as the

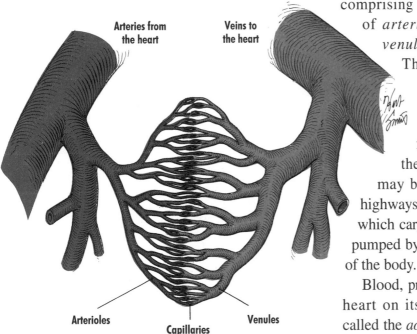

Arteries from the heart

Veins to the heart

Arterioles

Capillaries

Venules

Figure 3.1. From the heart, oxygenated blood passes from the arteries through smaller branches called arterioles into capillaries, where food and oxygen are supplied to the cells of the body and waste products are removed. After passing through the capillaries, the blood enters the small venules, which connect to the veins to return blood to the heart.

vascular or circulatory system. As William Harvey discovered, this system is a continuous network, connected with the heart, which serves as a pump. The blood vessels comprising the vascular system consist of *arteries, arterioles, capillaries, venules,* and *veins* (Figure 3.1). This is a closed system of vessels with a lining called the *endothelium.* The blood vessels transport the blood from the heart to the tissues of the body and back again; they may be compared to a network of highways, roads, and channels through which cargo (the blood) is continuously pumped by the heart to supply the needs of the body.

Blood, primed with oxygen, leaves the heart on its journey via a large artery called the *aorta.* From the aorta, the blood travels through smaller arteries and then arterioles to connect with a network of vessels known as capillaries. As blood moves from the heart to the capillary bed, the arteries become progressively smaller

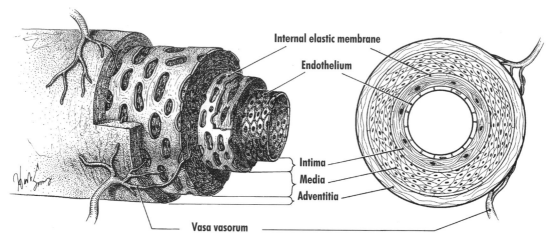

Internal elastic membrane

Endothelium

Intima

Media

Adventitia

Vasa vasorum

Figure 3.2. The different types of cellular components of the three layers that constitute the structure of an artery.

and more numerous. Their total cross-sectional area increases so that the rate of flow of the blood decreases as it travels farther away from the heart.

The arteries themselves range from a great superhighway, the aorta, with its one-inch diameter, down to the minute arterioles, whose width is only about 0.02 inch. The capillaries, the final pathways for the blood, are smaller than a single red blood cell, which must bend and squirm to pass through them. Along these avenues of transport lie many of the potential dangers of life.

An artery's wall may be divided into 3 layers or sections: the *intima,* the *media,* and the *adventitia* (Figure 3.2). The innermost layer of the artery is called the intima. At birth it is only one cell thick and consists of the endothelium, the lining that is in direct contact with the blood. Hardening of the arteries, referred to as *arteriosclerosis*

or *atherosclerosis*, probably begins with damage to the endothelial lining, permitting fatty substances and other toxic agents into the intima (see Chapter 13). A thin structure, the internal elastic membrane, separates the intima from a muscular coat, the media, of the artery's wall.

Large arteries nearer the heart are subjected to the strong pulsations generated as the heart contracts. These arteries are protected from the pounding action of the heart by virtue of their ability to recoil, a property that depends on the media's being relatively rich in elastic tissue (*elastin*). The pulsations decrease in intensity farther from the heart so that the smaller the artery, the greater its ratio of muscle tissue to elastin. The smooth muscle cells of the artery's media may play a key role in the development of arteriosclerosis. Atherosclerosis, a type of arteriosclerosis involving primarily the intimal section of the arterial wall, is the disease underlying most heart attacks and strokes. The outermost layer of the artery's wall, the adventitia, is rich in connective tissue, nerve fibers, and a special group of blood vessels called the *vasa vasorum,* which supply the artery itself. The vasa vasorum is a network of small vessels that provides oxygen-enriched blood for the walls of medium-sized and large arteries and veins. When the wall becomes thickened, as in the atherosclerotic vessel, the diffusion of oxygen to the center of the media may not be sufficient, and as a consequence, the cell dies, with further damage to the artery.

The state of contraction of muscular arteries is regulated by sympathetic nerve fibers, which are abundant in the adventitia, and by release of endothelial-derived relaxation factor (EDRF) or nitric oxide, which is a product that is released by the endothelial cells as well as by a chemical substance produced by platelets, called *prostacyclin.* Arterioles, the smallest of arteries, are of particular importance in determining the level of the arterial blood pressure. Relaxation or dilation of the arterioles decreases the resistance to blood flow and lowers the blood pressure. Vasoconstrictor nerve fibers, part of the sympathetic nervous system, release adrenaline and noradrenalin to regulate the contractile tone of the arterioles. EDRF has a paradoxical effect and causes contraction of an arteriosclerotic artery. Thromboxane A_2,

produced by platelets and endothelium, a peptide made by endothelial cells, also causes contraction.

An excessive degree of arteriole contraction is thought to be one of the important causes of high blood pressure (hypertension), in which the arterial blood pressure is persistently elevated. Substances that release calcium or move calcium from the smooth muscle cells will cause contraction. As will be evident from this oversimplified discussion, the state of relaxation or contraction of an artery's wall is extremely complex and involves a number of counteracting substances.

The smallest arterioles merge with capillaries of the same size, the distinction between these two types of vessels being the total absence of a muscular layer in the capillaries. Thus, the capillary consists of only a layer of endothelium surrounded by connective tissue.

Capillaries empty into venules, which in turn form veins. The vein has a larger *lumen* and a thinner wall with relatively less muscle and elastic tissue than an artery of the same size. The relatively larger lumen accounts for the slower flow of blood and lower pressure in the venous system.

If one were to tour the body, via the vascular system, the journey would begin with a departure from the left ventricle through the aortic valve. Just beyond the aortic valve are the *coronary arteries* and their network of branches that supply blood to the heart itself (Figure 3.3).

These arteries girdle the heart like a crown, hence the name "coronary." They account for 5 percent of the total blood flow, although their diameter at most equals that of a thick piece of twine or a soda straw. A healthy heart, particularly one developed through a regular program of exercise, shows an extensive field of blood vessels flowing from the coronary arteries.

Immediately beyond the exit of the coronary artery is the *aortic arch,* which forms the two major channels leading from the heart, one to the lower part of the body and the other to the upper part, especially the brain (Figure 3.4). The upper channel is formed by three major vessels that arise from the ascending aorta: the innominate, the left common carotid, and the left subclavian arteries. The *innominate* divides into the right subclavian and the right common carotid arteries. The *subclavian arteries* feed the left and right sides of the chest, shoulders, and arms through their branches. The left and right *common carotid arteries* carry blood to the neck and head.

Arteriosclerotic disease of the carotid arteries may lead to cerebrovascular disease and stroke. Some additional blood flows to the head through the vertebral arteries, which branch from the subclavians. Inside the skull, a vast network of arteries feeds the cells of the brain. The main arteries supplying the brain form a

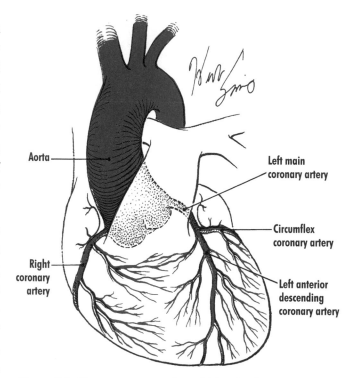

Figure 3.3. The coronary arteries, which arise from the aorta just above the aortic valve, provide blood for the various tissues of the heart.

circle at its base called the *circle of Willis.* This circle of arteries serves to provide all parts of the brain with relatively equal amounts of blood.

The arterial route to the lower half of the body starts at the downturn of the aortic arch. As the aorta passes through the diaphragm, it becomes the abdominal aorta (Figure 3.5). A series of crossroads fan out to supply organs and tissue along the way. Each major organ has its own route. Gastric arteries supply the stomach; the superior and inferior mesenteric arteries supply the small and large intestines; the

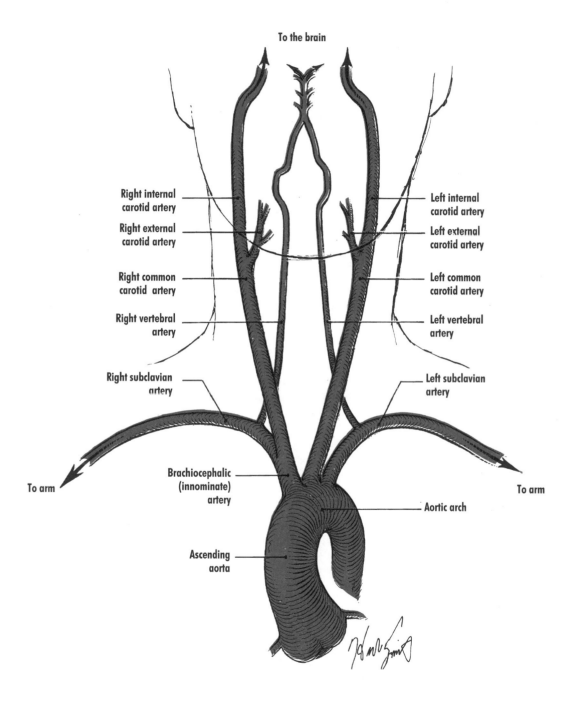

To the brain

Right internal
carotid artery

Right external
carotid artery

Right common
carotid artery

Right vertebral
artery

Right subclavian
artery

Brachiocephalic
(innominate)
artery

Ascending
aorta

Left internal
carotid artery

Left external
carotid artery

Left common
carotid artery

Left vertebral
artery

Left subclavian
artery

To arm

To arm

Aortic arch

Figure 3.4. Three major arteries—the innominate, left common carotid, and left subclavian—arise from the aortic arch to supply the head and arms with blood.

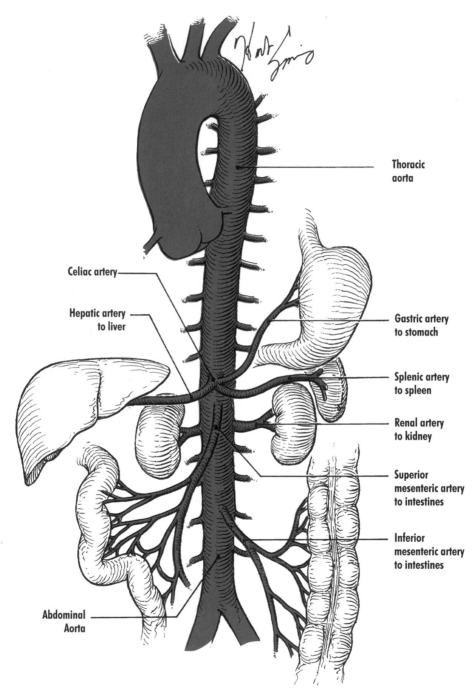

Thoracic aorta

Celiac artery

Hepatic artery to liver

Gastric artery to stomach

Splenic artery to spleen

Renal artery to kidney

Superior mesenteric artery to intestines

Inferior mesenteric artery to intestines

Abdominal Aorta

Figure 3.5. Branches arise from the aorta in the chest and abdomen to supply blood to the body wall and major organs.

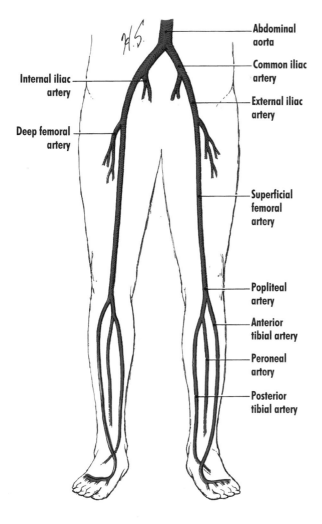

Internal iliac artery

Deep femoral artery

Abdominal aorta

Common iliac artery

External iliac artery

Superficial femoral artery

Popliteal artery

Anterior tibial artery

Peroneal artery

Posterior tibial artery

Figure 3.6. The abdominal aorta branches into the right and left iliac arteries to supply blood to the pelvis, thighs, and legs.

celiac has two major branches: the hepatic arteries, which supply the liver, and the splenic artery, which goes to the spleen; and the renal arteries feed the kidneys. The kidney has a special relation to the cardio vascular system, filtering about 150 quarts of blood every 24 hours to remove wastes from the system.

Below the stomach, the abdominal aorta branches into the right and left iliac arteries to supply the thighs and legs (Figure 3.6). Further subdivisions occur as the system extends to the lower legs, the feet, and finally the toes. Side roads from the arteries fan out into a maze of smaller and smaller blood vessels, until the arterioles and capillaries are reached. The capillaries pass through the spaces between cells where the delicate transfer of food and oxygen in exchange for waste occurs.

In the spleen and bone marrow, the capillaries may empty into tissue spaces. This is an exception, however, and the endothelium of the capillary is usually continuous with that of the venules and veins, which convey the blood back to the heart and lungs. Because the oxygen tension is low in the peripheral tissues, venous blood appears bluish (Figure 3.7).

During the early part of the trip, a strong pressure is generated by the contractions of the heart. The force is dissipated by the time the blood reaches the veins, and the outward rush of blood gives small impetus to the return flow. The push for the trip through the venous system comes from the normal use of the muscles of the leg, arm, back, and stomach that squeeze the veins whenever a human walks, writes, lifts, or even rolls over in his sleep. Because of the relative scarcity of muscle

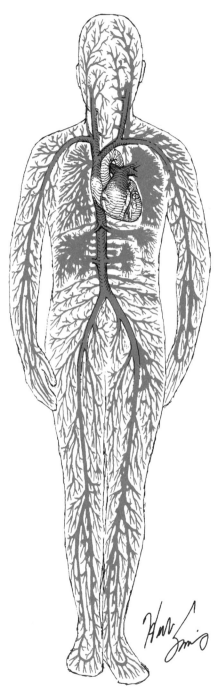

Figure 3.7. The venous system returns blood from the various tissues of the body to the heart.

and elastic tissue in its wall, a vein is more easily compressed by adjacent muscles and bones than is an artery. This phenomenon is important in promoting the return of blood to the heart from the limbs, since it must flow against the force of gravity, particularly when a person is standing.

In addition to the compressibility of the vein, the other significant factor in the anti-gravity flow is the presence of valves in veins. These one-way valves prevent blood from oozing backward (Figure 3.8). If the valves of the leg veins become impaired and allow a backward flow to occur, the blood tends to pool in the limb, distending the veins and resulting in varicosities. The presence of varicose veins is not, however, to be confused with arterial disease; these varicosities are unrelated to arteriosclerosis.

Normally, blood pressure, which is measured in millimeters of mercury during contraction of the heart (systole), reaches around 110 to 140 in a young adult. During the relaxed phase of the heart (diastole), pressure falls to 70 to 90. In 1733, an English parson, the Reverend Stephen Hales, performed the first experiment designed to measure blood pressure. He trussed up a horse, then inserted a glass tube, a primitive device for measuring fluid pressure, in an artery on the horse's neck. The column of blood rose to $7\frac{1}{2}$ feet, and Hales established that as normal blood pressure in a horse.

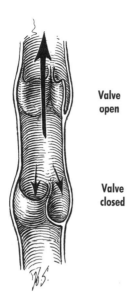

Figure 3.8. One-way valves in the veins prevent blood from flowing backward.

Valve
open

Valve
closed

Inconvenient for the physician, to say nothing of the patient (Rev. Hales sacrificed seven animals in the course of his experiments), the technique obviously required improvement. In 1828, Jean Marie Poiseuille succeeded at least in reducing the size of the tube by designing a U-shaped device filled with mercury, which is 13.6 times as heavy as water. Blood pressure could now be measured by the millimeter height of a column of mercury. Poiseuille also corrected one of Rev. Hales' errors. The clergyman concluded that blood pressure drops as arterial distance from the heart increases. Poiseuille constructed cannulas or tubes small enough to insert into the smaller arteries and discovered that arterial pressure maintains a steady level throughout the system.

Still, the need to open an artery in order to measure blood pressure restricted this valuable information to use in the experimental application. Practitioners in the second half of the nineteenth century began probing for methods that would enable them to determine how much pressure was required to obliterate the pulse beat in the radial artery at the wrist. In 1863, Etienne Jules Marey and Koming Dudgeon of France both built simple machines to record the frequency of pulse beats. A young British doctor, Frederick Akbar Mahomed, modified Marey's device. He measured the amount of thumbscrew pressure required to stop blood flow in the wrist. Some individuals whose pulse beat required excessive pressure were found to have *nephritis,* a kidney disease that produces acute elevation of blood pressure. But Dr. Mahomed's chief contribution was in showing a way to measure blood pressure without entering a blood vessel.

Others continued to improve machines to gauge the force of blood pumped through the heart. The device currently used is called a *sphygmomanometer*—the initial seven letters are derived from the Greek word for throb. There are several types, each named for the individual who devised it. One such device was designed in 1896 by the Italian physician, Scipione

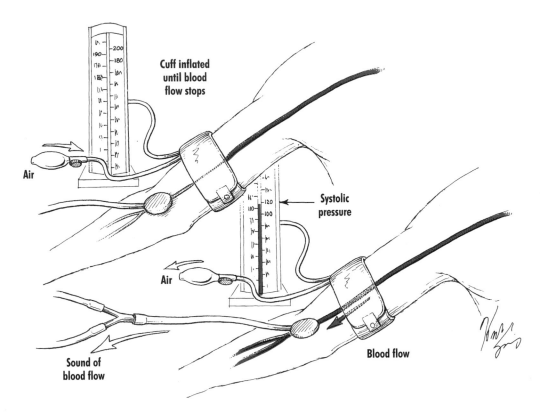

Cuff inflated until blood flow stops

Air

Systolic pressure

Air

Sound of blood flow

Blood flow

Figure 3.9. Blood pressure is determined by listening for certain changes in the sound of blood flowing through the artery as the pressure in the pneumatic cuff, which has been raised significantly to cut off arterial blood flow, is gradually decreased.

Riva-Rocci. An inflatable *pneumatic cuff* around the arm is used to constrict the brachial artery (Figure 3.9). Squeezing an inflatable bulb, the examiner raises the pressure in the cuff and listens with the stethoscope on the arm just below the cuff. While pressure in the cuff is lower than in the artery, some blood can flow through the vessel, and the sound of its turbulent passage can be heard through the stethoscope. Excessive pumping on the inflat-able bulb tightens the cuff enough to shut off circulation, and the sound stops. Gradually, air is released from the cuff. As cuff pressure drops below the level of arterial blood pressure, the examiner hears the distinct noise of renewed blood flow.

The cycle of sounds associated with the measurement of systolic and diastolic blood pressure was first described by Nicolai Korotkoff in 1905, and bears his name. These sounds are thought to be

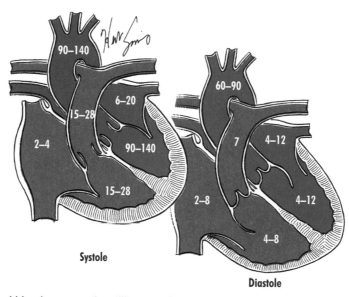

Figure 3.10. Normal blood pressure (in millimeters of mercury) in the various chambers of the heart.

caused by sudden distention of the arterial walls from a previous state of collapse, as the pressure in the pneumatic cuff is reduced. The height of the column of mercury when the pressure in the artery surpasses that of the inflated cuff is the systolic pressure. The diastolic pressure is registered as more air drains from the cuff and a change in the character of the sound is heard. Some observers record the pressure level at which these sounds disappear altogether. Mechanical or digitronic blood pressure devices are now available that are reasonably accurate and make the monitoring of blood pressure conveniently done at home.

Although an electrical impulse originating in the heart's pacemaker activates the heart's cycle of contraction and relaxation, the dynamics of the cardiovascular system depend on hydraulic pressure (Figure 3.10). During diastole, the period of relaxation of heart muscle and filling of the ventricles, blood pressure in the aorta is as much as 15 times that in the ventricle. It takes a tenth of a second for the cardiac muscle to contract enough to surpass the aortic pressure and force open the aortic valve.

While the blood pours from the heart in spasmodic spurts, it travels through the arterial system at a more even pressure, similar to water coursing through a hose. The intermittent flow of blood from the heart turns into a steadier stream because of the elastic muscle fibers that gird the arteries. As each beat of the heart pushes a greater volume of blood into the aorta, its fibers relax, an action that increases the cubic volume in which the blood circulates and lowers the pressure (Figure

3.11). During diastole, as the heart muscle relaxes, blood flow slackens, and the aorta shrinks its size to maintain pressure. Other large arteries possess the same flexible quality to keep pressure even. When a person becomes active and the tissues need more oxygen and other nutrients, the arterioles relax and resistance drops to help speed along the supplies through the capillaries.

More than 300 years ago, William Harvey proclaimed an appropriate conclusion for this chapter: "... by good leave of the learned and with due respect to the ancients, that the heart, as the beginning, author, source and organ of everything in the body and the first cause of life, should be held to include the veins and all the arteries and also the contained blood, just as the brain including all its nerves and sensory organs and spinal marrow is one adequate organ of sensation as the phrase is. If by the word 'heart' however, only the body of the heart be meant with its ventricles and auricles I do not believe that it is the manufacturer of the blood nor that the blood possesses vigor, faculty."

In fact, Harvey understated the case. With the limited knowledge of the time, he

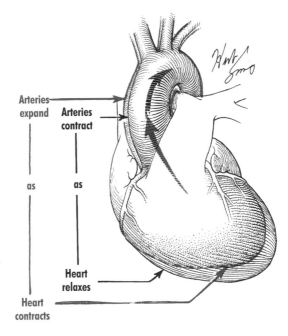

Figure 3.11. The arteries expand and contract to aid the heart in pumping blood throughout the body.

was unaware of roles played by the kidneys, liver, and lungs in "the first cause of life," and he was not cognizant of the cardiovascular system's role in causing strokes. He pointed the way, however, to understanding why we suffer cardiovascular disease and what can be done to protect our bodies and help us recover in the event of a heart attack.

CHAPTER FOUR

General Physical Examination

Physicians diagnose heart disease as detectives solve mysteries. Symptoms are the clues to identifying what the patient is experiencing; signs and results from the physical examination and diagnostic tests are the evidence. The doctor may suspect a diagnosis but must gather evidence to substantiate it. Sometimes the medical evidence is definitive; sometimes it is not. Also important to the physician is determining what the diagnosis is *not*, a process health professionals refer to as "ruling out." They rule out diagnoses in the same way detectives narrow down a list of suspects.

But the physician does more than just identify what is wrong or what is not wrong. Yes, the diagnosis is the central concern, but what caused the problem, how the problem may have changed the structure of the heart or its functioning, and what these changes mean in terms of the patient's life are all important issues that the physician must address.

In this process, the general physical examination is very important. A first-time visit to the cardiologist may proceed much

as the typical annual physical examination might, but the examination will intensify well beyond a blood pressure check and a review of family medical history. This process may take several hours and may require more than one visit.

The Medical History

Fundamental to proper assessment is a detailed personal medical history. You may be asked to fill out a questionnaire, or a technician, nurse, or physician's assistant may ask questions and record your answers. Inasmuch as most doctors use a team of professionals to provide health care, the physical examination may involve several people. Doctors rely increasingly on physician's assistants and nurse practitioners to perform parts of the examination.

One of the most important parts of a physical examination isn't physical at all. It's when the patient talks and the doctor—or someone else on the health care team—listens. Whether you are providing information with a pencil or with words, it is crucial that you communicate your problem clearly. Be sure to communicate not only what is asked, but also what you want the health care providers to know.

The history falls into three categories: current symptoms and problems, past medical profile, and history of risk factors for cardiovascular disease.

Describing the Symptoms

Only you know what the discomfort feels like, and yet explaining it to someone else can be difficult. But physicians need more to go on than "It hurts." They want to know where it hurts, the character of the pain, and other symptoms and signs that go along with the pain. A patient's attitude toward illness, toward treatment, or toward the health care team may hamper communication. Patients sometimes hedge in their descriptions out of embarrassment or fear; others exaggerate, hoping to show the problem is important. One way to provide a clear, honest description is to plan ahead: if possible (if your symptoms do not require that you go to the doctor or hospital immediately), keep a symptom diary for several days before your examination, and take the diary to your appointment.

To help you record information that is most helpful to the physician in diagnosing and treating the problem, here are questions you should answer to help your physician diagnose the problem.

Chest Pain

Is it localized to one area of the chest or is it diffuse? Does it radiate to your arm, neck, or jaw? Is it mild, moderate, or severe? Is it dull or aching? Does it feel tight or crushing? Does it burn or feel like indigestion? Is it constant, or does it come and go? How long does it last? Did it start suddenly or gradually? Do activities such as physical exertion, emotional stress, eating, having a bowel movement, or exposure to cold temperatures seem to trigger it? Do things such as rest, warmth, walking, or a prescribed nitroglycerin tablet relieve it? Are there any other symptoms with it, such as nausea, sweating, dizziness, shortness of breath, or anxiety? With the answers to these questions, the physician may be able to classify your ailment as a cardiac or pulmonary condition and to judge the degree of impairment. Chest pain may require *immediate* medical attention; see Chapter 17.

Breathing Problems

Do you become short of breath? Is it caused by certain activities? Does lying down make it worse? Do you wake up from sleep feeling as if you're fighting for air? Labored or difficult breathing, called *dyspnea,* is a common symptom in patients with cardiac disease or a respiratory ailment. The most common breathing problem experienced by patients with heart disease is *exertional dyspnea,* a shortness of breath detectable when the patient is active, and absent when the exertion ceases. Two others—*orthopnea* and *paroxysmal nocturnal dyspnea*—occur when the patient is in bed. A serious condition, orthopnea is breathing difficulty that prevents easy respiration when the patient is flat in bed. Also occurring when the patient is lying flat, paroxysmal nocturnal dyspnea is a nighttime attack of breathing difficulty in which the patient must sit upright or stand to overcome terrifying feelings of suffocation.

Heart failure may progress to the point that the lungs literally fill up with fluid. This is called *pulmonary edema* and demands emergency attention. Some have called these attacks *cardiac asthma* because of the wheezing heard in these patients.

Another unusual pattern of breathing, called *Cheyne–Stokes respirations,* is characterized by an alternating pattern of fast, deep breathing and slow, shallow breathing and occurs in some patients with severe failure of the left side of the heart. This type of breathing is not specific for heart failure and may be seen in other conditions, including stroke.

Fatigue

Have you noticed a progressive decrease in how well you tolerate activity? Are there any activities you have had to stop? When the heart cannot pump oxygen-rich blood fast enough to meet the metabolic demands of the body, the result is fatigue that seems to rob your body of all energy. A common complaint of patients with cardiovascular disease is excessive fatigue at the end of the day.

Palpitations

Does your heartbeat become rapid or seem irregular? Does it skip beats? Does it thump in your chest? What brings palpitations on? Patients may be overly conscious of their heartbeat and report palpitations when there is no arrhythmia, no cardiac problem, and no pathologic factor (excessive alcohol or exercise)—only a nervous or emotional problem. Conversely, some patients with verifiable heart disease may become so accustomed to cardiac rate and rhythm disturbances that they overlook them.

Leg Pain

Do you have pain in your foot, calf, thigh, or buttock? Is it localized, or does it radiate? Is it cramplike? Is there any burning, tingling, or numbness? Does walking or other activity cause it, or does it happen at night? Is it relieved by resting with legs up or by keeping them down? Painful muscle spasms can be caused by underoxygenation of limb tissues when damaged arteries may be unable to supply tissues with the oxygen they need.

Fainting

Have you fainted either during or shortly after physical activity or heavy work? Fainting, called *syncope* by physicians, indicates a dramatic and adverse occurrence in circulatory dynamics. It may be caused by a sudden slowing of the pulse (such as a vasovagal attack, a consequence of overactivity of the heart's inhibitory nerves), by a condition called heart block, by other forms of heart irregularity, or by stricture or stenosis of the aortic valve. There are, of course, many other causes of syncope, but these are a few of the common ones.

Past Medical Profile

It can also be helpful before visiting the doctor to jot down injuries, hospitalizations, surgeries, pregnancies, recent dental procedures, past and present illnesses, and any allergies. Make a list of all drugs you take now or have taken recently, and include the dosage and how often you take each one. (Better yet, do what doctors call "brown bagging," and take the containers with you.) The list should include both prescription and over-the-counter drugs such as pain killers, cold remedies, antacids, sleeping aids, vitamin or mineral supplements, herbal remedies, and any illicit drugs. Hiding illegal drug use can jeopardize your life.

Identifying Risk Factors

A family history of hypertension, heart disease, high blood cholesterol, stroke, or diabetes will let your physician know that you may be at risk of having one of these disorders. You will need to know the age and health of your grandparents, parents, brothers, sisters, and children and be able to report for deceased family members their age at death and cause of death.

Other questions concern lifestyle: your usual diet, any recent change in your weight, past or present use of tobacco, usual activities, alcohol and caffeine intake, and sleep patterns. Some questions may appear unrelated, but they are meant to help the physician assess the whole you, not just your medical status. Ask why some information is required, if it bothers you to supply it. Some of these lines of inquiry are psychological (family support, recent stress, such major life change as retirement or divorce, your own perception of your health problems), economic (resources, occupation), and cultural (educational, spiritual values). Questions may explore loss of control over factors in your life, anxiety, and various aspects of depression.

Finally, throughout the physical examination the doctor observes your demeanor—your tone of voice, body language, and emotional response to questions, to get a general impression of your state of health. Through this process, doctors often develop a hunch that directs further investigation, much in the same way a detective follows a hunch during an investigation.

The General Examination

A physical examination involves looking at, feeling, and listening to the body. This usually begins with an overall assessment of how the patient looks. Does he or she appear well? Acutely or chronically ill? Edematous? Extremely tense? Is the patient at ease, breathing comfortably and normally? The physician may then make a cursory examination of the skin and nails and pay attention to the skin's color, elasticity, temperature, and moisture. Physicians examine fingers and nails for abnormalities that occur in certain cardiovascular disorders. They look at the arms and legs to see if there are signs of peripheral vascular disease. Below are some of the characteristics the physician will evaluate.

Observing and Evaluating the Patient

Skin Color and Elasticity

Paleness (or pallor) may indicate poor oxygen supply. The wide range of skin tones among humans complicates this assessment. Usually, pallor is easy to see in a light-skinned person, but in a dark-skinned person, doctors rely on color changes of the tongue, whites of the eyes, the inside of the mouth, and the palms of the hands.

Pallor can be limited, or it can involve the entire body. Generalized pallor can be caused by several conditions, including anxiety, an overcool or underheated room, anemia, very low blood pressure, or extreme hypertension. To test circulation in the legs, the doctor may raise your legs to see if there is a change in color. In peripheral vascular disorders, the lower leg may appear mottled and pale when it is elevated for about half a minute.

Cyanosis, a blue tinge to the skin or nails, is caused by lack of oxygen in the blood. Cyanosis's occurring just in a foot or hand may be caused by failure of the circulation or of the lungs to maintain a normal supply of oxygen to the tissues. When it affects several areas, such as the nails and around the lips, it means oxygen is not being replenished efficiently. This could be caused by a congenital heart defect, myocardial infarction, or chronic obstructive pulmonary disease (such as emphysema).

Your body's water content is reflected in how elastic your skin is. To test elasticity, the doctor gently pinches up skin on the back of your hand. The skin fold should disappear in one or two seconds; if it stays pinched up longer, you may be dehydrated. Conversely, excessive fluid accumulation that causes edema may be an indication of a failing heart.

Temperature and Moisture

Normally, skin is warm and dry, and the temperature is about the same in all parts of the body. An extremity that feels cooler to the touch than does the rest of the body may suffer from poor circulation caused by blockage in a nearby artery; an area that's warmer may indicate an infection.

Increased sweating can occur with fever from an infection or may just reflect anxiety. When someone goes into shock because of circulatory collapse, the skin feels cold and clammy as a result of reduced circulation and increased sweating. Shock can occur after myocardial infarction, severe injury, or blood loss.

Fingers and Nails

Long-standing cyanosis changes the shape of fingertips and nails. The fingers look bulbous, like clubs; nails flatten out; and the skin at the bottom of the nail bulges. Peripheral vascular disease can cause pitting, dents, brittleness, and thinning of the nails.

Extremities

Peripheral vascular disorders usually involve the feet or legs, but occasionally the upper extremities are affected, so the examination includes evaluation of circu-lation in the hands and arms. Poor circulation can eventually cause hair loss on the extremity and skin that is thin, shiny, and smooth. If blood return to the heart is slowed down, the extremity may itch, look red and scaly, and develop brown spots. Varicose veins bulge when patients sit or stand, but when they lift their leg above the heart, the veins look normal.

The doctor may ask you to bend your knee and flex your foot. If this produces pain in the calf, you may have a blood clot in a vein (thrombophlebitis) and may experience tenderness along that vein.

It may be difficult to distinguish between a blood clot in a leg and an infection called *cellulitis*. A venous Doppler study or even a venogram may be necessary. In patients who have had saphenous veins removed from the legs in coronary bypass operations, these areas of old scars are occasionally sites where infections (cellulitis) occur. The infecting organism, usually a staphylococcal or streptococcal pathogen, enters the skin through cracks between the toes.

If you have any swelling in the lower legs, the doctor will try to determine how severe it is. Swelling can be a sign of *edema*, or too much fluid in the tissues. Edema can be caused by heart failure or by a local cardiovascular disorder such as a blood clot or an infection in the tissues. It can be subtle, however. To test for edema, the doctor presses a finger against the shin or ankle for several seconds. In some cases this pressure leaves no indentation, but often it does. Doctors call this *pitting edema.* If the indentation lingers for two minutes or longer, pitting edema is considered to be severe, but an imprint that disappears in seconds is considered mild.

Evaluating the Cardiovascular System

Pulse

When a nurse or physician says, "I'm going to take your pulse," most people assume he or she will hold the wrist while looking at a watch to estimate the number of times the heart beats in a minute. In a routine examination, the wrist is often the only place a pulse is assessed. But you also have easily accessible pulses in the neck, inside the elbow, behind the knee, near the groin, behind the ankle, and on top of the foot (Figure 4.1). If you have symptoms of a cardiovascular disorder, the doctor will want to compare findings at these different points to determine if the pulse varies. Because blood flow diminishes as it gets farther away from the heart, the pulse won't be as strong in the legs as it is in the upper body; however, an abnormally weak or absent pulse in an extremity is a sign of blockage. A pulse that alternates between weak and strong beats is called *pulsus alternans* and may signal a late stage of congestive heart failure.

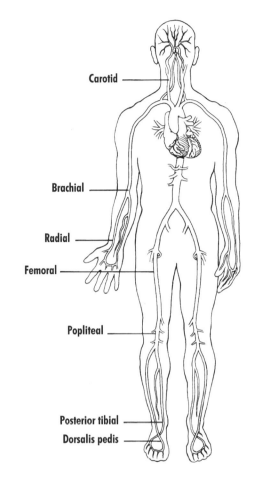

Figure 4.1. The 7 sites at which your pulse can be easily felt are the carotid, brachial, radial, femoral, popliteal, posterior tibial, and dorsalis pedis pulse points. The popliteal pulse is behind the knee, the posterior tibial pulse is behind the inner ankle, and the dorsalis pedis pulse is on top of the foot.

When taking your pulse, the doctor is paying attention to three characteristics: rate, rhythm, and strength. At rest, most adults' heart rates are 65 to 75 beats per minute, although conditioned athletes may have a lower rate. *Tachycardia,* a heart rate over 100, can occur with anemia, fever, an overactive thyroid, or poor heart performance. *Bradycardia,* a heart rate less than 50, can result from arrhythmias or other disturbances in electrical conduction. Normally, the heart has a regular rhythm, increasing slightly when you breathe in and decreasing slightly when you breathe out. Irregular rhythms or pauses between beats indicate a problem with the heart's electrical conduction system, although sinus arrhythmia is a normal variant.

With normal heart function, the pulse is easy to feel, symmetrical, strong, and steady. Cardiovascular disorders can produce a variety of abnormal pulses. For example, a pulse rate that is "thready"— that is, weak and varying in strength—can be caused by low blood volume, poor pumping action of the heart, or a stiff aortic heart valve. An unusually strong pulse may be the result of fever, stiff arteries, an overactive thyroid gland, or aortic insufficiency.

Blood Pressure

Since blood must travel through about 60,000 miles of vessels, the heart must pump with a great deal of force. The surge of blood creates a high-pressure wave through the arteries. The arteries expand to accommodate each surge and then relax between heartbeats. A blood pressure reading, measured in millimeters of mercury (mm Hg), is read as two numbers, such as "120 over 80" (written 120/80). The first number, called *systolic blood pressure,* is the highest measure of arterial pressure and is taken when the heart is contracting, or pumping blood to maintain circulation. The second is *diastolic blood pressure,* the lowest measure of blood pressure; it is measured when the heart is relaxed and filling with blood.

Heart

The physician will use observation, percussion (tapping), palpation (touching), and auscultation (listening) to evaluate the heart. Tapping on your chest will help the physician estimate the size and position of your heart. Pressing on your chest with fingertips, the physician will get more information about heart size and will try to detect any abnormal vibrations. With some types of heart failure, the size of the heart increases; with others, it remains the same. Using the stethoscope, the physician will strive to hear any abnormal heart sounds and will listen to the lungs, listening to determine what role pulmonary disorders play in the underlying condition or whether there is fluid accumulating in the heart. A third or fourth heart sound is called a *gallop rhythm.* A third heart sound is highly associated with a failing heart, but a fourth heart sound is less easily linked to a disorder. This heartbeat is normal in children but may signal high blood pressure, ischemia, or another disorder in adults.

Blood Vessels

To detect a blockage, doctors evaluate major arteries: carotid arteries in the neck, temporal arteries above the ears, the aorta in the trunk, renal arteries over the kidneys, femoral arteries at the groin, popliteal arteries behind the knees, posterior tibial arteries in the lower legs, and dorsal arteries of the feet. This evaluation includes palpation and, as far down as the groin, listening with a stethoscope. Normally, blood flow through healthy arteries and veins is silent. An obstruction alters this. A sound heard from a blood vessel is called a *bruit* (pronounced BREW-ee), derived from the French *braire* ("to bray," "to roar"). Bruits are caused by turbulent flow in arteries and veins, and often indicate the presence of atherosclerosis (although the sound may disappear when an artery becomes severely narrowed. Both the pitch and duration of bruits provide useful information to physicians.

The two major blood vessels in the neck—the carotid arteries and the jugular veins—are of special interest. High in the neck, under the jaw, specialized nerve fibers called *parasympathetic nerves* converge at the carotid artery. The parasympathetic nerves slow both heart rate and blood flow and can cause fainting through excessive stimulation of the vagus nerve. When the carotid artery is more than 30 percent to 40 percent obstructed, a bruit may be heard. Veins do not usually pulsate, but pressure changes in the right atrium can cause the jugular veins to pulsate. For this reason, the jugular pulse is a quick way to evaluate how well the right side of the heart is functioning. The jugular pulse is seen just above the collarbone but generally only when a person reclines, with shoulders propped up at about a 45-degree angle. A jugular pulse that is unusually strong (as measured by how high the vein rises at each pulse) may be caused by a leaky tricuspid valve or by high blood pressure in the lungs.

Noninvasively, carotid arteries are examined by Doppler ultrasound. Doppler ultrasonography is also used to determine the *ankle/brachial index* (also called the *systolic index*), which is the ratio of systolic ankle blood pressure to systolic brachial (arm) blood pressure. This index represents a simple early detection method for vascular disease of the lower extremities (peripheral vascular disease). The ratio should normally be greater than 0.9.

Other Evaluations

Chest X-rays

Structures with a high mineral content show up quite well on x-ray film. Bones, with their rich stores of calcium, are more visible on x-ray studies than organs, which contain only traces of minerals. On a standard x-ray, the heart and blood vessels are visible only as silhouettes. Even so, chest x-rays are valuable for showing the location and size of these structures. Because calcium deposits in organs are visible on x-rays, the doctor is able to see if there are calcifications on heart valves, coronary arteries, and great vessels.

Laboratory Tests

When a physician suspects that a patient has heart disease, certain laboratory tests may be ordered. These include a complete blood count, erythrocyte (red blood cell) sedimentation rate, prothrombin time, urinalysis, BUN (blood urea nitrogen), creatinine (kidney function), liver function, electrolyte, calcium, phosphorus, and thyroid-stimulating hormone values. Other thyroid function tests may be added. The patient's fasting blood lipid profile, including triglyceride and high-density lipoprotein, low-density lipoprotein, and total cholesterol values, is also important to delineate. If the patient is thought to have an infectious disease of the heart, blood cultures or serologic tests may be ordered.

Electrocardiography and Other Tests

Other diagnostic procedures, such as electrocardiography, which graphically represents the heart's electrical impulses; *echocardiography*, a method of detecting structural and functional changes using ultrasound; exercise testing; *angiography*; and cardiac catheterization, are also important in helping physicians understand the nature of a patient's heart ailment. (See Chapters 5 and 6 on noninvasive and invasive diagnostic procedures.)

Summary

The general physical examination of the patient by the cardiologist combines features of a standard annual examination and the specialty tests of the discipline of cardiology. Fundamental to expert diagnosis is the physician's ability to listen carefully to the patient, to observe the patient, to obtain a detailed personal and family history, and to perform an accurate physical examination. Evaluation of the patient with cardiovascular disease may incorporate many examinations necessary to provide the cardiologist with a clear picture of the patient physically, the physiological demands placed on the heart, and the expectation of cardiovascular performance in the future.

CHAPTER FIVE

Noninvasive Diagnostic Procedures

Many heart problems can be diagnosed with tests that are noninvasive, which means that the procedure does not require penetrating the body. Noninvasive tests are safe, rarely cause discomfort, and seldom have side effects. They are also generally less expensive than invasive tests.

Noninvasive tests are nearly always done by specially trained nurses or technicians. Some tests will probably be performed in your doctor's office, while others may be done at a hospital or other facility. Some of the tests use equipment that may look intimidating, but be assured they cause no harm. If you feel nervous because you do not know what to expect—or are simply curious—ask the technician to explain the machine and test. Most people are willing to talk about their work, and medical professionals are no exception. Test equipment video monitors may be a welcome addition to many patients, but others may be more comfortable thinking about other things. The tech-

nician can usually accommodate your preference.

Although technicians are expert in performing tests, interpreting the results should be left to a physician. Test films, scans, or other results are evaluated by specially trained doctors, who send a report to your cardiologist or primary care physician, usually the same day. Expect that it will be your cardiologist or primary care physician who will discuss the test results with you.

These noninvasive tests include clinical and ambulatory electrocardiography (ECG or EKG), exercise stress testing, echocardiography with and without exercise, Doppler ultrasonography, ultrafast computed tomography, positron emission tomography, magnetic resonance imaging (MRI), impedance plethysmography, scintigraphy or radionuclide angiography, thallium scanning with and without exercise, pyrophosphate technetium 99m scanning, and radionuclide ventriculography.

Clinical Electrocardiography

What it is: A recording of the heart's electrical activity.

Why it is ordered: To obtain a baseline reading of your heart's electrical activity. Results of this test help your physician diagnose and monitor arrhythmias; heart attack (whether in progress, a part of your medical history, or "silent"—one you were unaware of); thickening of the left ventricle (called *left ventricular hypertrophy*); enlargement of the left or right atrium; a shift of the heart's axis, suggesting abnormalities of the heart's intrinsic electrical conduction system; pericarditis; and coronary artery disease. This test is also used to monitor heart function at a routine physical examination.

Where it is done: Physician's office.

How long it takes: About 10 minutes. Actual recording time is three to five minutes.

An ECG machine has three main parts: electrodes, oscilloscope, and recorder. Electrodes are like microphones: they receive electrical current, which is transmitted to the machine through attached cords. To enhance reception, a technician first applies conducting jelly to the electrodes before placing them on your chest, arms, and legs. The oscilloscope is a monitor that shows electrical impulses of the heart. These impulses are translated into written form by the recorder, which produces a tracing on graph paper. Grids on the graph paper allow the doctor to measure speed (time) and electrical strength (voltage) of the impulse as it travels through the heart. (See pp. 30–36 for illustrations of electrocardiograms.)

Each electrical impulse is recorded as a wave form. The P wave shows the impulse as it leaves the sinoatrial node (the heart's natural pacemaker) and fans through the right and left atria. The R wave represents the initial activation of the ventricles. The interval between the P wave and the R wave normally takes between 80 and 110 milliseconds (about one-tenth of a second). The QRS complex reflects the electrical impulse's journey from the atrioventricular node through the right and left ventricles within about one-tenth of a second (or even faster). The segment between the S wave and the T wave is the "recovery" period, when electrical activity dissipates and the ventricles relax.

The ECG is a "snapshot" of your heart's performance during the test, and it can show irregularities in your heart's rhythm or rate. Such electrical impulse irregularities cause irregular heartbeats, or arrhythmias (see Chapter 9). However, when the ECG indicates that you do not have an arrhythmia, it does not rule out heart disease altogether. About 50 percent of people with coronary artery disease have completely normal results on electro-cardiography.

Ambulatory Electrocardiography

What it is: A continuous tracing is obtained from a portable ECG machine called a Holter monitor.

Why it is ordered: To evaluate heart rhythm. This test is also used to monitor the effectiveness of drug therapy for arrhythmias and to assess pacemaker function.

Where it is done: Outside the doctor's office.

How long it takes: Usually 12, 24, or 48 hours.

Sometimes symptoms are sporadic, so the standard ECG test may not show any abnormalities. The heart rhythm may be normal most of the time, becoming irregular only episodically. For example, physical exertion may bring on an arrhythmia that lasts for a few minutes and then disappears. Holter monitoring can detect such irregularities.

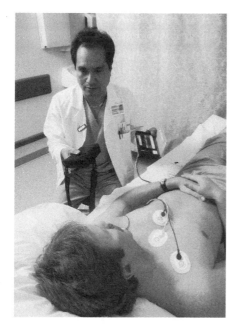

Figure 5.1. A patient is prepared to undergo ambulatory electrocardiography. The electrodes placed on his chest and connected to a portable recorder will provide his cardiologist with a record of his heart's electrical activity under normal daily stress.

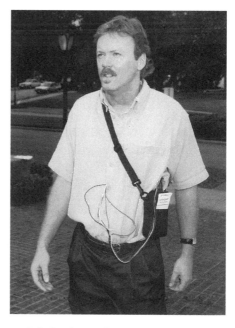

Figure 5.2. During Holter monitoring, the patient remains untethered to any stationary device. The recorder, weighing about 2 pounds, can be worn with a shoulder strap or attached to the patient's belt.

The Holter monitor's electrodes are connected to a 2-pound recorder that can be attached to a belt or shoulder strap (Figures 5.1 and 5.2). You are expected to continue with normal activities (unless the doctor instructs otherwise) with one exception: the equipment must not get wet, so you'll need to forgo showers and tub baths. You will be asked to keep a written diary of activities, emotional stress, symptoms, and any medications you take, including over-the-counter drugs.

Exercise Stress Testing

What it is: An ECG recording during exercise.

Why it is ordered: To diagnose the cause of chest pain and symptoms related to exercise. To evaluate the safety of starting an exercise program for people out of condition and patients recovering from heart attack or heart surgery. To note the effect of physical stress on the induction of arrhythmias. To assess the effectiveness of antiarrhythmia drug therapy.

Where it is done: Doctor's office or exercise lab.

How long it takes: Usually about 15 to 30 minutes.

Exercise stress testing (EST) is an extension of ECG. In addition to ECG monitoring, a technician takes blood pressure readings and evaluates your overall reaction to exercise. Most EST is done while you exercise on a treadmill (Figure 5.3) or stationary bicycle. EST falls into four general categories: single-stage, multistage, ministress, and maximal stress tests.

Single-stage tests, as the name implies, consist of repeating a single activity such as walking up and down a two-step staircase. These are the least demanding tests and they are rarely performed. Significant information about the functional capacity of the heart can be obtained if enough exercise is performed.

In *multistage tests*, the intensity of exercise is increased at intervals. For example, every three minutes both the incline and speed on a treadmill increase, forcing the heart to work harder.

Ministress tests are ordered for people recovering from heart attack to see whether it is safe to begin a walking program. Exercise is stopped after the person reaches a predetermined heart rate or develops symptoms.

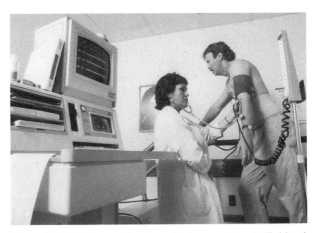

Figure 5.3. During exercise stress testing on a treadmill, blood pressure is monitored with a sphygmomanometer (right) and the heart's function with electrocardiography (left).

Maximal stress tests allow a person to continue exercising until either exhaustion or symptoms occur.

Wear comfortable exercise clothes and athletic shoes. You will be instructed not to eat for one or two hours before the test. Unless the doctor tells you otherwise, take prescribed medications as usual. During the test, tell the technician immediately if you experience such symptoms as chest pain or pressure, shortness of breath, leg pain, dizziness or a feeling of faintness, or mental confusion.

EST is not always accurate, and it is not unusual to have false-negative results (everything read normal during the test, but a heart problem existed) or false-positive results (some ECG abnormality was found, but there was actually no heart problem). For unknown reasons, the false-positive results occur more frequently in women.

Echocardiography

What it is: A means of producing a picture of the heart by sound waves.

Why it is ordered: To diagnose congenital heart disease, cardiomyopathy, congestive heart failure, pericardial disease, thrombosis, tumors, and valvular disease. To evaluate the left ventricle after heart attack.

Where it is done: Usually in a cardiology outpatient diagnostic laboratory.

How long it takes: About 30 minutes to an hour.

Echocardiography (sometimes called "echo" for short) is a diagnostic technique that relies on high-frequency inaudible sound waves known as ultrasound. It works much like sonar used on ships and submarines. Sonar locates objects underwater by recording how long it takes a sound wave to reach the object, bounce off, and return to the ship. Similarly, ultrasound records the position and the motion of internal structures of the heart and great vessels. A hand-held device called a *transducer* transmits and receives the ultrasound vibrations. The images from the transducer are fed back to a monitor (Figure 5.4).

To obtain an image, the technician uses a transducer, which looks like a short, fat wand. The technician applies gel to it to enhance sound transmission and presses the wand against the patient's chest. You will lie mostly on one side and will be asked to follow the technician's instructions to breathe in and out slowly or to hold your breath. Waves of ultrasound travel through the chest and ricochet off internal structures. The "echoes," or reflections, of the sound off the surfaces of the heart are converted into an image that can be displayed on a monitor.

Since it was developed in the 1970s, echocardiography has evolved dramatically. Formerly it produced a one-dimensional image that relied on the imagination of the physician to put "strips" of images together. It was like looking through a wrapping paper tube at a large canvas or sculpture, or trying to evaluate a piece of music presented in 10-second segments. Later, further development of ultrasound allowed the production of the two-dimensional, fan-shaped images familiar today. Further advances include a miniaturized transducer that can be attached to a flexible tube and inserted through the esophagus (blurring the line between noninvasive and invasive testing) and color-flow Doppler echocardiography. Stress echocardiography is now performed, sometimes with dobutamine administration. On dobutamine echocardiography, the development of regional-wall motion abnormalities or the loss of myocardial thickening has a high correlation with the presence of advanced coronary artery disease.

When the transducer is inserted through the esophagus, the technique is called *transesophageal echocardiography,* and exceptionally clear images are produced because the transducer is much closer to the heart. The health care team administers a sedative and numbs the throat. Patients generally tolerate the procedure well; however, complications have included esophageal puncture, arrhythmias, stroke, and even death. With Doppler ultrasound, sound frequencies that bounce off red blood cells are used to calculate the velocity of blood flow through the heart. Color Doppler studies convert different

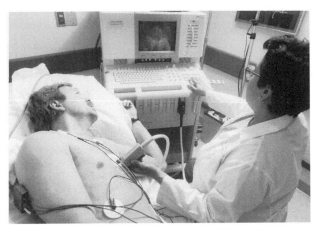

Figure 5.4. A patient undergoing echocardiography watches the monitor as the technician holds the transducer against his chest. The transducer emits sound waves, neither heard nor felt by the patient, that render the image visible on the monitor as they travel internally.

rates of blood flow into different colors. This graphic, moving picture of the heart's performance includes measures of the dimensions of the chambers, motion of the valves, and direction of the blood.

Doppler Ultrasonography

What it is: A measurement of blood flow through veins and arteries in the legs or through the carotid vessels in the neck.

Why it is ordered: To diagnose thrombosis and arterial insufficiency in the carotid arteries and vessels in the legs.

Where it is done: Usually in the physician's office.

How long it takes: About 30 to 45 minutes.

Normally, blood pressure in the legs is 10 percent lower than blood pressure in the arms. If there is an arterial blockage in the leg, blood pressure in the limb drops even lower. But it is hard to take a blood pressure reading because pulses in the foot and lower leg are difficult to hear with just a stethoscope. Doppler ultrasound works on the same principle as sonar and echo-cardiography—high-frequency sound waves bounce off soft tissues, and the echoes are converted to electrical impulses and displayed on a screen—with the added feature of magnified sound.

A blood pressure cuff is wrapped around the ankle and, instead of a stetho-scope, a transducer is placed over pulse points of the foot and lower leg. You may experience some discomfort from pressure of the cuff and transducer.

Another noninvasive method, ultrasonic duplex scanning, combines pulsed Doppler with ultrasound imaging methods. With it, it is possible to evaluate the velocity of blood traveling through the blood vessels and to measure it at selected points. More-over, it is possible to detect *venous thrombi* (blood clots in the veins) and arterial atherosclerotic lesions and to measure the extent of narrowing, which has proved important in detecting early lesions and in studying their development over time. Color ultrasonic images facilitate and expedite diagnosis. When duplex scanning is combined with plethysmography (see below), the physician has the ability to evaluate both superficial and deep veins.

Carotid Doppler ultrasound has become extremely valuable and widely used to evaluate plaque formation in the external and internal carotid arteries and in the carotid siphon (site of branching). When a bruit is discovered or a patient has symp-toms of transient ischemic attacks, carotid Doppler is routinely done. Both plaque and thrombus may be identified. Further-more, the intimal-to-medial thickness of the outer carotid wall is an indicator of carotid atherosclerosis and also a predic-tion of coronary events. It is favorably affected by blood lipid reductions.

Carotid Doppler is painless. A techni-cian places a transducer over the neck and the pattern of sound wave reflections is recorded and interpreted.

Ultrafast Computed Tomography

What it is: Scanning with electron beams that provides 17 scans per second. Sometimes called *electron-beam tomog-raphy,* this modality can provide movie-like, three-dimensional views of the beating heart and flowing blood that can be displayed on a television screen and matched in sequence to the ECG.

Why it is ordered: To evaluate coronary artery disease by determining if there are calcium deposits in the coronary arteries.

Where it is done: At a hospital or clinic.

How long it takes: Scanning takes less than a minute.

Ultrafast computed tomography (for short, ultrafast CT or CAT scanning) is very useful in delineating the coronary arteries and calcium deposits in them. Some patient groups may have a good deal of arterial calcification unrelated to the build-up of atherosclerotic plaque. These patients include those with hypercalcemia (a disorder in which there is an excess of calcium in the blood, which can lead to such symptoms as fatigue, depression, and nausea) and those with a condition that can lead to hypercalcemia (for example, hyperthyroidism or cancer). Another patient group in this category is the elderly, since arterial calcification tends to occur as a part of aging. In other patients, however, the calcium score provided by ultrafast CT has a high correlation with the presence of atherosclerotic plaque. That is, knowing the calcium score tells us a lot about whether atherosclerosis is present, so ultrafast CT can play an important role in risk assessment.

In contrast to schoolwork, a score of zero is a good score in this test. A higher score (say, 3 or 4) would indicate cause for concern: a motivator to adhere to the risk-reduction regimen prescribed by your physician. But remember that the results of this test, like any one test, are just a part of the whole diagnostic picture your physician is putting together. He or she will interpret the calcium score for you within the context of other assessments of your health.

Ultrafast CT is a relatively new imaging modality. Thus, scientists are still measuring its abilities and evaluating it against invasive and other noninvasive methods of gathering information about the heart.

Positron Emission Tomography

What it is: In cardiology, a method of producing three-dimensional, high-resolution images of the heart's blood flow, structure, and cellular metabolism by tracing the release of high-energy gamma rays from radioactive particles.

Why it is ordered: To diagnose coronary artery disease and to evaluate the status of the heart muscle.

Where it is done: At a hospital.

How long it takes: From an hour to an hour and 45 minutes.

Created by Louis Sokoloff in 1978, positron emission tomography (PET) is a diagnostic imaging technique able to provide biochemical and metabolic information. Its ability to produce high-resolution images and blood flow assessment are characteristics cardiologists cite as making this a superior diagnostic modality. With hollow rings of detectors and multiple x-ray sources encircling the patient, PET scanners detect the gamma radiation produced when positrons, marked with a radioactive tracer, collide with and are destroyed by electrons. The positrons are produced from short-lived isotopes, which require an expensive cyclotron or generator to prepare. With this information taken in multiple cross-sections, the scanner constructs three-dimensional images.

One of PET's uses is in the evaluation of acute or chronic injury to the heart's muscular layer (myocardium). Patients with heart failure, in whom the heart's pumping ability is waning, and those who have had a heart attack are excellent candidates for evaluation by PET. One crucial advantage PET scanning offers is the ability to tell the difference between myocardium that is "stunned" (temporarily not working but capable of functioning) and myocardium that will never work again because of irreversible cell death. Physicians can use the results of the evaluation to define myocardial status and to determine the best therapeutic approach. Because of its complexity and the high cost of acquiring, running, and maintaining the equipment, this technology is less widely available than others and usually used only in special cases.

Magnetic Resonance Imaging

What it is: A computerized method of scanning that uses radio waves and a powerful magnet to scan designated parts of the body.

Why it is ordered: In cardiology, to diagnose congenital heart disease, cardiomyopathy, congestive heart failure, pericardial disease, thrombosis, tumors, and valvular disease.

Where it is done: Usually at a hospital.

How long it takes: About 30 minutes.

The MRI scanner is a cylinder about 8 feet long with a tunnel running its length. MRI scanners are located in specially built rooms that shield the machine's magnetic field. No metal is allowed inside the room, so tell your doctor if you have a pacemaker, orthopedic pins, or other metal in your body. All jewelry, coins, and clothing with metal fasteners must be removed. You should also leave credit cards outside because the scanner can damage their magnetic strips. Do *not* undergo MRI if you have a cardiac pacemaker.

You will lie on a table that slides into the tunnel. To avoid distorting the images, do not talk or move during the procedure. Expect this to be a noisy experience: the machinery pings and bangs constantly. Some people feel claustrophobic, and many complain of boredom. MRI produces clear, cross-sectional images.

Impedance Plethysmography

What it is: A method to diagnose peripheral artery blockage. In Europe, this is its main use. What it is not, generally speaking, is a method to diagnose venous disease. Doppler ultrasonography has replaced both uses.

Why it is ordered: To diagnose thrombosis and thrombophlebitis, although its use is rare.

Where it is done: Usually in the doctor's office.

How long it takes: About 15 minutes.

Plethysmography records changes in blood volume and vessel resistance. The information is displayed on a monitor and recorded on ECG graph paper. A blood pressure cuff is wrapped around the leg above the knee. Around the calf, four encircling electrodes are placed in pairs, two near the knee and two near the ankle. The cuff is inflated to a point above venous pressure and below arterial pressure (about 40 to 60 mm Hg), causing the blood pressure to drop in veins below the cuff and venous blood to collect in the limb. The instrument measures the increase in leg volume while the cuff is inflated, and then measures the decrease when the cuff is deflated.

This measure indicates how efficiently the veins can return to normal. With this information, the physician can evaluate the possibility of an obstruction. Peripheral veins are normal when blood pressure returns to the initial reading within 10 seconds. A delay indicates reduced circulation. Although plethysmography is usually painless and risk free, people with aching or throbbing legs may find the test increases their discomfort. This procedure may be used by those who are experienced in its application and interpretation.

Radionuclide Angiography

What it is: A method of visualizing vessels and the heart. A radioactive pharmaceutical is injected into a vessel, and a scanning camera takes a series of pictures of the heart.

Why it is ordered: To diagnose thrombosis, tumors, and valvular disease. To evaluate the heart after myocardial infarction.

Where it is done: Usually in a hospital's nuclear medicine department.

How long it takes: Scanning takes about 30 minutes to an hour. May be repeated.

Radioactive isotopes emit gamma rays. They are used to "label" certain compounds that are known to localize in particular tissues when injected into the body. When a heart-targeting radiopharmaceutical is injected into the bloodstream, some of it travels to the heart to be deposited. Some radiopharmaceuticals collect only in damaged tissue, and others congregate only in healthy tissue. A scanning (scintillation) camera that detects gamma rays is passed over the body and produces a series of pictures showing the isotopes' journey. This method of testing is also called *scintigraphy*. Substances used in the radionuclear assessment of cardiovascular disease include thallium, pyrophosphate technetium 99m, and fibrinogen iodine 125.

The nuclear scanning equipment includes a control panel with a video screen, dials, keyboard, and video recorder. A scanning camera, suspended above a table, resembles an x-ray machine. You will lie on the table while the camera passes back and forth over you. Expect to hear clicks, bumps, and electronic hums as the automated machine moves.

Nuclear scanning is not dangerous and exposes the patient to roughly the same amount of radiation as a chest x-ray. Only a tiny amount of isotope is used, and the radioactive material is completely gone from the body within a few days.

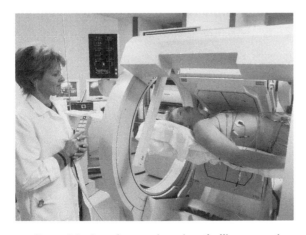

Figure 5.5. **A patient undergoing thallium scanning lies still while the equipment is positioned.**

Thallium Scanning

What it is: A radiopharmaceutical is injected into a vessel, and a scanning camera takes a series of pictures of the heart. A thallium scan is often done in conjunction with an exercise stress test.

Why it is ordered: Thallium scanning is used to evaluate perfusion and uptake by normal tissue, which may be altered by conditions such as coronary artery disease.

Where it is done: Usually in a hospital's nuclear medicine department.

How long it takes: About 30 minutes to an hour. The scan is done immediately after injection and repeated about four hours later.

Thallium collects in tissue that is functionally normal and has an intact blood supply. Thallium scans are usually done in conjunction with ECG and a stress test. As soon as the stress test ends, the thallium is injected and you resume exercising for about one minute, which gives the heart's muscular wall, or myocardium, time to absorb it. When patients are unable to exercise or to obtain an adequate heart rate, for example, from beta-blockers, adenosine may be administered intravenously to increase the heart rate. This is sometimes called the adenosine–thallium stress test. One scan is done immediately, and another is performed four hours later (Figure 5.5). Since thallium does not collect where blood flow is poor or where scarring is present, ischemia shows up on the scan as dark areas, or "cold spots." The second scan helps physicians tell the difference between areas that are scarred and those that are ischemic.

Pyrophosphate Technetium 99m Scanning

What it is: A scanning method in which a radiopharmaceutical is injected into a vein and a camera takes a series of pictures of the heart.

Why it is ordered: To evaluate the heart after heart attack, among other uses.

Where it is done: Usually in a hospital's nuclear medicine department.

How long it takes: The scan is done about two or three hours after the injection; scanning takes about 30 minutes to an hour.

Pyrophospate technetium 99m is used for bone scans because it binds to calcium. Calcium is also deposited on diseased valves and on tissue damaged by myocardial infarction. Tiny calcium deposits appear within 12 hours of a heart attack and normally disappear within a week. For this reason, pyrophosphate technetium 99m scans are generally repeated over several weeks to be certain no further damage occurs.

Radionuclide Ventriculography

What it is: A nuclear scanning technique that can provide information about the heart's function and the flow of blood through it.

Why it is ordered: To determine if the ventricles are functioning properly.

Where it is done: Usually in a hospital's nuclear medicine department.

How long it takes: Scanning takes about 30 minutes to an hour.

Unlike an x-ray film, which shows only structure, a radionuclide ventriculogram is a tracing of the flow of blood through the heart and part of the bloodstream. Special scanning cameras measure the small amount of radioactive material injected into the circulation, and then a computer uses the information to create an image and calculate the ventricles' size and shape. Physicians study this information to determine if the ventricles are functioning efficiently.

The physician may pair this type of scanning with stress or exertion. The test is run while the patient is at rest, and then at increasing levels of exertion. Comparisons are made with the pumping function of a normal heart at those levels, and conclusions can be drawn about the function of the heart being tested. Physicians want to know how much blood the ventricle ejects during one pumping cycle (*stroke volume*) and in one minute (*cardiac output*), and what percentage of the blood that fills the ventricle is actually pumped out per heartbeat (*ejection fraction*).

CHAPTER SIX

Invasive Diagnostic Procedures

Sometimes a diagnosis cannot be made with noninvasive tests because the physician needs more information in order to select the best treatment. Though many noninvasive tests are providing more and more information, results may require confirmation before a treatment regimen is recommended and initiated. Symptoms may or may not be present. Patients may be without any symptoms but have evidence from noninvasive tests of coronary artery disease, or patients may have accelerating symptoms, increasing in severity or frequency. Physicians may suspect a blocked artery in the heart (coronary artery), the neck (carotid artery), or the leg (peripheral artery). Or they may want to test for an aortic aneurysm or a valvular or congenital disease.

An invasive procedure is usually undertaken when surgery, angioplasty, or a vascular repair procedure is being considered. The invasive procedure allows the physician to establish a precise diagnosis, to define the extent of the disease, to make a determination about the need for surgical or medical intervention, and to plan the exact procedure to be performed. These are only a few of the many instances in which invasive diagnostic testing is necessary. The good news is that these invasive diagnostic procedures are relatively safe, although from the patient's point of view, any hospital-based procedure and the illness it implies can be perceived as major interferences in a normal life.

In recent decades, medical technology has brought invasive cardiovascular procedures a long way. The equipment is more precise; physicians are better trained to use it and more experienced with it; and procedures are safer than they formerly were. Risks, though clear, are few and rarely serious, and the doctor will want to discuss them with the patient before the procedure. Physicians review a patient's history and health status very carefully before deciding what tests are necessary and how they should be done. It may be reassuring to know that complications occur in less than 2 percent of patients and that cardiac catheterization, the technique making these diagnostic tests possible, is routinely performed on an outpatient basis.

If you are a candidate for invasive diagnostic testing, do not be intimidated by having to sign consent forms or by the precautions physicians and hospitals take. Consent forms are the physician's and facility's explanation to you of the procedure and risks, and you acknowledge the risks with your signature. Take the forms seriously, and get explanations for any sections you do not understand. Conducting the tests should be experts who hold your well-being foremost and who are skilled enough to remedy any untoward response. Careful patient assessment and screening are fundamental. Only unusually high risk situations require reserving an operating room and having a surgical team on call. Hospitals with in-house cardiovascular surgery can provide such facilities and personnel should an emergency develop during a diagnostic procedure.

Cardiac catheterization and angiography, though they go hand-in-hand, are not identical. Catheterization is a technique by which angiography is performed. The term *angiography* encompasses the x-ray visualization of any blood vessel, including aortography, arteriography, and pulmonary angiography. Catheterization also makes electrophysiologic studies, hemodynamic monitoring, and venography possible.

Cardiac Catheterization

What it is: Cardiac catheterization is a technique used to evaluate the heart, including its blood vessels, valves, and muscular wall.

- With angiography, it provides a view of the heart's chambers, great vessels, and coronary arteries, using x-ray technology.
- With a balloon-flotation catheter, it provides hemodynamic monitoring.
- With other specially designed catheters, it allows physicians to perform a biopsy of heart tissue and other evaluations.

In cardiac catheterization, a cardiologist inserts a *catheter,* a long, flexible tube, into a blood vessel, usually in the arm or groin, and guides it into the heart using a guide wire. After the catheter is maneuvered into place, the guide wire is removed and contrast solution is injected through the catheter so that the heart and its major vessels will be clearly visible on the x-ray. Injecting the contrast solution makes angiography, or the recording of the blood vessels on film, possible. The *angiogram,* or picture of the blood vessels, can reveal congenital defects and indicate clogged arteries. Though angiography is only one use of cardiac catheterization, the terms are sometimes used interchangeably

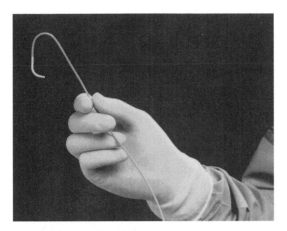

Figure 6.1. In cardiac catheterization, physicians use a long, thin tube called a *catheter* to enter and evaluate the cardiovascular system. Physicians use catheterization to assess coronary artery disease, evaluate defects and congenital anomalies, define valvular disorders, and retrieve specimens on which to perform specific tests. Specialized catheters carry minute instruments, are used to administer drugs or contrast solution, and enhance visualization with minute cameras.

(and the description below incorporates angiography). Besides being a route for contrast solution, catheters can be used to retrieve blood samples, administer drugs, enhance visualization with fiberoptics, and insert other instruments for a variety of diagnostic tests. During the procedure, one catheter may be removed and another inserted to evaluate different structures or to perform various tests. Special catheters have been manufactured for specific uses (Figure 6.1).

Why it is ordered: Cardiac catheterization has many uses: assessing coronary artery disease, including causes of angina and complications following myocardial infarction, and evaluating congenital heart defects, the heart wall, and valvular disor-

ders. To evaluate arrhythmias, physicians sometimes use an electrophysiologic study (see below). Cardiac catheterization can also be employed therapeutically (see Chapter 4).

Before the procedure: If you are scheduled for cardiac catheterization, you will not be allowed to have anything to eat or drink for six to 12 hours before the procedure. You will be asked to sign a consent form after the risks and benefits of the procedure are explained. Cardiac catheterization is safe, but as with any invasive procedure, there are risks. If you have a history of allergic reactions, the doctor may order medications to prevent or minimize a reaction to contrast solution.

You will be awake, though relaxed, during cardiac catheterization so that you can follow instructions from the health care team to assist in the procedure. Expect very little discomfort. About an hour before the procedure starts, you will be given a sedative such as diazepam (Valium) to take by mouth to help you relax. An intravenous (IV) line is inserted into a vein, and IV fluids are started. If medications are ordered to prevent a reaction to contrast solution, they will be injected through the IV line.

How it is done: The cardiac catheterization laboratory, or fluoroscopy suite, is equipped with an x-ray camera, video monitor, electrocardiography unit, and other monitoring equipment. Some rooms are set up with an automated camera that moves around the table; others have a stationary camera, and the table moves from side to side. In either case, the patient is strapped securely to the table. All the physicians, nurses, and technicians will be wearing surgical gowns, caps, and masks to prevent infection.

ECG electrodes are taped onto the patient's chest, and the area where the catheter will be inserted is shaved and disinfected. Sterile towels, draped around the area, may block the patient's view of what is going on. A local anesthetic is injected, and after the site is numb, a small incision is made in the blood vessel. Expect to feel a slight pressure as the catheter is inserted.

Physicians watch the video monitor as a guide to moving the catheter through the blood vessels and positioning it in the heart. When the contrast solution is injected, you may feel a warm flush for about 15 to 30 seconds. From time to time you may be asked to hold your breath, breathe deeply, or cough. Holding your breath during picture taking ensures better photographic quality, and coughing helps move the contrast solution through the chambers and vessels. If you feel any chest pain during the procedure, say so.

The procedure takes from half an hour to two hours, depending on what studies and how many tests are needed. Most procedures are now done by direct femoral puncture and the catheter is removed with pressure applied over the vessel until hemostasis is achieved. The physicians and nurses monitor patients continuously throughout the procedure and observe them for several hours afterward.

After the procedure: Even when cardiac catheterization is done in an outpatient surgery unit, you will be kept in a recovery area and monitored for several hours afterward. The arm or leg with the incision is immobilized for two to four hours. Nurses check your pulses and blood pressure regularly, and your heartbeat may be monitored by an ECG unit. Pain medication is available if you need it. Nurses will want you to drink extra fluids to encourage the elimination of the contrast solution through the kidneys. To allow bladder emptying during immobilization, a Foley catheter or external catheter may be used, or you may need to use a bed pan.

If the catheter was inserted through a vein, you will be asked to stay in bed for four to six hours. If it was inserted through an artery, you will be asked to maintain strict bed rest for six to eight hours, with your head raised about 30 degrees. A cold pack may be placed over the dressing to reduce swelling.

Before you go home your physician will discuss the results of your tests with you and let you know whether treatment or more tests or both will follow. Ask the physician or nurse supervising your care any questions you have.

When you return home: When you return home following the catheterization, follow any written instructions the hospital gives you. Unless your doctor says otherwise, you may resume regular activities the next day. The incision area will be sore for several days. Call your doctor if the wound bleeds or if there is any sign of infection—swelling, redness, increased pain, drainage, or fever. There may be a lump, but it will disappear gradually.

As mentioned above, complications from cardiac catheterization are rare. Bruising sometimes occurs around the incision, but it disappears. Such serious complications as myocardial infarction, arrhythmia, and puncture of the heart or arteries occur rarely. Complications that may appear days or weeks later include stroke, thrombosis (development of a blood clot), lung embolism (the blocking of a vessel serving the lung by a clot or other material carried by the blood current), and infection.

In some medically underserved areas, cardiac catheterization mobile vans have been developed, sometimes operating under the aegis of a large hospital (perhaps as part of a university hospital). The van is parked next to a local hospital when procedures are performed. Free-standing catheterization clinics have also emerged. Few data exist about the safety and self-regulation practices of these nontraditional providers, prompting professional medical organizations and supporting groups in the early 1990s to refuse to recommend services at free-standing clinics.

Angiography

What it is: Angiography, encompassing aortography, arteriography, coronary angiography, pulmonary angiography, and ventriculography, is the x-ray study of the heart and blood vessels during cardiac catheterization. Its purpose is to delineate on x-ray film structures of the circulatory system. As described above, contrast solution containing iodine is injected through the catheter into the heart, making it and nearby structures visible on x-ray. Depending on where the catheter is positioned, different areas are studied: the aorta and aortic valve (aortography), coronary arteries (arteriography), blood vessels in the lungs (pulmonary angiography), and the right or left ventricle and atrioventricular valve (ventriculography). Cineangiography produces a motion picture, and serial angiography produces still images taken in rapid sequence.

Why it is ordered: Different types of angiography serve different purposes. Coronary angiography is used to diagnose coronary artery disease. Plaque build-up is important to locate and evaluate, because if it succeeds in dramatically limiting blood flow, a heart attack can result. Aortography can help physicians identify abnormalities of the aorta and assess the aortic valve. Pulmonary angiography may be ordered to evaluate congenital heart disease or pulmonary embolism. Ventriculography can detect abnormalities in ventricular contraction. Other vessels—those in legs or arms or those serving the brain or specific organs, for example—can also be studied with angiography.

Before the procedure: If you have any allergies or have ever had a reaction to contrast solution, the doctor may order medications to reduce the chance that a reaction will occur during the procedure.

During the procedure: When the contrast solution is first injected, expect to feel a flushing sensation and nausea. Usually this passes within a few seconds. If it does not, you may be having a reaction to the contrast solution. Express your discomfort because the physician can administer a medication to relieve the discomfort quickly. (Sometimes people become hypersensitive to iodine unexpectedly, but there is no way to predict if this will happen.)

After the procedure: You will need to drink plenty of liquids for about eight hours to flush the contrast solution out of your system. You may eat a regular diet unless the doctor orders otherwise.

Electrophysiologic Study

What it is: Electrophysiologic studies evaluate the heart's electrical conduction system. Electrophysiologic studies require cardiac catheterization such that electrodes within a catheter are passed through the right atrium, through the tricuspid valve, and into the ventricle. Once there, these multiple electrodes stimulate different areas of the heart's electrical conduction system. The goal is to pinpoint the exact origin of an irregular heartbeat, or arrhythmia, by stimulating its production while monitoring the heart. In addition, these studies are used to assess how well antiarrhythmia drugs correct the problem.

Why it is ordered: Electrophysiologic studies are ordered under highly selected circumstances when it is necessary to explain an irregular heartbeat, rapid heartbeat, previous cardiac arrest, and fainting.

During the procedure: For electrophysiologic studies, the cardiac catheter is usually inserted through the femoral vein in the groin. During the procedure you may feel your heart speed up, slow down, or skip beats. Changes in rhythm during testing are normal; however, report any chest pain or other discomfort you experience.

After the procedure: You will be asked to remain in bed for four to six hours. A continuous ECG recording will be made during this time. You may be sent to a cardiac unit for close monitoring for a longer period of time.

Hemodynamic Monitoring

What it is: Hemodynamic monitoring is a continuous recording of heart function. In cardiac catheterization, the catheter is usually inserted in the right side of the heart; for hemodynamic monitoring, a second catheter is inserted into an artery in the arm. The catheters are equipped with fiberoptics and electronic devices that measure blood gases (oxygen and carbon dioxide), the amount of blood pumped through the heart, and pressure inside the arteries.

Why it is ordered: Hemodynamic monitoring is usually done in a critical care unit. It is used to monitor patients with heart failure, respiratory failure, shock, and other life-threatening illnesses. It is also used during and after some surgeries.

How it is done: The procedure is similar to cardiac catheterization, but the equipment is generally much less elaborate. Typically, the catheter is inserted in a large vein in the neck just above the collarbone, advanced through the right atrium and ventricle, and into the pulmonary artery. The pressure and other variables measured in the pulmonary artery reflect the status of the right side of the heart and venous circulation. The catheters are called *flow directed.* When wedged against the pulmonary capillaries the catheter measures the *wedge pressure*, which is the same as the pressure in the left atrium on the left side of the heart. A small balloon at the tip holds the catheter in place. Catheters used in hemodynamic monitoring have four or five lumens, or channels. These branches allow several procedures to be done at the same time. Drugs can be injected through one lumen without interrupting monitoring. A second catheter may be placed in an artery some distance from the heart, usually in the arm.

The cardiac catheter is connected to IV fluids, a monitor and oscilloscope, and a pressure-sensitive transducer that converts pressure readings to electrical signals. In critical care units where patients may be catheterized for routine monitoring, the information is transmitted to a central area such as a nurses' station. Monitors are watched at all times, so any abnormalities that develop can be investigated immediately.

Patients and visitors sometimes believe that physicians and nurses pay more attention to the machinery than to the patient.

This impression may arise because both the procedure and the equipment are complex. The equipment needs frequent checking to be sure it is working correctly, and the importance of these measures as indicators of well-being can hardly be overestimated.

Venography

What it is: Venography, or phlebography, allows the visualization of veins through the use of contrast medium. It enables viewing the location of blood clots (thrombi) in the extremities. A catheter is inserted into the vein, and contrast solution is injected. X-rays are taken serially over time to observe how the contrast solution disperses through the vein.

Why it is ordered: Phlebography is performed to diagnose venous thrombosis.

Before the procedure: The contrast solution contains iodine, which causes an allergic reaction in some people. Be sure you tell the doctor if you have a history of allergies or hay fever, or if you have ever had a reaction to contrast solution. Also, the doctor may prescribe a sedative such as diazepam (Valium) to help you relax.

During the procedure: If the area where the catheter is to be inserted is very hairy, it will be shaved. The area is cleaned and a local anesthetic is injected to numb the skin. A small incision is made and the catheter is inserted. When the contrast solution is injected, expect to feel a warm, flushing sensation in your arm or leg. You may also feel this sensation throughout your body, as well as some nausea, but these feelings disappear quickly. When the procedure is finished, the catheter is removed and a bandage is placed over the area.

After the procedure: You will be kept on bed rest for two to four hours, with the extremity immobile. Drinking plenty of fluids will help flush the contrast solution from your system quickly. Ask for pain medication if you need it. The incision area will be sore for a few days, but unless your doctor says otherwise, it is safe to resume normal activities the following day. Notify the doctor if you experience swelling, redness, pain, or fever.

Summary

Cardiac catheterization offers a technique for performing diagnostic procedures meant to confirm or refine diagnoses obtained from clinical or other technologic evaluation. Patients, awake during the procedure, experience little pain or inconvenience with cardiac catheterization. They benefit enormously from the information concerning heart and vessel structure and function it provides, whether it is employed as a diagnostic tool in the catheterization laboratory or as a monitoring tool in the cardiac care unit.

CHAPTER SEVEN

Risk Factors for Coronary Heart Disease

Coronary heart disease, also called *coronary artery disease,* is atherosclerosis of the coronary arteries, that is, the blood vessels that supply blood to the heart muscle itself. As we discuss later, in Chapter 13, exactly how atherosclerosis arises remains speculative, even though the disease process, including its consequences in such events as angina pectoris (chest pain), heart attack, and stroke, is a very familiar one. Since we have not yet defined the precise mechanism of atherosclerosis development, it is fortunate that we can identify factors that determine people's risk for development of the disease. We do not have to know the exact mechanism for the development of a disease to be able to reduce risk for it. For example, the exact mechanism of lung cancer is not known, but the great majority of cases of lung cancer could be prevented through smoking cessation.

A risk factor is defined as any trait or habit, whether genetic or environmental (which includes lifestyle factors), that can be used to predict an individual's probability of developing a particular disease. Atherosclerotic disease has two major groups of risk factors: those that can be changed or controlled by an individual and those that cannot be changed or controlled. Those risk factors over which we have control largely concern dietary and other lifestyle choices, and these choices are powerful over a lifetime. Much of the decline in the coronary heart disease death rate in the United States over the past three decades has been attributed to lifestyle modifications, specifically, less tobacco use and the reduction of saturated fat and cholesterol in the diet. However, coronary heart disease is still the leading cause of death and disability in the United States, both for men and for women, and a large part of the problem is that many people continue in habits that are conducive to the development of atherosclerotic disease.

The wise course of action is to modify cardiovascular risk factors *before* the disease has had the opportunity to develop or to progress. Information on reducing risk for atherosclerotic disease is provided in Chapter 26.

For a quick estimate of your risk for a heart attack or other coronary heart disease event, complete the "Coronary Heart Disease Risk Chart" on page 81 (Table 7.1). This chart is based on the major modifiable risk factors except diabetes (see Table 7.2). A low score does not necessarily mean that you are safe from heart disease, and a high score does not mean that you will definitely have a heart attack. Completing the quiz does not substitute for a complete medical workup by your physician. You are at higher risk if you already have evidence of atherosclerotic disease (if, for example, you have had angina, a heart attack, a stroke, transient ischemic attacks—temporary strokelike attacks—or peripheral vascular disease) or if you have diabetes. The particular database used to develop the chart did not include aging and a family history of early coronary heart disease; these factors, too, increase your risk (see Table 7.2).

If you have a high score, do not despair. You can decrease your risk by (1) following a diet low in saturated fat, cholesterol, and sodium; (2) controlling your weight, including losing weight if necessary; (3) increasing your physical activity; (4) not smoking; and (5) taking the medications your physician has prescribed. Excellent drug therapy is available to improve your blood lipid profile, lower blood pressure, or control diabetes when lifestyle changes alone are not enough. These interventions are discussed further in Chapter 11 (on blood pressure), Chapter 26 (on reducing risk from other lifestyle risk factors), and Chapter 27 (on medications, including lipid-lowering drugs).

Major Risk Factors for Heart Disease

The National Cholesterol Education Program (NCEP), a National Institutes of Health program that issues guidelines for assessing and treating high blood cholesterol, has determined 10 specific risk factors, shown in Table 7.2, that have been strongly associated with coronary heart disease risk. These major risk factors also apply to atherosclerotic disease at other locations in the body, although their relative contributions to risk may vary somewhat according to the anatomic site (for example, lowering high blood pressure affects stroke risk more dramatically than heart disease risk). Having two or three of these risk factors does not simply double or triple cardiovascular disease risk. For example, data from the Multiple Risk Factor Intervention Trial (MRFIT, or "Mr. Fit") showed that a male cigarette smoker with high total blood cholesterol and

Table 7.1. Coronary Heart Disease Risk Chart

Category	Level of Risk	Points	Your Score
Cigarette smoking	Never smoked or stopped three or more years ago	1	
	Never smoked but live or work with smokers	2	
	Stopped smoking within the last three years	3	
	Smoke regularly	4	
	Smoke regularly and live or work with smokers	5	
Systolic blood pressure (mm Hg)[a]	Less than 120	1	
	120 to 139	2	
	Don't know	3	
	140 to 159	4	
	160 or higher	5	
Total blood cholesterol (mg/dl)	Less than 160	1	
	160 to 199	2	
	Don't know	3	
	200 to 239	4	
	240 or higher	5	
HDL-cholesterol ("good" cholesterol) (mg/dl)	Over 60	1	
	56 to 60	2	
	Don't know	3	
	35 to 55	4	
	Less than 35	5	
Body weight	Within 10 pounds of desirable weight	1	
	10 to 20 pounds above desirable weight	2	
	21 to 30 pounds above desirable weight	3	
	31 to 50 pounds above desirable weight	4	
	More than 50 pounds above desirable weight	5	
Physical activity	Highly active	1	
	Between moderately active and highly active	2	
	Moderately active	3	
	Between inactive and moderately active	4	
	Inactive	5	

Your total points

SCORE

Total Points	Heart Attack Risk
6 to 13	Low
14 to 22	Moderate
23 to 30	High

You are at higher risk if you already have evidence of coronary heart disease or other atherosclerotic disease (for example, stroke) or if you have diabetes. Other major risk factors are age and a family history of premature coronary heart disease (see Table 7.2).

SOURCE: Adapted from the American Heart Association's brochure "What's Your Risk of Heart Attack?"
[a] Systolic blood pressure is the first value in a blood pressure reading (for example, 120 in 120/80). Blood pressure should be confirmed by measurement on several occasions.

Table 7.2. Major Risk Factors for Coronary Heart Disease

Risk Factor	Notes
Uncontrollable	
Personal history of coronary heart disease or other atherosclerotic disease	For example, angina pectoris, heart attack, need for coronary artery bypass surgery or angioplasty, transient ischemic attacks, stroke, peripheral vascular disease
Age	Men 45 years or older; women 55 years or older, or women who have undergone premature menopause without estrogen-replacement therapy
Family history of premature coronary heart disease	Father, brother, or son who suffered a heart attack or sudden coronary death before age 55, or mother, sister, or daughter who had a heart attack or sudden coronary death before age 65
Controllable	
Current cigarette smoking	It is never too late to stop smoking.
High blood pressure	Systolic blood pressure 140 mm Hg or higher or diastolic blood pressure 90 mm Hg or higher (confirmed by measurements on several occasions), or taking medication to lower blood pressure
Elevated LDL-cholesterol ("bad" cholesterol)	See Tables 7.4 and 7.5, pp. 92, 93.
Low HDL-cholesterol ("good" cholesterol)	Below 35 mg/dl. See Table 7.6, page 94.
Diabetes mellitus	Blood sugar before eating breakfast of 80 to 120 mg/dl; blood sugar at bedtime of 100 to 140 mg/dl.
Obesity	Body mass index of 27 or higher. See Table 7.8, page 102.
Physical inactivity	Talk with your physician before starting an exercise program.

elevated diastolic blood pressure is 14 times more likely to die over a six-year period of coronary heart disease than a male nonsmoker with lower cholesterol and diastolic blood pressure. Decreasing multiple risk factors can greatly lower coronary heart disease risk.

Risk Factors That Cannot Be Changed

The NCEP's first group of risk factors are factors that cannot be changed. These are uncontrollable. Foremost among these risk factors is a personal history of angina, a heart attack, a stroke, or other evidence of atherosclerotic disease. Such a medical history places an individual in the highest risk category for a future coronary heart disease event such as a heart attack or need for bypass surgery. Another unmodifiable risk factor is simply growing older. The third risk factor in this category is a family history of early-onset coronary heart disease. *Early onset* means that evidence of disease occurred before age 55 in men and before age 65 in women.

But just because these risk factors cannot be changed does not mean that risk cannot be lowered in patients who have them. Reducing risk from the factors that can be changed is even more important for those people known already to have athero-sclerotic disease, for the elderly, and for those with a family history of disease.

Clinical research studies have shown, for example, that individuals with a history of coronary heart disease have excellent results in lowering their rates of future coronary events by decreasing their blood cholesterol levels. In the Scandinavian Simvastatin Survival Study, called the *4S study,* conducted in men and women who had had angina or a heart attack, choles-terol lowering through the use of a drug called an HMG-CoA reductase inhibitor (or statin) not only reduced rates of disability and death from coronary heart disease but also reduced rates of death from all causes. Another large trial that used a statin, the Cholesterol and Recurrent Events (CARE) study, showed that patients who have survived a heart attack and who have relatively normal cholesterol levels can benefit from cholesterol lowering. Cholesterol lowering also decreases the rate of progression (or growth) of athero-sclerotic lesions in the coronary arteries, as discussed in the following pages.

The major risk factors for coronary heart disease and other atherosclerotic disease are still very important beyond age 60, and even beyond age 70, in both men and women. Low-density lipoprotein (LDL) cholesterol and high-density lipoprotein (HDL) cholesterol levels, for example, have been shown to be predictors of heart disease disability and death well into the 80s. In the 4S study, risk for death from any cause and risk for a coronary event were significantly reduced in patients above and in patients below 60 years of age.

If you are at increased risk for heart disease because of your family history, consider appropriate lifestyle changes to reduce your overall risk. Also, you can help members of your family make changes to reduce their risk.

Personal History of Atherosclerotic Disease

Risk for a heart attack is higher if you have already had a heart attack or stroke or other atherosclerotic disease. American Heart Association statistics show that within six years of a heart attack, 23 percent of men and 31 percent of women will suffer another heart attack, and 13 percent of men and 6 percent of women will die suddenly of heart disease. Men who have evidence of coronary heart disease (for example, men who have experienced angina) are five to seven times more likely to have a heart attack than men with no evidence of heart disease. The rate of sudden cardiac death is four to six times higher among men and women who have had a heart attack, compared with the general population. Because of their high risk, people known to have atherosclerotic disease have a lower LDL-cholesterol goal than people without evidence of such disease (see Tables 7.4 and 7.5).

It may seem confusing that stroke or peripheral vascular disease (that is, atherosclerotic disease of the legs or arms) can indicate greater likelihood of coronary heart disease until one remembers that atherosclerosis tends to develop in vessel beds throughout the body (see Chapter 13). High cholesterol, smoking, high blood pressure, or another risk factor may damage, for example, the arteries leading to the brain as well as those serving the heart. Coronary heart disease is the leading cause of death after transient ischemic attacks have occurred, as well as after surgical repair of an abdominal aortic aneurysm (in one group of patients, 86 percent with this type of aneurysm had significant coronary heart disease). Within 30 days after a stroke, stroke itself is the most common cause of death; thereafter, cardiovascular disease is the leading cause of death. One study found that only 8 percent of patients with peripheral vascular disease had normal coronary arteries; the presence of large vessel peripheral vascular disease increases disability and death from heart disease 2.4 times in men and 3.6 times in women. Another study found that 40 percent of patients with carotid artery disease also had angiographically visible coronary heart disease. The good news, however, is that reducing risk factors for coronary heart disease helps decrease risk for all these disorders.

Age

Risk for atherosclerotic disease increases with the aging process, in part because such factors as systolic blood pressure, blood cholesterol, and body weight tend to increase with age. The NCEP reports that a 62-year-old man is 500 times more likely than a 22-year-old man to die of coronary heart disease during the next year. In people 45 to 64 years old, about one in six American men and one in seven American women have been affected by heart attack or stroke; that risk soars to one in three after age 64. In fact, about five of six Americans killed by cardiovascular disease are 65 years of age or older. In 1993 the number of Americans who died of cardiovascular disease increased significantly, in part because the population of older people increased. In 1900 only one in four Americans lived beyond age 65, while in 1985 about 70 percent lived past age 65 and about 30 percent lived to age 80 or beyond.

Even though risk for heart disease increases continuously with age, coronary heart disease events such as heart attack or need for bypass grafting are fairly uncommon among men until they are in their mid-40s. Events are delayed about six to 10 years in nondiabetic women because of the relative cardioprotection afforded by premenopausal status. (Women's cardiovascular health is the subject of Chapter 25.) Therefore, the NCEP considers age 45 years or greater as a major risk factor for men. For women, a major risk factor is age 55 or greater, or premature menopause (whether natural or surgical) without estrogen-replacement therapy. You have probably heard that being male is a risk factor for heart disease. The NCEP accounts for this risk by setting a lower age limit as a risk factor for men than for women.

Since the prevalence and incidence of coronary heart disease are highest in people older than 65 years of age, this group has the most to gain from risk factor intervention.

Family History of Early Coronary Heart Disease

Coronary heart disease tends to cluster in families, and a family history of early-onset heart disease is predictive of the development of heart disease, even after factors such as elevated blood cholesterol, high blood pressure, and diet are taken into account. The NCEP defines a family history of heart disease as having a father, brother, or son who suffered a heart attack or sudden coronary death before age 55, or a mother, sister, or daughter who had a heart attack or sudden coronary death before age 65.

Knowing major illnesses and risk factors of relatives, as well as age at death and cause of death for those who have passed away, can help you and your physician gauge whether risk for certain conditions is increased.

To prepare a family medical history, list everyone in your family, including your parents, siblings (that is, brothers and sisters), children, grandparents, aunts, uncles, and cousins (Table 7.3). Everyone listed should be a blood relative. Include family members in earlier generations if you have any medical information about them. First-degree relatives (that is, your parents, brothers, sisters, and children) are very important because they are the people with whom you share the most genes. For each relative, list major illnesses and risk factors (for example, high blood cholesterol, high blood pressure, or smoking) and the age when symptoms first appeared (onset). For people who have died, list the cause of death and the age at death. You may be able to obtain information from older relatives, medical records, and death certificates. Include any unusual occupational exposures. You can share your written report (which should be clear and brief) not only with your physician but also with other members of your family. If you do not have time to research your

family medical history, even a list prepared in a few minutes can be helpful.

Risk Factors That Can Be Changed

Of the 10 major risk factors the NCEP identified, seven can be changed by the individual. While you cannot modify your personal or family history or your age, you *can* control your medical future by making changes in these seven factors. Many of these controllable risk factors are interrelated, so that making a change in one risk factor can also affect another. For example, lowering fat intake not only can improve your blood cholesterol, but also can help in weight control and therefore aid in lowering blood pressure. All these changes can work together to lower heart disease risk. Discussed elsewhere in this book are lifestyle changes to decrease your risk for coronary heart disease (Chapter 26) and changes to lower blood pressure (Chapter 11).

Smoking

Smoking is the single most important preventable cause of death in the United States. Cigarette smokers' risk of heart attack is almost twice that of nonsmokers, and their risk of sudden cardiac death is two to four times that of nonsmokers. Cigarette smoking is estimated to be responsible for 20 percent of all deaths due to heart disease and 30 percent of all deaths due to cancer. Smokers are practically the exclusive sufferers of peripheral vascular disease, in which vessels carrying blood to the arms and legs narrow and fail to deliver the oxygen and nutrients these limbs need. Cigarette smoking is also a major risk factor for stroke. On average, cigarette smoking cuts about seven years from an individual's life expectancy. Smoking is a particular concern for Hispanic-Americans: the smoking rates among Mexican-Americans, Cuban-Americans, and Puerto Ricans range from 42 to 45 percent for men and 24 to 34 percent for women, compared with rates of 27 percent for white men, 33 percent for black men, 24 percent for white women, and 20 percent for black women in the United States.

Any surgeon can attest to the startling difference between the blackened, shrunken lung tissue of heavy smokers and the pink resiliency of healthy lungs. Other changes that the smoker doesn't see include reduced blood clotting time, increased blood thickness, increased platelet adhesiveness and decreased platelet survival, and the entry of carbon monoxide into the blood, which reduces the amount of oxygen that can reach the body's cells. Also, the nicotine in tobacco smoke leads to increases in blood pressure.

As noted above, risk factors for atherosclerotic disease do not just add up: they multiply one another's power. Thus, an individual who has, for instance, high cholesterol, high blood pressure, and diabetes has risk for a heart attack or stroke multiplied severalfold over the additive risk. Combining smoking with taking oral contraceptives multiplies risk considerably.

Cigarette smoking has a dose–response relation to heart disease—that is, the more cigarettes you smoke each day, the higher your risk. *But any level of cigarette smoking increases your risk, and don't expect smoking "low-yield" cigarettes to decrease the excess risks.* Smoking a pipe or cigars also increases risk, and people who have switched to a pipe after quitting cigarette smoking have higher death rates than people who quit smoking altogether. Some studies have shown pipe smokers to have the same excess death rate as cigarette smokers. Many pipe and cigar smokers are unaware of how much smoke they are actually inhaling. Since tobacco use is a key risk factor for head and neck cancers such as tongue cancer and laryngeal cancer, tobacco products that are not inhaled (snuff, chewing tobacco) must be avoided as well.

There is evidence that passive smoking—inhaling the smoke produced by smokers in the immediate environment—increases the risk of dying from heart disease. Children are the most dramatic victims. These "involuntary smokers" suffer in the

Table 7.3. Family Medical History

Prepared by:

Date prepared:

List only blood relatives. Information about first-degree relatives is the most important (additional information optional).

Family Member (Name and current age or age at death)	Major Illness or Condition		Heart Disease Risk Factors (See Table 7.2)		Other Information	Death	
	Condition	Age at Onset	Factor	Age at Onset		Cause	Age
First-degree relatives							
You						N/A	N/A
Your mother							
Your father							
Your siblings							
Your children							

Other relatives								
Mother's mother								
Mother's father								
Father's mother								
Father's father								
Mother's siblings								
Father's siblings								
First cousins on mother's side								
First cousins on father's side								

womb, and their newly formed respiratory systems are extremely vulnerable to smoke in their new home environment. Also, a pregnant woman who smokes is more likely to suffer a miscarriage than a woman who does not.

If you are a smoker, it may help you quit if you know that your increased risk for heart disease and stroke disappears within two or three years after quitting. Studies have shown that this appears to hold true regardless of how long you smoked or how many cigarettes you smoked daily. The American Heart Association's directive is clear: "If you smoke, quit now. And if you don't smoke, don't start."

High Blood Pressure

High blood pressure, or hypertension, threatens healthy blood vessels and raises the risk of coronary heart disease, congestive heart failure, and stroke. High blood pressure demands that the heart increase its pumping, and the heart may enlarge to meet that demand. The arteries and smaller arterioles lose their elasticity and harden from the scarring caused by the pressure, generally becoming less able to supply the tissues they serve with needed blood. High blood pressure is considered to be present when systolic blood pressure (the first number in a reading) is 140 mm Hg or higher, or diastolic blood pressure (the second number in a reading) is 90 mm Hg or higher, based on readings at several points in time. About one-fifth of the U.S. population suffers from it. Blacks, Puerto Ricans, Mexican-Americans, and Cuban-Americans are more likely to have high blood pressure than Anglo-Americans. As a group in the United States, blacks develop high blood pressure at an earlier age than whites, and their blood pressure elevation is more severe in any decade of life. They have a 1.8 times greater rate of fatal stroke, a 1.3 times greater rate of nonfatal stroke, and a 1.5 times greater rate of heart disease deaths, probably in part because of higher rates of high blood pressure.

What causes high blood pressure remains unknown in most cases, but physicians have several types of medications they can prescribe to reduce it. Nondrug therapy for reducing high blood pressure or preventing it includes (1) avoiding obesity and maintaining a healthy weight, (2) banishing the saltshaker from the table and reducing sodium intake in prepared foods, (3) limiting alcohol intake, and (4) increasing physical activity.

Blood Lipids

Lipids are fat and fatlike substances. Lipids in the blood that are known to affect risk for atherosclerosis are cholesterol (a fatlike substance) and triglycerides (which are fats).

Measuring Cholesterol and
Triglyceride Levels

All adults should regularly have their cholesterol levels measured. The NCEP recommends that cholesterol levels be checked every five years, beginning at age 20. The blood test should include measurement of both total cholesterol and HDL-cholesterol ("good" cholesterol) levels. Although both may be measured in a nonfasting blood sample, a fasting blood sample will be needed for many people, such as those who are at increased risk for heart disease or who already have heart disease. A fasting blood sample will allow the physician to measure triglyceride and to calculate LDL-cholesterol level by the following formula:

$$LDL = \text{total cholesterol} - HDL - (\text{triglyceride} \div 5)$$

Determination of total blood cholesterol, HDL-cholesterol, LDL-cholesterol, and triglyceride levels is called a *full lipid profile*. Some physicians prefer to have a full lipid profile on all of their patients, even those who are not at increased risk for heart disease. Values are generally reported in milligrams of lipid per deciliter of blood, that is, mg/dl (a measure of weight per unit of volume). Values may also be reported in millimoles per liter (mmol/l), which are international units (molecules per unit of volume). To convert total cholesterol, LDL-cholesterol, or HDL-cholesterol values in mmol/l to mg/dl, multiply by 38.7. To convert triglyceride values in mmol/l to mg/dl, multiply by 88.6. Lipid levels in the blood are usually determined from a sample of blood drawn from a vein in the arm. (Tests based on a few drops of blood from your finger may be less reliable.)

The NCEP recommends that blood lipid levels be measured in children and adolescents who have a family history of early cardiovascular disease; who have other risk for heart disease, such as smoking, diabetes, hypertension, obesity, or physical inactivity; or who have a parent with high cholesterol. Also, lipid monitoring may be needed when a young person is receiving drug therapy, such as isotretinoin (given to treat acne) or steroids, that can alter lipid levels, or if the family history is unknown. It is important to assess and manage risk factors in young people because atherosclerosis begins in childhood. Unless a genetic disorder is suspected, blood lipid levels are usually not measured until after the second birthday. Before age 2, more calories as fat are needed for growth; after the second birthday, cholesterol levels are reasonably consistent. (The heart healthy diet recommended for the general population applies to people aged 2 years or older. See the Step I Diet on pp. 421–423.)

If you are going to have either a nonfasting or fasting blood test, do not change what you typically eat or drink before having the test. Changing your diet can give your physician inaccurate test results on which to base his or her recommendation. If you are going to have a fasting blood test, fast for 10 to 12 hours before the test, that is, do not eat anything and do not drink anything except plain water or coffee or tea without whitener. If you eat, your total cholesterol and HDL-cholesterol readings will be accurate, but your triglyceride reading will be inaccurate. Most people find it easiest to fast overnight and have a fasting blood test performed in the morning. Classifications of total cholesterol, LDL-cholesterol, HDL-cholesterol, and triglyceride levels for adults, children, and adolescents are given in Tables 7.4 to 7.7. LDL-cholesterol goals are lower for people already known to have atherosclerotic disease because of their high risk.

Cholesterol

Elevated blood cholesterol has long been recognized as a significant coronary heart disease risk factor. Early in the twentieth century, a Russian physician named Nikolai Nikolaevich Anichkov determined

Table 7.4. Classification of Total Cholesterol and LDL-Cholesterol Levels in Adults Without Evidence of Atherosclerotic Disease

Classification	Value (mg/dl)
Total cholesterol	
Desirable	Below 200
Borderline-high	200 to 239
High	240 or higher
LDL-cholesterol	
Desirable	Below 130
Borderline-high	130 to 159
High	160 or higher

that atherosclerosis developed in rabbits that were fed cholesterol. In the 1950s, researchers in the Seven Countries Study discovered that differences in blood cholesterol levels and saturated fat consumption played a significant role in the fact that countries such as Japan, Greece, and Italy had lower rates of coronary events than did countries such as the United States and Finland. The Ni-Hon-San Study found that when lifestyles and disease rates in men of Japanese descent living in Japan (Nippon), Honolulu, and San Francisco were compared, dietary fat, blood cholesterol levels, and the incidence of coronary heart disease events all increased as lifestyles became more "American," that is, as the men ate more fat and cholesterol. Other population studies, including the Framingham Heart

Study initiated in 1948, offer strong data to verify that elevated blood cholesterol levels play an important part in increasing coronary heart disease incidence. Many large clinical research trials have determined that lowering blood cholesterol can lower heart attack rates, and have established that, in general, each 1 percent decrease in total blood cholesterol leads to a 2 to 3 percent decrease in risk for coronary heart disease events.

In the Framingham Heart Study, about 20 percent of people who had a heart attack had total cholesterol concentrations below 200 mg/dl. Thus, elevated cholesterol, even though it is a major risk factor, is not required for a heart attack, just as obesity or high blood pressure is not required. Those 20 percent of heart attack victims may have had risk from other

Table 7.5. Classification of LDL-Cholesterol Levels in Adults Known to Have Atherosclerotic Disease

Classification	Value (mg/dl)
Acceptable LDL-cholesterol	100 or lower
Higher-than-acceptable LDL-cholesterol	More than 100

NOTE: It is recommended that LDL-cholesterol always be determined in individuals who already have evidence of atherosclerotic disease (for example, angina, heart attack, stroke, or peripheral vascular disease) because LDL-cholesterol is a better measure of risk than total cholesterol.

known risk factors, for example, a described genetic predisposition, smoking, their age, diabetes, or other blood lipid risk factors such as low HDL-cholesterol plus increased triglyceride (as occurs in metabolic syndrome X, described below). Coronary heart disease doubtless also is related to risk factors scientists have not yet recognized.

Although a full description of cholesterol's generation, function, and effects is beyond the scope of this book, it is important to know that cholesterol is manufactured by the body, primarily in the liver, and is required for the human body to function properly. An essential part of cell membranes, some hormones, and other body components, cholesterol also is needed for the manufacture of bile acids, which are necessary for the absorption of fat. Many cells and tissues in the body manufacture their own cholesterol, usually in quantities sufficient for their own function. One exception is the adrenal gland, which derives a substantial amount of cholesterol from HDL particles, which it then uses to make steroid hormones.

In addition to manufacturing cholesterol in the body, an individual can take in cholesterol by eating cholesterol-containing foods. Any food of animal origin, including meat, seafood, poultry, and dairy products, provides cholesterol. Egg yolk and organ meats are especially rich sources of dietary cholesterol. But most people do not have to eat any cholesterol at all to get the cholesterol that their bodies require for good health, for the body usually can make all the cholesterol it needs. Yet while dietary cholesterol can increase blood cholesterol levels, the main dietary contributor to raising blood cholesterol levels—and, in particular, LDL-cholesterol levels—is saturated fat, which is usually consumed as animal fat.

In the arterial wall, cholesterol can exist in several forms. It may be present as unesterified (free) cholesterol or cholesteryl ester in the soft, mushy lipid core of an atherosclerotic plaque, or it may occur

Table 7.6. Classification of HDL-Cholesterol and Triglyceride Levels for All Adults

Classification	Value (mg/dl)
HDL-cholesterol ("good" cholesterol)	
Low (increased risk for heart disease)	Below 35
Acceptable	35 or higher
High (protective level of HDL)	60 or higher
Triglyceride	
Normal	Below 200
Borderline-high	200 to 400
High	400 to 1,000
Very high	1,000 or higher

NOTE: Triglyceride must be measured after fasting for 10 to 12 hours.

in a crystalline form. Cholesterol crystals are typically seen when a pathologist examines the arterial wall in and around an atherosclerotic plaque. Nevertheless, cholesterol is only one substance, just as water—whether encountered as a liquid, as steam, or as ice—is one substance.

When we speak of the "types" of cholesterol in the blood, such as LDL-cholesterol or HDL-cholesterol, we are referring to the way in which cholesterol and other lipids are "packaged" for transport through the blood. Since cholesterol and triglyceride are not water soluble, they are transported in a soluble form in the blood by being made into a complex with proteins (called *apolipoproteins*) and phospholipids. This complex is called a *lipoprotein*. Lipids are continually being delivered

throughout the blood stream by plasma lipoproteins. Lipoproteins vary in size, density, and lipid content. Each type of lipoprotein has a particular job to do. Total cholesterol (or "blood cholesterol") is a measure of all the cholesterol in a blood sample, regardless of its packaging.

LDL-Cholesterol. Most of the cholesterol in the bloodstream (about 60 to 80 percent) is carried to the body's cells in packages called *low-density lipoproteins*, or LDL particles. "Low-density" refers to the fact that the lipoprotein is composed primarily of lipid (which is buoyant), with relatively little protein. LDL-cholesterol is the cholesterol that is packaged in LDL particles. LDL-cholesterol is often called "bad" cholesterol because an elevated

Table 7.7. Classification of Total Cholesterol and LDL-Cholesterol Levels in Children and Adolescents (2 to 19 Years)

Classification	Value (mg/dl)
Total cholesterol	
Acceptable	Below 170
Borderline	170 to 199
High	200 or higher
LDL-cholesterol	
Acceptable	Below 110
Borderline	110 to 129
High	130 or higher

NOTE: Low HDL-cholesterol is the same as in adults: below 35 mg/dl. A fasting triglyceride level above 150 mg/dl is considered quite elevated in children and adolescents. Triglyceride is considered moderately elevated at about 120 mg/dl in boys and 130 mg/dl in girls.

LDL-cholesterol level is strongly linked with the development of atherosclerosis.

Elevated LDL-cholesterol in our society most often results from eating too much dietary fat, especially saturated fat. Some diseases, such as hypothyroidism (underactive thyroid) and chronic kidney disease, also can lead to elevated LDL-cholesterol, and treatment of such an underlying disease can often lead to normalization of blood lipid levels. (Hypothyroidism is a common cause of lipid problems in the elderly.) Individuals may also have a genetic predisposition to elevated LDL-cholesterol levels (or other lipid problems), although in most of these cases lifestyle factors such as diet and physical inactivity play an important role in the expression of the disorder. In other words, *an inherited tendency toward elevated blood cholesterol may be activated because of lifestyle habits.* "Purely genetic" lipid disorders are uncommon. For example, in homozygous familial hypercholesterolemia (which occurs in only about one in one million people), individuals have no functional LDL receptors and their total cholesterol levels reach 700 to 1,200 mg/dl, leading to widespread atherosclerosis and, usually, early death (some patients die of heart attacks in childhood).

Small, Dense LDL. A subclass of LDL particles termed *small, dense LDL* may be particularly likely to lead to atherosclerosis and may underlie some family predispositions to coronary heart disease. These LDL particles have a higher proportion of protein than normal LDL particles, which are more buoyant because of a higher lipid content. Groups of people who have a preponderance of small, dense LDL (LDL pattern B) rather than a preponderance of buoyant LDL (LDL pattern A) have been found to be three times more likely to have a heart attack. Which LDL pattern you have has a genetic basis, but it is modified by factors such as aging, obesity (in particular, having central obesity, usually referred to as being "apple shaped"), physical inactivity, and completing menopause (all of which can shift the LDL pattern to a more atherogenic pattern). People with diabetes are more likely than nondiabetics to have LDL pattern B, and small, dense LDL has been linked to metabolic syndrome X and to familial combined hyperlipidemia (FCH), a genetically based disorder characterized by an elevated LDL-cholesterol level or an elevated fasting triglyceride level (or both) and associated with an increased risk for coronary heart disease.

The formation of small, dense LDL appears to be closely linked to the metabolism of triglyceride-rich lipoproteins. It is thought that small, dense LDL particles may play a greater role in the development of atherosclerosis because they are more susceptible to oxidation (an important step in the contribution of lipids to atherosclerosis) or may more easily enter the vessel wall because of their small size.

LDL subclasses at this time remain a research issue, but modification of the subclass may be a treatment approach in the future. Some clinical studies have shown treatment with a fibrate or nicotinic acid (which are both lipid-lowering drugs) to shift LDL pattern B toward the normal LDL pattern A, perhaps through lowering the triglyceride level. Increased physical activity and weight loss may also help normalize the LDL pattern. Also, several recent studies have shown that LDL subclass may influence response to lipid-lowering treatment. When patients with elevated cholesterol followed a low-fat diet, those with pattern B had greater reductions in LDL-cholesterol than those with pattern A. Patients with pattern B rather than A had greater reductions in triglyceride when they lost weight.

Lipoprotein[a]. An LDL-like particle also linked to increased risk for coronary heart disease when its levels in the blood are elevated is lipoprotein[a], abbreviated as Lp[a] and often referred to as "lipoprotein little a" or "Lp little a." Lp[a] is identical to an LDL particle except for the addition of a special protein termed *apolipoprotein[a],* or *apo[a]* ("apo little a"). Apo[a] resembles plasminogen, which is a substance important to preventing blood clots. Lp[a] appears to promote not only atherosclerosis but also thrombosis (that is, the formation of blood clots), the latter through competing to take plasminogen's place without performing its functions (plasminogen is a precursor of plasmin, which dissolves clots). Both atherosclerosis and thrombosis are important in the occurrence of heart attacks and strokes.

Although Lp[a] was discovered in the 1960s, the evidence linking Lp[a] elevation and atherosclerosis risk is not yet nearly as extensive as evidence linking elevated LDL-cholesterol and risk, so elevated Lp[a] has not yet entered clinical risk assessment guidelines. Also, measurement of Lp[a] is not yet standardized, although in general a level higher than 30 mg/dl is considered elevated. Some physicians, however, may choose to order Lp[a] determinations, especially in patients who already have atherosclerotic disease. Interestingly, Lp[a] levels vary greatly among ethnic groups: for example, black Americans typically have Lp[a] values twice as high as white Americans. Standard lipid-lowering therapies, including diet and drugs, have generally been ineffective against elevated Lp[a] values, although among major lipid-lowering drugs nicotinic acid has shown some effectiveness. Limited recent evidence suggests that Lp[a] may cease to be a risk factor when LDL-cholesterol levels are low enough.

HDL-Cholesterol. HDL is the lipoprotein that is thought to carry excess choles-terol away from cells to be delivered to the liver for reuse or eventual excretion from the body. *High-density* refers to the fact that the lipoprotein contains a great deal of protein and a relatively small amount of lipid. HDL-cholesterol is the cholesterol that is packaged in HDL particles. HDL-cholesterol frequently is called "good" cholesterol because an elevated level of HDL-cholesterol is strongly linked with a *decreased* risk for atherosclerosis. In population studies, risk for coronary heart disease decreases about 2 percent in men and 3 percent in women for each 1 mg/dl *increase* in HDL-cholesterol. HDL-cholesterol appears to be a somewhat stronger risk factor in women, and women typically have higher HDL-cholesterol levels than men.

Low HDL-cholesterol levels often result from physical inactivity, obesity, or smoking. A low HDL-cholesterol level also can be a result of diabetes mellitus and is associated with high levels of triglyceride. Some very rare cases of low HDL-cholesterol are due to genetic disorders ranging from "fish-eye" disease (in which the corneas of the eyes become cloudy) to Tangier disease (in which the tonsils may turn orange). (Tangier disease is so named because it was first discovered in people living on Tangier Island in Chesapeake Bay.) Interestingly, a number of these rare genetic disorders characterized by low HDL levels are not associated with the premature development of athero-sclerotic disease.

The ratio of total cholesterol to HDL-cholesterol can be useful in estimating risk for coronary heart disease. It is obtained by dividing your total cholesterol value by your HDL-cholesterol value, and it de-scribes how much of your total cholesterol value is attributable to "good" cholesterol. A high ratio—generally defined as more than 5 for individuals without atheroscle-rotic disease and more than 4 for individ-uals with atherosclerotic disease—indi-cates increased risk. For example, if your total cholesterol is 210 mg/dl and your HDL-cholesterol is 80 mg/dl, your ratio of 2.6 does not indicate increased risk. If you have the same total cholesterol of 210 mg/dl but an HDL-cholesterol of 35 mg/dl, your ratio of 6.0 indicates increased risk. With this, as with any approximation of risk, however, you need to discuss your complete risk picture with your physician, including both lipid and nonlipid risk factors.

Triglycerides

Triglycerides are yet another type of lipid. Whereas cholesterol is a building block for cells, triglycerides are used by the body for energy. Triglycerides contain fatty acids that are delivered through the bloodstream to be used by the muscles or stored in fat for use as energy in the future. Triglycerides are transported through the bloodstream primarily through two lipoprotein classes: the large chylomicron, which is manufactured in the intestinal wall by using fats and dietary cholesterol; and the very low density lipoprotein (VLDL), which is manufactured in the liver. While both LDL-cholesterol and HDL-cholesterol levels have been defini-tively linked to coronary heart disease risk, the role of fasting total triglyceride level is not as well defined, although an elevated fasting triglyceride level has been associ-ated with increased risk in many research studies. It is believed that triglyceride-rich lipoproteins may cause lipid deposits to form in the arterial wall in much the same way that LDL causes such deposits to form. While elevated blood levels of VLDL and its remnant, intermediate-density lipoprotein, have been associated with increased risk for atherosclerotic disease, elevations of chylomicrons have not been. However, partial breakdown products of chylomicrons called *chylomi-cron remnants* appear to accelerate athero-sclerosis. Like HDL-cholesterol, fasting triglyceride level may be a somewhat stronger risk factor in women than in men.

Elevated triglyceride levels can result from eating a diet that is high in saturated fat and/or simple carbohydrate. Elevated triglyceride levels also can be due to other causes, including obesity, excessive alcohol usage, use of estrogens, diabetes mellitus, and pregnancy. All of these factors can bring to light a family predisposition to elevated triglyceride. As with cholesterol disorders, "purely genetic" triglyceride disorders are uncommon. Some familial disorders of triglyceride elevation (for example, familial combined hyperlipidemia and type III hyperlipidemia) are associated with premature atherosclerosis, while others are not. Very high triglyceride levels (above 1,000 mg/dl) increase risk for pancreatitis, an inflammation of the pancreas that can be life-threatening. Some cases of very high triglyceride represent a rare genetic disorder called *familial chylomicronemia,* in which the triglyceride-rich chylomicron particle level is very elevated. Blood plasma in which the triglyceride level exceeds 1,000 mg/dl usually has a milky appearance.

Syndrome X

Dr. Gerald Reaven and his associates have described a condition known as *metabolic syndrome X*, which may account for a significant number of cases of atherosclerosis in which there are relatively normal levels of total cholesterol and LDL-cholesterol. (Metabolic syndrome X should not be confused with cardiologic syndrome X, which is the finding of angina pectoris or anginalike chest pain in the presence of a normal coronary angiogram.) Insulin resistance or hyperinsulinemia appears to be the cornerstone of this condition (which is also called *insulin-resistance syndrome*). The condition is also characterized by elevation of triglyceride level, a low HDL-cholesterol level, elevation of blood pressure, glucose intolerance, and the presence of small, dense LDL particles (see above). Some investigators believe that central obesity is also an integral part of the syndrome. Further investigations are under way regarding the genetics of metabolic syndrome X, its diagnosis and management, and its overall contribution to coronary heart disease in the U.S. population.

Lipid-lowering Trials

Large clinical trials for more than two decades have clearly shown that lowering elevated levels of total cholesterol and LDL-cholesterol reduces disability and death from coronary heart disease. The excellent results—for example, fewer heart attacks, reduced angina, reduced need for bypass or angioplasty, and fewer deaths—have been achieved by both lifestyle interventions (including diet) and drug therapies, and in both patients with and without a history of heart attack or other evidence of coronary heart disease. Many clinical trials have also shown that lipid lowering can slow, halt, or sometimes even reverse the progression of atherosclerosis (see pp. 191–192).

The 4S study found that lowering cholesterol decreased not only coronary events, but also the overall death rate in patients with a history of heart problems. The 4,444 men and women aged 35 to 70 years who took part in the study were randomly assigned to receive either a placebo or a powerful cholesterol-lowering drug called an HMG-CoA reductase inhibitor, or statin, as part of their treatment regimen. After five years, those who took the drug not only had lowered their LDL-cholesterol levels, but also had suffered 42 percent fewer heart attacks and had a 30 percent lower overall death rate than those in the placebo group.

The West of Scotland Coronary Prevention Study (WOSCOPS) showed that the benefit of lipid lowering in reducing total death rate extends to patients without evidence of coronary heart disease. A 22 percent reduction in total death rate, a 28 percent reduction in coronary heart disease death rate, and a 31 percent reduction in either nonfatal heart attack or coronary heart disease death were achieved with statin therapy in the WOSCOPS patients, who were all men without symptoms of coronary heart disease. (For more information on statin therapy, see pp. 451–452.)

In the CARE trial, a study completed in the United States and Canada, men and women who had experienced a heart attack and who had average levels of cholesterol and LDL-cholesterol (as opposed to high cholesterol levels) were shown to benefit from statin treatment. Although this study was not statistically powered to show differences in total death rate, the primary endpoint of nonfatal heart attack or coronary heart disease death was decreased by 24 percent. All the patients in the CARE trial began the study with total cholesterol levels below 240 mg/dl.

These new findings from 4S, WOSCOPS, and CARE are very important. Their conclusions, combined with the results of other studies in which patients have been observed over long time periods, indicate that lowering blood cholesterol levels can help people live longer as well as decrease coronary heart disease events. Also, 4S and WOSCOPS provided strong evidence against an argument, derived from weaker data, that low cholesterol may increase deaths from noncardiovascular causes such as cancer. In neither study was there any increase in deaths from any cause.

Diabetes

Diabetes mellitus is a syndrome in which insulin production or processing is faulty, thereby impairing the body's ability to process glucose, its main source of energy. It occurs in two forms. Type I diabetes mellitus, or insulin-dependent diabetes mellitus (once called *juvenile-onset diabetes*), usually begins in childhood or adolescence. It has a peak age of onset of 12 years, although it can develop at any age. Onset is abrupt, and insulin must be taken to sustain life. Type II diabetes mellitus, or non-insulin-dependent diabetes mellitus (formerly called *adult-onset* or *maturity-onset diabetes*), develops more gradually. It may occur any time after adolescence, although the peak age of onset is 50 or 60 years. Control of this type of diabetes can often be achieved through lifestyle adjustments, in particular diet and exercise, with or without oral medication, although some patients require insulin injections.

Both types of diabetes significantly increase risk for both microvascular (small blood vessel) and macrovascular (large blood vessel) disease. In the days before insulin and oral therapy for diabetes, most people with diabetes died of causes such as coma, renal failure, and infection. Today, atherosclerotic disease accounts for 80 percent of all deaths in diabetic patients. Coronary heart disease is responsible for 75 percent of the atherosclerotic deaths; the remainder result from stroke and peripheral vascular disease. When a comparison is made with people of the same age without diabetes, the likelihood of dying from coronary heart disease is three to 10 times higher in people with type I diabetes and two to three times higher in men and four to six times higher in women with type II diabetes. Moreover, coronary heart disease occurs at an earlier age in people with diabetes. Risk is also high in diabetes for disorders of the eyes, kidneys, and nerves, although controlling glucose levels so that they are near normal can decrease these risks.

Why do people with diabetes have earlier and more atherosclerotic disease? In part, the additional risk can be attributed to the multiple major risk factors that characterize most cases of diabetes. For example, about one third of people with type I diabetes and up to half of people with type II diabetes have high blood pressure. In type II diabetes, as many as 80 percent of patients are obese, and more than 60 percent may have elevated triglyceride, elevated LDL-cholesterol, and/or low HDL-cholesterol levels. Elevated triglyceride and low HDL-cholesterol levels are the most common lipid problems in diabetes, and people with diabetes are twice as likely to have LDL pattern B. LDL particles from individuals with diabetes are more susceptible to oxidation, and diabetic individuals are more likely than those who are not diabetic to have elevated lipoprotein[a]. However, such risk factors do not account for all of the excess risk for atherosclerosis in diabetes. There is something about diabetes itself that contributes to risk—a puzzle scientists are still investigating.

Control of risk factors, including the diabetes itself, to reduce risk for heart disease, stroke, and peripheral vascular disease is very important in people with diabetes. Risk factor control includes a prescribed meal plan, exercise, weight control, and glucose control. Smoking significantly increases risk for death from cardiovascular disease in people with diabetes, even smoking less than one pack of cigarettes per day. Some medical experts recommend that risk factor goals be lower in diabetic patients because of their high risk. These include, for example, a fasting triglyceride level below 150 mg/dl (rather than 200 mg/dl) and an LDL-cholesterol level below 100 mg/dl for adults, regardless of whether atherosclerotic disease is already known to be present.

Obesity

If you look at photographs of people taken during the 1930s at county fairs or other public gatherings, you notice imme-diately that the clothes and hairstyles are different from those of today. But something else is different also. It is how people look. Most are slender. In the 1990s, 61 million Americans are considered obese, representing an increase of 36 percent over the 1960 figure.

Obesity is defined as having a body mass index (BMI) of 27 or higher. Body weights at different heights that define overweight or obesity are shown in Table 7.8. If you wish to calculate your exact BMI, use the formula

BMI = weight in kg ÷ (height in meters × height in meters).

Table 7.8. Classifying Persons as Overweight or Obese According to Body Mass Index (BMI)

Height	Body Weight in Pounds Corresponding to	
	BMI of 25 (Overweight)	BMI of 27 (Obese)
4'10"	119	129
5'0"	128	138
5'2"	136	147
5'4"	145	157
5'6"	155	167
5'8"	164	177
5'10"	174	188
6'0"	184	199
6'2"	194	210
6'4"	205	221

NOTE: To use the table, find the height nearest your height in the column on the left. If your body weight is lower than the weight shown in the BMI 25 column, you are not overweight. If your weight is that shown in the BMI 25 column, you are considered overweight. If your BMI is 27 or higher, you are considered obese.

One pound equals 0.454 kilograms (kg), and 1 inch equals 2.54 centimeters, or 0.0254 meters. A 5'6" individual who weighs 170 pounds has a BMI of 26.7, since

66 inches $\times$ 0.0254 = 1.7 meters

170 pounds $\times$ 0.454 = 77.2 kilograms

77.2 $\div$ (1.7 $\times$ 1.7) = 26.7

About one-third of American adults are obese. The prevalence of obesity increases with age, particularly in women. Black and Hispanic Americans are more likely than white Americans to be obese. These groups are also more likely to have high blood pressure.

In addition to high blood pressure, some of the medical hazards entailed by obesity are insulin resistance, diabetes, elevated triglyceride level, decreased HDL-cholesterol level, elevated LDL-cholesterol level, gallbladder disease, some types of cancer, sleep apnea, and degenerative joint disease. Having central, or abdominal, obesity (the "apple" rather than the "pear" shape) worsens many of these risks. Much of obesity's contribution to risk for atherosclerotic disease and death from atherosclerotic disease arises from its effects on risk factors such as blood pressure, lipid levels, and diabetes. *Maintaining a healthy weight throughout life appears to have the greatest correla-tion with living longer.* Some evidence has shown that even moderate weight gain can significantly increase risk for premature death. About 300,000 deaths each year in the United States can be attributed in part to excess weight.

Unfortunately, children and adolescents share the burden of obesity. In the 1980s, the Center for Adolescent Obesity at the University of California estimated that 20 million American youngsters were over-weight. During the same decade, the federal government reported that 40 percent of U.S. children four to eight years of age already had risk factors for heart disease.

Physical Inactivity

Americans are becoming increasingly sedentary: 60 percent do not get enough exercise daily to stay healthy, and 25 percent do no physical activity at all. This is surprising since regular moderate exercise, which is easy and inexpensive (or free), provides so many health benefits: among them, reduced risk for heart disease, diabetes, arthritis, osteoporosis, and some cancers (such as colon cancer); lower blood pressure; improved circulation; an improved blood lipid profile (often most dramatically a higher HDL-cholesterol level, but also lower LDL-cholesterol and triglyceride); weight control (in part through naturally curbing the appetite); decreased shortness of breath; improvement of mood, concentration, alertness, and productivity; relief of anxiety; better digestion; increased energy; stronger muscles; and longer life. Low physical fitness is one of the most powerful predictors of early death: as powerful as cigarette smoking, according to some studies. Those who are physically inactive are 1.5 to 2.5 times more likely to develop coronary heart disease and 30 to 50 percent more likely to develop high blood pressure. Also, exercise can improve individuals' sense of well-being, self-esteem, and body image. The benefits of exercise on risk for coronary heart disease result in part from the direct effect of exercise on the blood vessels and heart, and in part from effects on risk factors, such as control of body weight and blood pressure, improvement of the blood lipid profile, and moderation of insulin levels.

Mounting evidence shows that only moderate exercise is required to achieve most of these benefits, including reduced heart disease risk and increased longevity. Exercise is a preventive and a remedy. Experts recommend that everyone be physically active for 30 minutes or more on most, and preferably all, days of the week. It is possible to become moderately fit in only 10 weeks through engaging in activities such as the following on most days: 30 minutes of brisk walking; 15 minutes of jogging; 30 minutes of lawn mowing, raking, or gardening; or bicycling 3 miles

in 30 minutes. But the activity need not be performed all at once to achieve the benefit: what is important is the total amount of activity performed, whether 10 minutes here or 10 minutes there, for example, taking the stairs instead of the elevator or parking a little farther away when conditions are safe. An earl of Derby was quoted as saying, "Those who think they have no time for bodily exercise will sooner or later have to find time for illness."

Trigger Effect of Strenuous Activity

Another important benefit of regular exercise is that it reduces risk for having a heart attack or sudden cardiac death triggered by strenuous exercise. Sudden, vigorous activity by people who are unaccustomed to it can end in tragedy. The temporary risk period is the time spent exercising and about one hour afterward, a period that may account for about one in 20 heart attacks (some studies have shown as many as one in 10). The reasons behind this phenomenon are unknown, but some scientists speculate that the exercise may induce disruption of atherosclerotic plaques. Also, in sedentary people, but not active people, strenuous activity leads to changes in platelet activity that could contribute to or initiate thrombosis (the formation of blood clots). The excess risk is limited for the most part to people who do not exercise regularly: studies have shown little or no additional risk in groups of people who exercise at least four or five times a week. *The trigger effect underscores why it is very important to discuss an exercise regimen with your physician, and to begin any program of increased physical activity gradually.* While the risk for heart attack or sudden cardiac death from physical exertion is small in the population as a whole, it can be high for any given individual.

Other Risk Factors for Heart Disease

One researcher has calculated that more than 250 risk factors for coronary heart disease have been described, including such odd predictors as earlobe creases and short stature (both of which lack adequate scientific confirmation). The 10 risk factors selected by the NCEP as major risk factors (Table 7.2) were recognized because of the strong, extensive scientific data linking them to the development of coronary heart disease. Many well-designed studies over the years have confirmed the importance of these major risk factors. For the risk factors not included by the NCEP, findings to date may be weaker or contradictory, measurement of the risk factor (such as a laboratory value) may not be standardized or readily available, or the risk may be accounted for by one of the factors listed (for example, LDL-cholesterol level may approximate

the risk contribution of apolipoprotein B level). This section discusses just a few of the "leading contenders" among other risk factors that have been described.

Alcohol

Alcohol consumption has a U-shaped relation to coronary heart disease risk: moderate drinkers have less risk than nondrinkers, and heavy drinkers have increased risk. Moderate alcohol intake is defined as a maximum of 1 ounce of pure alcohol (ethanol) per day, which roughly equates to two drinks. Each of the following is considered one drink:

- 12 fluid ounces of regular or light beer
- 5 fluid ounces of table wine
- 3 fluid ounces of fortified wine, such as port, sherry, marsala, or Madeira
- 1 fluid ounce of 100-proof liquor or $1^1/_2$ fluid ounces of 80-proof liquor

How moderate alcohol intake decreases risk for coronary heart disease may relate in part to its effects on blood lipids, including an increase in HDL-cholesterol.

Chronic alcohol use, however, entails many health hazards, among them liver disease, some cancers, injuries from accidents, malnutrition, brain damage, fetal damage, pancreatitis, impotence, and, because of loss of judgment, increased rates of sexually transmitted diseases. Therefore, it is generally not recommended that people start to drink to lower their risk for coronary heart disease. In fact, chronic alcohol consumption has been associated with a variety of other cardiovascular problems, including hypertension, high triglyceride levels, stroke, arrhythmias, heart failure, and sudden cardiac death. It is the leading cause of secondary cardio-myopathy, a heart muscle disease. Smoking can further increase many of these risks.

Homocysteine

An elevation of homocysteine, which is an amino acid, can damage muscles and predispose blood factors to form clots rather than to inhibit them. As many as one-third of people with atherosclerosis have elevated blood levels of homocysteine, and major studies such as the Framingham Heart Study and the Physicians' Health Study have linked elevated levels of homo-cysteine with increased risk for heart attack and stroke. Interestingly, risk appears to arise from increases as small as 20 to 30 percent in homocysteine, which is found in very small amounts in the blood (about 1/1000 of the concentration of cholesterol).

Folic acid, which is a vitamin of the B-complex group, is very important to main-taining normal homocysteine metabolism; vitamins B^6 and B^{12} play roles as well.

Whether reducing homocysteine levels will decrease risk for atherosclerotic disease has not yet been demonstrated, but people should make sure they are getting enough folic acid (also known as folate) in their diet. Also, adequate intake of folic acid is very important in reducing a woman's risk of giving birth to a baby with a neural tube defect, such as spina bifida or anencephaly. Four hundred micrograms (mcg) per day, which is the reference daily intake of folic acid, appears to be adequate for maintaining normal homocysteine levels.

It is best to obtain adequate folic acid through a balanced diet. Rich sources include fortified oatmeal, wheat germ, spinach, broccoli, turnip greens, Brussels sprouts, lettuce, oranges, cantaloupes, strawberries, and legumes. (The name folic acid was derived from the Latin folium, which means "leaf.") These foods provide many other health benefits besides their folic acid content, including antioxidants, other micronutrients, and roughage. The guidance of a physician is advised if folic acid supplementation is used, since high folic acid levels may decrease the absorption of zinc and may mask pernicious anemia.

Fibrinogen

The protein fibrinogen is a coagulation factor in the blood—that is, it plays a role in the clotting process. Elevated fibrinogen in the blood has been described by many studies as a strong risk factor for heart attack and stroke. Thrombosis (that is, clot formation) plays an important role in the development of a vascular event such as a heart attack or stroke. How fibrinogen contributes to heart attack and stroke risk is complex, apparently involving not only coagulation effects but also effects on such processes as platelet aggregation and endothelial cell injury.

Fibrinogen levels are higher in women, in smokers, in people with diabetes or hypertension, and in people who are obese or sedentary. Elevated fibrinogen may be a component of metabolic syndrome X, which is defined by a constellation of risk factors for atherosclerosis. The lifestyle change that is key to lowering fibrinogen levels is smoking cessation. Lesser effects are achieved by weight loss, increased physical activity, and perhaps stress reduction. Remember that increases in physical activity should be undertaken only after checking with your physician. No drugs selectively lower fibrinogen, although some (notably, the lipid-lowering drugs called *fibrates*) lower fibrinogen in conjunction with achieving other effects. Estrogen-replacement therapy and omega-3 fatty acids (found, for example, in fish oils) may also lower fibrinogen. However, measurement of fibrinogen has not yet been standardized, and clinical evidence is not yet available to show that lowering elevated fibrinogen will lower risk for heart attack or stroke.

There is also some evidence linking other coagulation factors to risk for atherosclerosis. Factor VII has been associated with coronary heart disease, and factor VIII with stroke. (Fibrinogen is factor I.)

Psychosocial Factors and Coronary Heart Disease

It is observed in the Apocrypha that "envy and wrath shorten the life" (Ecclesiasticus 30:20), and many people believe that mental stress or a pattern of aggressive behavior causes coronary heart disease. In fact, there are two aspects of this question: first, whether like high blood cholesterol or smoking, psychosocial factors are risk factors for the development of atherosclerotic heart disease, and second, whether a stressful event can trigger a coronary event such as angina, a heart attack, or sudden cardiac death.

Scientific results regarding psychosocial characteristics as risk factors for the development of coronary heart disease are very mixed. Among the multitude of studies that have been performed, some have been positive and some have been negative. The strongest data suggest a relation between hostility or anger and coronary heart disease, but no clear conclusions can yet be drawn. Examining this question is difficult, since measuring stress or anger is not as simple as measuring blood pressure or a blood cholesterol level. Stress is very individual, and what disturbs one person may not bother another. Still, some studies have correlated factors such as isolation or occupational stress with risk for heart disease. Marriage and pet ownership, for example, have each been shown in some studies to reduce risk for coronary heart disease or increase survival after a heart attack. Some studies have linked anxiety, repressed anger, and submissiveness to high blood pressure, but despite many years of research there is still no clear evidence that a "hypertensive personality" exists.

Also, it is important to remember that stress can indirectly increase risk for heart disease through causing people to smoke, overeat, drink excessively, or stop exercising. Smoking, eating a diet high in fat, drinking too much alcohol, inactivity, and obesity then each increase risk directly.

Most people have heard of the *type A personality*, also called the *coronary-prone behavior pattern*. This personality or behavior pattern, initially described more than 30 years ago, is characterized by competitiveness, time urgency (or a feeling of being pressured or rushed), and aggression. But despite the 30 years of research, it cannot be concluded that personality type predicts or influences the development of coronary heart disease; neither can it be concluded that the idea is misguided. In contrast, data supporting increased blood cholesterol, increased blood pressure, and smoking as risk factors are very powerful. It should be borne in mind that the recent declines in coronary heart disease rates have not accompanied widespread decreases in aggression or life stress, whereas they have accompanied public health measures to control smoking, blood pressure, and blood cholesterol, as well as improvements in cardiologic therapies and techniques. The aggressiveness of peoples throughout history has not been related to the development of heart disease. In fact, there was a decline in coronary deaths in Europe during World War II; dietary deprivation was the likely explanation.

The idea that personality type generates certain diseases is an ancient one. For example, in ancient Greece and Rome, the human body was believed to be composed of four humors—blood, phlegm, black bile, and yellow bile—roughly corresponding to four temperaments—sanguine (cheerful), phlegmatic (impassive or stolid), choleric (bilious or peevish), and melancholic (depressed)—vulnerable to characteristic disorders. Science has enabled us to replace mysticism with microbes, to attribute particular diseases to pathogens rather than personality. Remarkably, we have known for only a few years that nearly all stomach ulcers are due to a bacterial infection (and thus can be successfully treated with antibiotics); it was previously believed that stress played the major role in many cases. Nevertheless, there is scientific evidence of a connection between psychological stress and immune response. Studies have shown that long-term stress tends to suppress immune response at the cellular and humoral levels, whereas short-term, or acute, stress tends to enhance it (as does exercise). But whether this alters susceptibility to particular diseases remains to be shown, and how important the influence is needs to be established.

It is clear that there is no simple connection between illness and life events, and no doubt there are large individual differences in susceptibility. Stress may lead to illness in some people. But it is very important to remember that attributing illness to personality or weak psychological coping skills unfairly places the blame on the patient and can be little different from the idea that illness is a punishment.

Stress as a Trigger

Another role that mental stress or the anger or grief to which it leads might play in heart disease is as a trigger of an acute event such as angina, a heart attack, or sudden cardiac death. The great eighteenth-century anatomist Dr. John Hunter, mentioned in Chapter 1, understood that emotional fervor can bring on painful chest pains and one day died suddenly, collapsing after a dispute with colleagues. He had predicted the manner of his own death, saying that his life, because of his angina and temper, was at the mercy of any rascal who chose to upset him.

Studies have sought to make sense of the link between stressful events and cardiovascular events. One study, for example, showed risk for a heart attack to be increased 14 times on the day after the death of a close relative or friend. Another found risk for having a heart attack to be more than doubled during the two hours after an episode of anger. Several studies have identified an informant-described increase in life stress immediately before sudden cardiac death or in the weeks preceding the event. On January 17, 1994, the day of the Northridge, California, earthquake, there was a sharp increase in the number of sudden cardiac deaths in Los Angeles County: 24 deaths, as opposed to a daily average of 4.6 deaths during the week preceding the earthquake. Only three of the 24 deaths were related to unusual physical exertion. Similarly, sudden cardiac deaths increased among the Israeli civilian population during the first 10 days of the Gulf War in 1991.

How mental stress might lead to a cardiac event is complex, but it may involve an increased demand by the heart muscle for oxygen through an increased heart rate and blood pressure. This is a role for stress in an ischemic event: the demand for oxygen from the blood is not met and anemia of part of the heart muscle (ischemia) occurs, which may cause pain (angina) or lead to death of that part of the muscle (a heart attack). Some studies have shown that the people most likely to experience this effect are those who already have coronary atherosclerosis—that is, acute stress may precipitate coronary events in people predisposed to them. One study examined 43 cases of stress-related sudden death. The stress was fear in 15 cases, an altercation in 21 cases, sexual activity in three cases, and police questioning or arrest in four cases. Subjects ranged in age from 20 to 92 years. Thirty-eight of the deaths were due to cardiac causes, and 27 of those to atherosclerotic heart disease. Autopsy findings led the investigators to conclude that stress-related sudden death occurs primarily in individuals with severe heart disease, especially atherosclerotic heart disease.

Some researchers have suggested that mental stress is a trigger in the well-documented early-morning increases in heart attacks, sudden cardiac death, and stroke. (There are also seasonal variations, with heart attacks more likely to occur in winter.) Why these events are more likely to occur shortly after people awaken and arise remains unclear. There is also a circadian (that is, 24-hour) variation in blood pressure and heart rate, among other factors. Blood pressure and heart rate both rise rapidly during the morning hours and then decrease throughout the day, to a low point around three o'clock in the morning. It has been hypothesized that mental stress, like strenuous physical activity, may lead to the rupture of atherosclerotic plaque and the formation of blood clots, and indeed both beta-blockers and aspirin (which act to prevent clotting) have been shown to blunt or abolish the morning peak of onset of heart attacks. More limited research has shown an excess of heart attacks on Monday mornings among the working population, a finding that suggests a role for mental stress but one that requires confirmation.

In laboratory experiments, scientists have found that mental stress can induce ischemia of the heart muscle in as many as 80 percent of volunteers, although some experiments have shown no such effect. One recent study used radionuclide ventriculography, a sensitive imaging test, to determine whether mental stress induced ischemia in volunteers with coronary heart disease. The volunteers were asked to complete five potentially stressful tasks, such as quickly performing mental arithmetic or speaking, with only one minute of preparation, to an audience. Also assessed was whether ischemia was induced by exercise on a stationary bicycle. The patients were then followed up by mail or telephone for up to five years. The investigators found that the patients who were vulnerable to mental stress–induced ischemia had nearly three times the relative risk for having a cardiac event such as a heart attack or for dying, compared with the patients who did not show the stress vulnerability. Also, the mental stress tests were better predictors of eventual outcome than the exercise test. The investigators concluded that modifying the response to stress may reduce the risk for cardiac events.

Also, a single severe stress episode may trigger arrhythmia (an irregular heartbeat) or a disturbance of the heart's electrical stability, which can lead to sudden death. Catecholamines, which are chemical compounds produced by the body that mimic the activity of the nervous system that controls the heart muscle, increase in the blood, preparing the body for fight or flight. They are also increased in the heart muscle and in the circulation during myocardial ischemia or a heart attack.

Beta-blockers, as a kind of "antidote to overdrive," help block this effect. The stress hormones that flood the bloodstream during the "fight or flight" response may represent an outdated survival mechanism. But it may be possible to interrupt the cycle of stress through avoiding stressful situations or learning how to cope with them.

Effects of Stress Reduction

Attempts at managing chronic stress have been very successful, and type A behavior can be modified through fairly simple procedures such as relaxation training. Whether such stress reduction or behavior modification will reduce risk for heart disease remains unclear. However, one study conducted in almost 900 heart attack survivors showed that risk for another heart attack was reduced almost 50 percent in patients who received training to reduce "coronary-prone" behavior such as hostility, as opposed to patients who did not. And, as noted above, some studies have shown that risk for coronary heart disease may be decreased by attachment to other human beings or pets. But whether or not stress reduction decreases risk for heart disease specifically, it can help an individual achieve an overall sense of well-being and has not been associated with any health hazards. Also, stress reduction may help in the management of other risk factors such as smoking, overeating (and thus obesity), and alcohol abuse, which, as noted above, can be responses to stress. Even though science has not as yet been able to describe the exact relation between specific psychosocial risk factors and heart disease risk, the mind–body connection is important. No doubt with time, research will delineate its significance with greater clarity.

CHAPTER EIGHT

Heart Failure

Heart failure, a chronic condition that can cause a lifetime of debilitating symptoms, is the diagnosis most frequently listed on patients' records when they are discharged from U.S. hospitals—875,000 in 1993. Two to three million Americans live with congestive heart failure every day, and the number is steadily increasing. In the United States annually, heart failure contributes to about 230,000 deaths. Managing heart failure costs Americans between $10 and $15 billion annually.

The death rate from coronary artery disease has decreased as patient survival has increased with the use of long-term medication, coronary angioplasty, bypass surgery, and thrombolytic therapy and as salvage from acute coronary events has improved. The result has been an increase in the number of patients who develop and die of chronic heart failure. Claude Lenfant, M.D., director of the National Heart, Lung, and Blood Institute, has described this phenomenon as one of the future frontiers or challenges in cardiovascular medicine.

In part, then, heart failure is the dark side of the good news about surviving a heart attack caused by coronary artery disease. Many patients who survive a heart attack must live with the result—a damaged or worn-out heart that cannot pump enough blood to meet the oxygen and nutrient demands of the body adequately. For these and others with impaired heart function, treatment can keep heart failure's debilitating symptoms at bay until late in life. But for many patients, it is a condition that must be accepted and accommodated.

Defining Heart Failure

Heart failure is the inability of the heart to supply the oxygen needs of the body. This mechanical failure, which may be due to malfunctioning or to diseases affecting the heart valves, the coronary arteries, the muscular tissue of the heart (myocardium), or other causes, is characterized by fatigue, shortness of breath, and swelling. It is associated with reduced exercise tolerance and a high incidence of ventricular arrhythmias. When both sides of the heart are affected and fluid invades the lungs and the legs and ankles, making tissues swell, the condition is called *congestive heart failure*. Fifty to sixty-five percent of patients with this condition die within four years of receiving their diagnosis. The World Health Organization calls heart failure "common, costly, disabling, and deadly" and recognizes it as a major, growing public health concern worldwide.

Causes

Any kind of heart disease can result in heart failure, but the two most common causes of heart failure are coronary artery disease and high blood pressure (hypertension). Patients with heart failure frequently have both. Disorders unrelated to problems of the coronary arteries, the valves, or high blood pressure, whose cause often remains unknown, can also cause heart failure. They are called *idiopathic cardiomyopathies*, which means "diseases of the heart muscle with unknown cause." Here the discussion will be restricted primarily to the two causes first mentioned.

When your arteries become blocked by atherosclerosis, your heart may suffer because it may not get the oxygen and nutrients it needs. Blood may be withheld dramatically (heart attack) or chronically. This deprivation can impair the ventricles, whose function it is to fill with blood and to send it out to circulate. Or the heart itself may be unable to function fully and may down-regulate in reaction to the inadequate blood supply, pumping the blood less vigorously.

Another major cause of heart failure is high blood pressure (hypertension). In the United States, high blood pressure affects more than 50 million people, and more people receive prescription medication for it than for any other condition. It is a major risk factor for heart attack and stroke as well as for heart failure. By making adjustments, the heart can continue to function properly, despite the effects of the increased workload it must perform because of the increased blood pressure. But eventually, as the heart's strength fades, it is unable to compensate.

High blood pressure can result in a type of cardiomyopathy. The heart becomes enlarged and unable to contract sufficiently. Other types may be caused when the heart is infected by viruses or injured by diabetes or excessive alcohol intake. The heart may also suffer from the effects of aging or from congenital malformations that may become known as early as infancy or as late as old age.

Symptoms

Shortness of breath (dyspnea), fatigue, and swelling in the legs, ankles, and feet are the complaints patients with heart failure make to their physicians. Sometimes their breathing difficulty may extend to nighttime occurrences of waking up breathless (paroxysmal nocturnal dyspnea) or be characterized by a cough. Lying flat in bed can cause problems in breathing or prompt a dry, hacking cough to begin.

Feeling tired or weak may be explained by the insufficient supply of oxygen-rich blood circulating. Related symptoms include feeling faint or dizzy, as if objects are moving around you. Some patients experience nausea, pain, and abdominal tenderness.

Swelling may be what sends the patient to the doctor, especially in patients who do not exert themselves by exercise or other activity enough to recognize the limits on their physical abilities. Swelling, due to *edema* (fluid accumulation), occurs when the heart fails to pump the blood forcefully enough to keep the circulation moving properly. And swelling in or around the lungs will be what the physician will look for. Fluid fails to be carried along and seeps from the vessels into tissues and body cavities. Gravity pulls the fluid downward, and it collects in the feet and ankles (Figure 8.1). When patients are confined to bed, this type of swelling from fluid accumulation may be detected in the lower back as well as in the legs, ankles, and feet. When this kind of swelling occurs in the lungs, it prevents deep inspiratory breathing, thereby causing shortness of breath. Swelling in the bowels can interfere with proper absorption.

These symptoms are the broad brushstrokes of clinical heart failure, but they can also be associated with other ailments completely unrelated to the heart or its arteries. Respiratory disease or obesity, for example, can cause feelings of fatigue and shortness of breath. So that means for your doctor to diagnose heart failure, he or she needs not only the presence of these symptoms but also evidence that they are the consequence of heart disease. Furthermore, heart failure can be symptomless and detected unexpectedly during examination undertaken for other reasons.

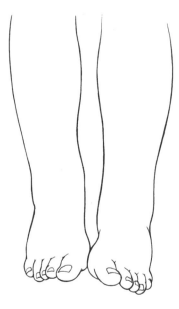

Figure 8.1. When heart failure causes fluid retention, the feet, ankles, and legs may swell. During the physical examination, the physician may press on these areas to see how far the swelling can be indented. It a pit remains after the pressure is removed, physicians call it *pitting edema*.

Diagnosing and Evaluating Heart Failure

To understand the reasons a patient is experiencing shortness of breath, fatigue, and swelling and to delineate any underlying heart disease, a physician will obtain a medical history, perform a physical examination, and have other studies done, such as chest x-ray, echocardiography, electrocardiography, blood tests, and perhaps radionuclide ventriculography. These tests document the impairment of the heart's functioning, and understanding that impairment is essential to providing successful therapy.

Medical History

Putting the puzzle pieces of your symptoms into the right places to create an accurate picture, or diagnosis, will require understanding your personal medical history as well as exploring the medical history of your siblings, parents, and grandparents. Besides characterizing the three symptoms described above, your doctor's questions will probably follow along these lines: Have you ever had a heart murmur or a heart attack? Do you sometimes have chest pain (angina)? Do you have high blood pressure? Have you had rheumatic fever (or any other disease that would have affected the valves of your heart)? What is your lifestyle, and what is your activity level? Do you use alcohol, tobacco, or recreational drugs?

By these questions, the physician is trying to identify aspects of your medical history, family history, or lifestyle that might put you at higher risk for heart failure. Personal risk factors include coronary artery disease, high blood pressure, previous heart attack, angina, diseases of the heart valves, and a history of rheumatic fever.

Physical Examination

In the physical examination, the doctor will be paying particular attention to your heart, your lungs, and your jugular veins. Examinations vary from physician to physician, but below are some evaluations you might expect.

Inspection and palpation (touching) are the initial parts of the examination. The physician will visually inspect you in an orderly fashion, though if you are answering questions during the inspection, you may not realize it. After the visual inspection, physicians use their hands to take the pulse, assess blood pressure, and detect the apex beat of the heart by pressing on the chest, and then to examine by touch the chest area. The physician may press arteries in your neck, near your armpit, and in your groin to better understand the pumping rhythm of your heart.

When the doctor checks the heartbeat in the jugular veins, he or she will try to gauge whether the venous pressure is normal and to characterize the type of heart failure you might have. The physician may test for increased jugular pressure, indicated by distention of the jugular vein, which can be made manifest by pressing on the liver in the right upper quadrant of the body (hepatojugular reflux). If the increase is persistent, the function of the right ventricle may be impaired. The physician will also check to determine if the liver is swollen and if the extremities exhibit signs of swelling.

The doctor will listen to your heart as you lie on the examining table on your back and on your left side. Pulse and heartbeat variations that are specific signs of heart disease may be detected using the stethoscope. The aim is to identify any abnormal or muffled sounds indicating dysfunction in the left ventricle, a heart murmur, or both. Listening to your lungs

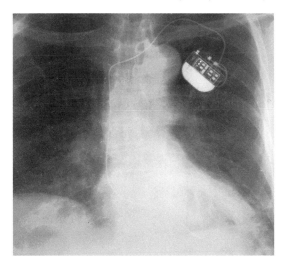

Figure 8.2. This chest x-ray shows cardiac enlargement, the heart's response to weakened contractions causing low pumping ability. The pacemaker in the pectoral area is evidence of the complexity of the heart ailments.

will also be part of the examination. Abnormal sounds at the base of the lungs, when combined with certain other measures, can indicate heart failure. The doctor will also be listening for sounds of congestion and looking for swelling around the lungs.

Chest X-ray Examination

When heart failure is a possibility, chest x-ray examinations are performed to see if the heart is enlarged (Figure 8.2) and to determine if the lungs are congested. Although the range of sizes of the normal heart makes it difficult to judge size on an x-ray, it may be possible to identify a specific chamber that is enlarged. Having an enlarged heart indicates meaningful cardiac disease, but x-rays cannot precisely disclose the underlying cardiac problem.

Echocardiography

Because the left ventricle is so often involved in heart failure, getting a picture of how it works is essential to accurate diagnosis. Echocardiography, an imaging method that relies on high-frequency inaudible sound waves (ultrasound), can tell the physician how big the ventricle is, how thick its walls are, and how well it is contracting in specific areas and overall. Echocardiograms also show valves and their abnormalities, and can provide information about the aorta and the aortic valve. The test is noninvasive, safe, and fast, and with portable equipment, it can be performed bedside or in a doctor's office. More than four million echocardiographic examinations are performed annually in the United States. (See Chapter 5 for more information about echocardiography.)

Electrocardiography

An electrocardiogram may show a heart irregularity in patients with heart failure. Physicians know how to recognize the changes and interpret them for diagnosis. Variations in the QRS wave and ST segment can indicate that the patient has had a heart attack. Heart rate–related problems can show up as atrial fibrillation or changes in the speed of heartbeats.

Radionuclide Ventriculography

For characterizing the function of the ventricles during contraction of the heart (systole), physicians sometimes rely on radionuclide ventriculography. This nuclear imaging technique uses radioactive material injected into the bloodstream that can be detected with special scanning cameras to calculate the size and shape of the ventricles and to evaluate how they are functioning. Radionuclide ventriculography can be paired with stress or exertion testing to compare the heart's performance at rest and when challenged.

Blood Tests

Measures of blood hemoglobin or hematocrit, serum electrolytes, blood lipids, and liver and renal function should be a part of the laboratory studies ordered for patients who are thought to have heart failure. These assessments can be valuable in identifying coexistent disease and in providing baseline values against which to compare measures obtained during therapy. Physicians may also want to rule out anemia and thyroid or liver dysfunction as causes of symptoms.

Confirming Heart Failure and Determining the Underlying Condition

Heart failure is confirmed when the physician links the symptoms with a heart condition (Table 8.1). These underlying conditions include the following:

- *Myocardial systolic failure*
  The heart fails to contract properly.
- *Myocardial diastolic failure*
  The heart fails to relax properly after contracting.
- *Severe valvular disease*
  The valves fail to operate properly.
- *Pericardial disease*
  The sac surrounding the heart becomes stiff or fills with fluid, adversely affecting heart function.
- *Endocardial disease*
  The inside surface of the heart toughens with fiberlike growth that restricts the heart.

Table E.1. Therapy for Heart Failure by Diagnosis

Diagnosis/Evaluation	Definition	Therapy	Aim
Myocardial systolic failure	Muscular layer of heart fails to contract and pump properly; left ventricle abnormally enlarged. Causes include previous heart attack, long-standing hypertension, viral infection of the heart, Chagas' disease, and heart disease caused by alcoholism.	Angiotensin-converting enzyme (ACE) inhibitor, diuretic, and/or digoxin. Alcohol consumption ended.	To improve health status and heart's pumping action.
Myocardial diastolic failure	Muscular layer of heart enlarged and fails to relax properly. Occurs most often in elderly. Causes include hypertension.	No standard therapy identified. Therapy for identifiable conditions, such as hypertension; diuretic.	To reduce enlargement of heart, to reduce fluid retention.
Severe valvular disease	Severe dysfunction of heart valve due to abnormality or aging.	Surgery, including valve replacement or balloon valvuloplasty; vasodilators.	To restore function or relieve symptoms.
Pericardial disease	Pumping function of heart impeded by changes in the tissue surrounding the heart. Causes include tuberculosis, viral disease, or bleeding within the sac surrounding the heart that results in compression (cardiac tamponade).	Pericardiectomy (surgery), pericardiocentesis (fluid aspiration).	To relieve compression.
Endocardial disease	The inner lining of the heart enclosing the blood becomes overgrown with excess tissue; sometimes inner and middle layers of heart (endomyocardium) are affected.	No standard treatment because mechanisms are not clearly defined. Diuretics and digoxin for relief of symptoms.	To relieve symptoms.
Congenital heart disease	Failure of heart function due to defect present at birth; dysfunction may become evident in infancy, in childhood, or in late years of life.	Medical and surgical treatment.	To relieve condition.
Metabolic heart disease	Dysfunction of heart due to problems in physical or chemical processes; causes include thyroid disease, thiamine deficiency (beriberi), and iron overload.	Nutritional, hormonal, or metabolic factor adjustment.	To cure.

- *Congenital heart disease*
  A defect present from birth may cause dysfunction.
- *Metabolic heart disease*
  A dietary deficiency or metabolic or hormonal abnormality causes malfunction.

The condition most commonly resulting in heart failure is myocardial systolic failure of the left ventricle. When the heart cannot pump at its normal level, it compensates by enlarging. Once enlarged, the heart can pump the same amount of blood as before by taking in more. The enlarged profile can be observed on x-ray examination. This mechanism works for a while, but the pumping continues to weaken and, of course, the heart cannot continue to enlarge.

Important to consider is the severity of the heart failure. Shortness of breath and fatigue are the most common symptoms, and peripheral edema is the most common sign of heart failure. The New York Heart Association classifies heart failure into four categories, based on the patient's sense of how the disease limits physical activity:

CLASS I: No limit on physical activity. No unusual fatigue, shortness of breath, palpitations, or pain in the chest accompanies normal activities.

CLASS II: These same characteristics—fatigue, shortness of breath, palpitations, and angina—may appear singly or in some combination in a mild form with ordinary activity. Disease places slight limit on activities.

CLASS III: These characteristics occur with less than ordinary activity levels, placing dramatic limit on activity.

CLASS IV: Discomfort exists even at rest and increases with any increase in activity. Symptoms related to cardiac insufficiency or anginal syndrome may be experienced at rest.

Some problems can be treated with lifestyle adjustments, some with medicine, and others with surgery, but treatment must be individualized and take into account the severity of the symptoms, the presence of other illnesses, and the underlying conditions resulting in the heart disease. Treatments for heart disease are not interchangeable or simple, and optimal success with drugs requires cooperation between the patient and his or her physician and other members of the health care team.

Treating Heart Failure

Optimal heart failure treatment depends on careful identification of the underlying problem. Heart failure is classified according to degree of severity, and patients whose disease is the least severe may require no intervention except following heart healthy dietary guidelines and exercise recommendations. Other patients may require both medical and surgical treatment. As more and more patients survive initial heart attacks, and as a large segment of the population moves toward that period of life when heart disease is most often diagnosed, the number of heart failure diagnoses is rising, making intervention strategies gain increasing importance in cardiac care. Physicians work to retard or reverse the disease's progression. Their goals are to prolong life and to improve its quality.

Therapy Without Drugs

Nonsurgical treatment of heart failure without drugs encompasses dietary and other lifestyle recommendations.

Recommendations for changes in diet are aimed at reducing the workload of the heart, regulating fluid intake, and improving nutritional status overall. Because being overweight increases the strain on the heart to pump blood to the body's tissues, reaching and maintaining an optimal weight reduces the work the heart has to do. Limiting calories can help you bring your weight within guidelines (see Chapter 26). Reducing your weight may also help prevent or delay other cardiovas-

cular problems. It is especially important if you have high cholesterol or triglyceride, high blood pressure, or coronary artery disease. Ask your doctor for advice and consult *The New Living Heart Diet* for specific recipes and guidelines for reducing calories, fat, and sodium (salt). Controlling sodium intake will help prevent the symptoms of heart failure from worsening.

Sodium usually makes a person thirsty and tends to make the body retain fluid. Patients with heart failure often experience an intense thirst, but daily fluid intake should be limited to the amount recommended by a patient's physician. When blood flows too weakly through the body, fluid tends to collect in the tissues and the tissues swell. Too much salt or fluid intake can worsen this condition. Fluid restriction is often ineffective, however, in patients who are not hyponatremic (*hyponatremia* means a deficiency of sodium in the blood).

Limiting alcohol or eliminating it from the diet is recommended because of the damage it can do to the middle layer of the heart wall (myocardium) and because of its ability to cause arrhythmias. And it is possible, even in cases of cardiomyopathy caused by alcohol, that symptoms will moderate or largely disappear when the patient stops drinking alcohol.

Regular coffee, once considered necessary to eliminate from the dietary list, is no longer viewed as taboo. In moderation, say,

Congestive Heart Failure and Dietary Sodium

When congestive heart failure slows circulation, the organs, which need blood to work, cannot keep up their former pace. Without a fully functioning heart muscle, kidneys are unable to effectively clear the body of excess fluid and the sodium it carries. Therefore, sodium fails to be swept from the body, and it instead collects in the tissues. The diuretics physicians prescribe help reduce the swelling by removing fluids and their sodium load from the system. To further assist in decreasing sodium saturation and to reduce reliance on diuretics, physicians will also sometimes restrict the amount of sodium a patient can take in through diet. When heart failure requires hospitalization, the sodium restriction may be 1,000 to 2,000 mg/day.

Once home, patients will become their own sodium gatekeepers. Physicians or dietitians can supply lists of foods that describe which ones are recommended and which ones should be avoided. Your doctor will probably recommend that you eat all the fresh and frozen vegetables that you want but warn you to avoid canned vegetables unless the label is marked "low sodium." Food and drug manufacturers are bound by laws defining the amount of sodium allowable when using specific terms. "Sodium free" or "no sodium" means less than 5 mg per serving, "very low sodium" 35 mg or less per serving, and "low sodium" 140 mg or less per serving. Other labels are less reliable. "Reduced sodium" means that sodium has been reduced from the usual level by 25 percent. "Unsalted," "no salt added," and "without added salt" mean that no salt was added when the manufacturer was preparing the food. They do not mean there is no sodium in the food because the restriction is on only what the manufacturer added and does not account for sodium that naturally occurs in the food. Even "salt-free" refers only to whether sodium was added during processing. The best way to determine the amount of sodium you are getting from food is to add up the milligrams per serving (shown on the food label). The sodium values for more then 1,000 foods, plus low-sodium recipes and information on selecting low-sodium food at home and away from home, appear in *The New Living Heart Diet* (see the last page of this book).

Nonprescription drugs and other products typically purchased in a drugstore (cough medicines, laxatives, toothpastes, and powders) can add substantially to sodium intake. Some antacids can add up to 7,000 mg per day. Inspect the labels. Those containing more than 80 mg of sodium per dose may be worth mentioning to your doctor.

Salt substitutes should not be taken without consulting your physician. These are usually made of potassium chloride. Though the potassium is in most cases helpful—it compensates for the potassium many diuretics eliminate and may help offset the threat of digitalis toxicity—in certain cases excess potassium is dangerous. Your physician will determine if the use of salt substitutes is advisable.

two cups daily, coffee is acceptable. Research by Harvard cardiologists found that in patients who already had irregular heart rhythms (arrhythmias), 200 mg of caffeine (about the amount in two cups of coffee) failed to set off additional irregularities.

Smoking should be abandoned. The World Health Organization advises that smoking should be "avoided at all costs" by patients with heart failure. Inasmuch as smoking is a risk factor for not only cancer but also pulmonary problems that so frequently exacerbate cardiovascular problems, it is difficult to imagine a persuasive argument for its continued practice. The functioning of the lungs is affected by increased tension in the lungs' venous system caused by heart failure. The mechanical relation between the flow of blood and ventilation with fluid removal is altered, resulting in the most common symptom of heart failure—shortness of breath. Smoking only further compromises the lungs' ability to do their job. Also, nicotine has a deleterious effect on coronary blood flow, which is a major problem in congestive heart failure.

Balance between rest and activity is a goal in patients with heart failure. After acute heart failure particularly, bed rest is essential, though getting moving again at some level is a high priority early in treatment. Walking or biking around the neighborhood can improve your spirits as well as your cardiovascular system. Swimming

is also excellent and spares the bones from jarring contact with pavement. Gardening may be a good way to make a transition from rest to higher activity levels. Finding the right pace for an activity and building on it are fundamental to improvement.

Therapy with Drugs

Some physicians begin therapy for heart failure without drugs, but some others believe all patients should begin a combination of diet modification and drug therapy. Most often that first line of drug therapy includes drugs that reduce fluid build-up in the tissues (diuretics), strengthen the heartbeat (inotropic agents), and increase the inside diameter of the blood vessels (vasodilators). (See Table 8.2.)

Diuretics

Along with restricting sodium and fluids in the diet, doctors prescribe *diuretics* for long-term therapy for heart failure. Diuretics help patients reduce the fluid in their bodies by causing a loss of sodium, which may lead to increased urination. When prescribed and taken properly, a diuretic drug effectively reduces swelling in the ankles and legs and improves the patient's ability to breathe more deeply.

The most commonly prescribed of these drugs are the thiazide diuretics, which are mild and also help control high

Table 8.2. Treating Heart Failure with Diuretics, Inotropic Agents, and Vasodilators

Generic Name	Brand Name	Function	Precaution
Diuretics			

Thiazide diuretics
  Chlorothiazide
  Hydrochlorothiazide
 	
  Metolazone
	Diuril
	Esidrix, HydroDIURIL,
	Oretic, Thiuretic
	Diulo, Microx, Zaroxolyn
		All the diuretics decrease swelling and blood pressure by prompting removal of fluid by kidneys.	For any diuretic, report irregular heartbeat, rash, loss of hearing.

Loop diuretics
  Furosemide
 	
  Ethacrynic acid
  Bumetanide
	Fumide MD, Lasix,
	Lo-Aqua
	
	Bumex		

Potassium-sparing diuretics
  Amiloride
  Spironolactone
  Triamterene
	Midamor
	Aldactone, Spironazide
	Dyrenium		

Inotropic Agents			

Digitalis agents
  Digoxin
  Digitoxin (digitoxin is
    uncommonly used)
	Lanoxicaps, Lanoxin
	Crystodigin
		Strengthen the heartbeat and improve irregular heart rhythms.	Serious problems can occur in a small percentage of patients, including arrhythmias and low levels of potassium.

Sympathomimetic agents Dopamine		Fortifies heartbeat and helps stabilize patients with hypotension.	Monitoring of hemodynamic and electrocardiographic values essential.
Dobutamine	Dobutrex	Strengthens heartbeat, dilates vessels, and increases cardiac output.	Report increase in heartbeat.

Phosphodiesterase inhibitors
  Amrinone
  Milrinone
	Inocor
	Primacor
		Strengthen heartbeat and dilate vessels.	Monitor for hypotension, arrhythmias, and low level of platelets.

Continued on next page

124

Table 8.2. *Continued*

Generic Name	Brand Name	Function	Precaution
Vasodilators			

Angiotensin-converting enzyme (ACE) inhibitors
  Captopril
  Enalapril
  Lisinopril
  Quinapril
	
	Capoten
	Vasotec
	Prinivil, Zestril
	Accupril
		Lessen constriction of vessels, improve blood supply to vital organs, lower risk that salt and potassium levels will fall, and moderate swelling.	Monitor kidney function and watch for rash or wheals on the skin and changes in the sense of taste; monitor laboratory values.

Nitrates
  Erythrityl tetranitrate
  Isosorbide dinitrate
	
	Cardilate
	Isordil, Sorbitrate
		Reduce effect of pulmonary symptoms and dilate coronary arteries, but drug tolerance may preclude long-term use; given with hydralazine, shown to decrease mortality rate in patients with heart failure.	Monitor for hypotension.

Hydralazine	Alazine, Apresoline, Novo-Hylazin	Reduces effect of regurgitant valve disease; dilates vessels.	Monitor for fast heartbeat and lupuslike symptoms.

Adrenergic receptor antagonists
  Alpha
    Prazosin
    Doxazosin
	
	Minipress
		Dilate vessels and help control hypertension.	

Beta (still under study for some patients)
    Atenolol
    Metoprolol
	
	Tenormin
	Lopressor
		Improve symptoms in patients with certain underlying conditions.	

Calcium channel antagonists
  Amlodipine
  Felodipine
	
	Norvasc
	Plendil
		Prevent calcium from entering myocardial cells; promote diastolic relaxation; improve exercise tolerance.	The early calcium channel antagonists did not prove as successful in treating heart failure as those developed more recently have.

NOTE: The listing of brand names is for informational purposes only, and inclusion or exclusion here represents neither endorsement nor rejection of any drug.

blood pressure. Loop diuretics are stronger and are used more frequently in patients with severe heart failure. A third type, potassium-sparing diuretics, do what their name states: help reduce fluid retention without reducing potassium levels in the body to below normal. These are most often paired with one of the other two types rather than used alone. Loop and thiazide diuretics are also sometimes paired. These may all be given by mouth and are sometimes given by injection or by intravenous drip. Careful monitoring of weight and of some laboratory measures is necessary to prevent depleting the blood and to ensure that levels of potassium, sodium, and magnesium do not fall dangerously low.

Inotropic Agents

Inotropic agents are drugs that affect the performance of muscle (*ino* is the Greek combining form meaning "to turn" or "to influence," and *tropic* is a word ending meaning "tending to turn or change"). Thus, these drugs change the heart, influencing it to contract more forcefully.

Digitalis drugs are well known for their roles in cardiac therapy. The most commonly used digitalis drug is digoxin, which, like digitalis, was originally derived from leaves of foxglove plants. It increases the ability of the muscular layer of the heart to contract and pump properly. Because it is useful in slowing the heart-beat, digoxin is most effective in patients in whom the action of the atrium is out of sync with that of the ventricle (atrial fibrillation), the left ventricle is enlarged (dilated), or systolic function is impaired.

Digoxin probably has its major effects in heart failure through correcting neurohumoral imbalance, in addition to the effects on heart rate in atrial fibrillation. As a mild inotropic agent, it also fortifies the pumping action of the heart, improving the ability of the blood to meet the nutritional and oxygen needs of the body. It is most effective in patients with severe heart failure, and studies have shown that digoxin improves patients' ability to tolerate exercise. Patients on digoxin are carefully monitored because too much digoxin can cause irregular heartbeats (arrhythmias), low levels of potassium and oxygen in the blood, and other complications.

A study, involving about 7,000 patients with heart failure and normal sinus rhythm, conducted at 302 centers in the United States and Canada between 1991 and 1995 found no difference in mortality rate between the portion of those patients taking digitalis and the portion taking a placebo (an inert medication). Drug administration did reduce risk for hospitalization and improved quality of life in this Digitalis Investigation Group (DIG) trial. Despite digoxin's inability to alter the natural history of heart failure, it remains, for most patients, a safe, effective, and inexpensive choice for symptom relief. Thus, it is usually prescribed for symptoms that persist despite treatment by agents that do reduce risk for death (for example, ACE inhibitors and beta-blockers).

Other inotropic agents include the sympathomimetic agents dopamine and dobutamine, and the phosphodiesterase inhibitors amrinone and milrinone. All these drugs improve the heart's ability to pump and most dilate the blood vessels. They are administered by infusion, and patients are carefully monitored by electrocardiography and measures of blood pressure and heartbeat.

Vasodilators

When the work of the heart outpaces the ability of the arteries to supply the blood it needs, physicians call on vasodilators to

Old Mother Hutton's Secret Ingredient

Digitalis was discovered to be the active ingredient of the foxglove plant by the English physician William Withering (1741–1799). Withering was the only son of an apothecary in Shropshire, and trained as an apothecary before studying to become a doctor. Thus, he was familiar with the preparation of herbal medicines, and throughout his life he pursued botanical investigations in addition to his busy Birmingham medical practice. Foxglove (originally, "folksglove," with reference to the plant's shape of a finger in a glove) had been a popular folk remedy for at least two centuries in England, used for such conditions as skin diseases and epilepsy. Reference to foxglove as an external medication goes back as far as thirteenth-century Wales. Withering discovered foxglove to be the essential ingredient of a secret recipe of many components used to treat dropsy (now known as *edema*) by a locally renowned herbalist in Shropshire known as "Old Mother Hutton." He misattributed the benefits in dropsy to the drug's diuretic effects, not recognizing the cardiotonic action. But his 1785 publication—*An Account of the Foxglove and Some of Its Medical Uses*—is one of the cardiologic classics. Withering administered the drug as the dried leaf or an infusion of leaves, and was successful in reducing its toxicity, giving one grain twice a day mixed with opium.

Digitalis was derived from the *Digitalis purpurea* plant (purple foxglove). (*Digitus* is Latin for "finger," and *digitalibum* is Latin for "thimble." In German, the plant is called *Fingerhut*, which means "thimble.") Digoxin is the digitalis drug most often used today; it was first extracted in 1930, from *Digitalis lanata*. Another well-known digitalis drug, but one little used today, is digitoxin, originally derived from *D. purpurea*, *D. lanata*, or other *Digitalis* species. Digitalis has also been known as a poison, because of the toxic effects with overdose; Withering describes a man who "narrowly escaped with his life" when his wife (with good intentions) gave him a potent foxglove brew for his asthma. Victims have often been "done away with" by foxglove, or digitalis, in mystery fiction, including works by Agatha Christie and Dorothy Sayers.

increase the luminal space, or opening of the blood vessels, throughout the body so that passage through them is easier for the blood. These vasodilators help reduce the resistance the circulating blood meets within the vessels and thereby lower blood pressure and improve heart rate.

Called the cornerstone of heart failure therapy, vasodilators have been fine-tuned to reduce demands on the heart before or after pump action, or at both times. The best known of the vasodilators are the angiotensin-converting enzyme (ACE) inhibitors. Captopril, enalapril, lisinopril, and quinapril are ACE inhibitors that are prescribed to be taken by mouth and may follow other vasodilators administered intravenously during hospitalization when patients are unable to take medications orally.

Nitrates are also helpful in relieving venous and pulmonary congestion and high blood pressure. In combination with hydralazine, they promote survival.

In the 1970s, researchers realized that the slowing down of the heart's contractility is a compensatory action on the part of a heart in distress, working to conserve energy. Alpha- and beta-adrenergic receptor antagonists work against this compensatory activation of the sympathetic nervous system. They appear to improve survival rates, as well as relieve debilitating symptoms, by enhancing cardiac pumping and relaxing mechanisms.

Mechanical Support for the Circulation and Cardiac Transplantation

When pharmacologic therapy fails to improve a patient's heart failure to a satisfactory level, it may be necessary to assist the circulation mechanically or to evaluate the feasibility of transplantation. Patients who may need mechanical support include those whose heart failure produces blood pressure so low that it is life threatening and whose vital organ function is endangered by lack of blood transport. Some patients whose heart needs time to recover proper function require support. Some patients whose condition requires more serious intervention such as transplantation need help until that intervention can be undertaken. Two types of devices—the intra-aortic balloon pump and ventricular assist devices—can be used to mechanically assist pumping (Figure 8.3 shows an external device that assists both ventricles). Technical advances in these devices are enabling support for longer periods and increasing survival rates. (A fuller discussion of these devices and cardiac transplantation, mentioned below, is in Chapter 24.)

When the damage to the heart is significant and treatment yields no hope of improvement, the patient may be identified as a candidate for heart transplantation. Prospects as well as need characterize the optimal candidate. These patients ideally have no condition that would prevent them

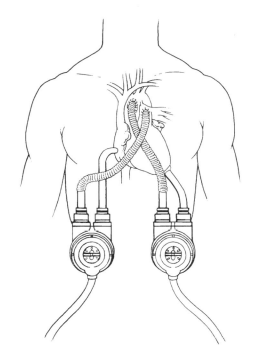

Figure 8.3. Biventricular external assist device.

from recovering fully or predispose them to complications. Unfortunately, each year many U.S. patients die waiting for a donated heart.

Other Treatments for Heart Failure

Other treatments for heart failure include valvuloplasty and relief of problems with the pericardium, or sac, surrounding the heart. Of the four valves in the heart, the mitral and aortic valves on the left side of the heart are the ones that most commonly cause heart failure and require repair or replacement. Problems may include a hardening or calcification that prevents the valve from opening fully

or the inability of the valve to prevent blood from backing up. *Valvuloplasty* is a type of valve repair and encompasses dilating the valve with a balloon through a catheter or repairing the valve surgically. Valve replacement may be with a mechanical artificial valve, or with a valve taken from an animal or a human who has died. Rejection is not an issue in valve replacement, but infection is a concern, no matter whether the replacement is made of metal, synthetic materials, or tissue.

In heart failure, fluid may accumulate not only in limbs or near lungs but also in the *pericardium* surrounding the heart, compressing the heart within it and preventing it from pumping as it should. Called *cardiac tamponade,* this condition requires draining the fluid from the sac through a needle (*pericardiocentesis*). In some cases, surgical incision (*pericardiotomy*) may be the preferred method for relieving the tamponade. Another type of ventricular impairment is produced when inflammation of the sac occurs and produces constrictive pericarditis, requiring surgical removal of the pericardium (*pericardiectomy*).

Managing Heart Failure

To help you live better with heart failure, your physician will probably demand some changes in your diet, your physical activity level, and other aspects of your lifestyle. Treatment will probably include certain of the medicines described above, usually with what one writer called 3-D medicines—diuretics, dilators, and digitalis. These aim to reduce swelling, to increase the inner diameter of the blood vessels to improve blood flow, and to ensure proper heartbeat. Sometimes surgery is also required. To improve blood flow to the heart, your physician may recommend coronary artery bypass or percutaneous transluminal coronary ("balloon") angioplasty. Repairing or replacing one or more heart valves may be another way to correct all or part of the problem.

These treatments are designed to help you feel better, reduce or eliminate further damage to your heart and blood vessels, and minimize the negative effect of your disease on your life. You will want to discuss any questions you have with nurses or physicians involved in your care. Determine what restrictions apply to your plans to work or to participate in sports or other leisure activities. Patients often have questions about whether sexual intercourse is risky or overtaxing for someone with heart failure. Your physician should help you resolve these questions.

Besides wanting you to reduce risks for additional heart disease, your physician will probably ask you to reduce your risk for lung infections. Having an annual flu shot and getting a vaccination against pneumonia are good preventive measures to take.

To support you in your effort to live as fully as possible within the confines of your illness, enlist your family and friends in your treatment. Being diagnosed with heart failure, beginning drug therapy or undergoing surgery, and making many lifestyle changes can be overwhelming. Don't think you have to go through your illness by yourself. Adjusting to these changes and accepting yourself as you are may pose emotional challenges that may best be overcome with help from those you love and trust. Many times these loved ones want to help but need direction. Be open with them. Remember that changes you have to make may affect them, too, so working together can serve you all.

Beyond your family and friends, you may want to secure other help to bolster your response to your diagnosis and treatment. A professional counselor, clinic or hospital social worker, or support group can provide opportunities for you to express your feelings and examine them. These professionals and groups also can provide additional information about your ailment that can help you manage it. People respond differently to health challenges: some can never gather enough information, and others want to know as little as they can without jeopardizing their treatment. Recognize what approach will make coping easier for you, and help your health care team and family understand it.

Considering the Future

The outlook for patients with heart failure depends on many factors, including age, the type and severity of the underlying condition, its potential for reversibility, and problems associated with it. For those who make adjustments, follow medication schedules, and generally work at improving, the prognosis is generally better than for those who haphazardly or inadequately follow therapeutic recommendations. Sometimes lack of motivation, knowledge, or money can keep patients with heart failure from following their treatment plans. Sometimes cultural practices also prevent patients from being comfortable in making large-scale dietary, other lifestyle, and drug-taking changes. Tell your physician about any problems you foresee so that as many obstacles as possible can be removed from following the treatment meant to relieve symptoms and prolong life.

If you are a patient living with severe heart failure, hospitalization can loom large in your view of the future. Emergency transport to the hospital can be important to plan for—whom to call, whom to ask to monitor the house or household, whom to expect to perform daily household maintenance.

Advance directives, prepared as a legal document with specific instructions about how you would like your care handled in an emergency, set down in writing your wishes about lifesaving measures in case you are unable to express them at the time of an emergency. State laws dictate how advance directives can be used. Talk to your attorney, your family, and your health care team about how you can make decisions about your care through advance directives.

The medical community's commitment to alleviating the burden of heart failure is seen in American Heart Association conferences on the subject and in National Heart, Lung, and Blood Institute endeavors, including a 1992 task force that laid the groundwork for five Specialized Centers of Research in heart failure and a special emphasis panel of 1996. The 1996 panel found much reason for optimism for soon reaching improved understanding and treatment of the condition. New directions include transgenic mouse models available for research, the feasibility of transplants from larger, genetically altered animals, the strategy of cell transplants to improve cardiac function, novel gene vector development, and the identification of endogenous regulators contributing to pathologic conditions.

Summary

Impaired heart function may result from many causes, and its treatment is highly individualized. The mainstay of treatment is drug therapy. Quality of life can often be greatly enhanced for patients who watch their diet, aid their circulation with appropriate exercise, and follow the drug therapy prescribed by their physician. Congestive heart failure may require both medical and surgical treatment, yet even these may not prevent the long-term prognosis from remaining ominous. Cardiac transplantation serves only a small percentage of patients with heart failure; nonetheless, survival rates show this uncommon operation can effectively extend life. Attempts at matching marginal recipients and donors are expanding its usefulness. Meanwhile, those with heart failure must follow the advice of their physicians, find ways to incorporate more healthful habits into their lifestyle, and ease the burden of illness with advance planning and by sharing their concerns with those they love.

CHAPTER NINE

Arrhythmias

The heart is more than a tireless muscle, more than a powerful pump. It is also an amazing electrical device, one that typically runs for more than 70 years with neither a tune-up nor major repairs.

The heart's electrical conduction system is where it all begins. Electrical impulses travel through the heart along pathways of specialized muscle cells, setting in motion the rhythmic beating of the heart. Beginning in the sinoatrial node (also called the *sinus node*), these impulses race along an established route, triggering contraction of each of the heart's chambers.

Any deviation from this orderly signal transmission has the potential to cause an arrhythmia—an abnormal heart rate or rhythm. Cardiac arrhythmias range in seriousness from the insignificant to the life threatening. They can be set in motion by many external and internal factors. Some of the external factors that can set off heartbeat irregularities are extreme fatigue, physical exertion, emotional stress, cigarette smoking, heavy drinking, and inges-

tion of stimulants (such as caffeine, decongestants, and cocaine). Even some of the medicines used to *treat* arrhythmias can *trigger* arrhythmias.

Physiologic conditions that increase the risk of arrhythmias include congenital heart defects, imbalances of electrolytes (potassium, magnesium, and calcium), thyroid disorders, inflammatory diseases, and problems in the autonomic nervous system, which carries nerve impulses from the brain and spinal cord to the heart.

The most important factor contributing to arrhythmias, however, is acquired heart disease. Coronary artery disease, heart attack (*myocardial infarction*), and high blood pressure (hypertension) all damage the heart—as can heart surgery and other invasive procedures. Scar tissue and areas of "dead" muscle can redirect electrical waves and set off an abnormal rhythm. Cardiac arrhythmias become more common with age.

To understand how arrhythmias develop—and ultimately what can be done about them—let's first review how the heart's normal rhythm is set and maintained.

A Finely Tuned Device

The rhythmic filling and contraction of the heart's four chambers are set in motion by electrical signals originating within the heart itself. Normal signal transmission begins in the sinoatrial (SA) node, located in the ceiling of the right atrium. The SA node is the heart's primary pacemaker. When the SA node fires an electrical impulse, it sets the rate of rhythmic signal transmission and triggers a wavelike, top-to-bottom contraction of the atria. This wave of electrical activity then passes from the right atrium to the heart's secondary pacemaker, the atrioventricular (AV) node. At the AV node, the impulse slows—delayed for about one-fifth of a second—before passing through to the ventricles. This split-second pause allows the ventricles to fill completely with blood squeezed through from the atria.

After the impulse passes through the AV node, it accelerates and spreads through the *His–Purkinje system*. The His–Purkinje system is a network of specialized fibers that comprises the *bundle of His,* which branches into a *right bundle branch* and a *left bundle branch,* and the *Purkinje fibers,* which ultimately trigger contraction of the ventricles.

The impulse fired from the SA node terminates in the Purkinje fibers. It completes its journey in less than a second. In that brief instant, the heart fills and empties a portion of its contents—takes blood sapped of its life-giving cargo, sends it through the lungs for replenishing, and propels it out into the far reaches of the body. Under normal circumstances in an adult, the SA node fires an electrical impulse about 65 to 75 times every minute. Barring a disturbance, this orderly process continues in relative synchrony, minute after minute, day in and day out for a lifetime.

But sometimes the normal heart rhythm gets out of sync. Any number of conditions and external factors can set the stage for an arrhythmia to develop. The mechanisms that actually derail the electrical signals fall into three general categories: *focal arrhythmias, reentry arrhythmias,* and *heart block.*

Focal arrhythmias (often referred to as *ectopic* or *automatic arrhythmias*) arise when a group of cells or an area of tissue (an abnormal *focus*) begins firing electrical impulses independently. Muscle cells throughout the conduction pathway have the ability to generate their own electrical activity. This allows them to act as a remote pacemaker if the SA node malfunctions or signal transmission breaks down somewhere else along the regularly traveled route. Although this amazing backup plan can be lifesaving, it also can override the SA node, taking control of heart rhythm and producing an abnormal heartbeat.

Reentry arrhythmias are the cardiac equivalent of a short circuit. Electrical impulses get stuck along a pathway and then detour into a subsidiary or bypass pathway. Here the impulses keep "reentering," in effect, circling around and around.

Heart block is the third mechanism that can alter normal impulse transmission. (The term heart block is also used to describe a category of conduction abnormalities.) In heart block, electrical impulses fired from the SA node hit roadblocks along the conduction pathway, slowing or even halting transmission of the signals needed to maintain a strong and rhythmic heartbeat. With communication from the SA node cut off, backup cells in the ventricles begin firing their own electrical impulses to maintain ventricular contractions. This backup pacemaker sets a different rate from the original, firing only 30 to 40 times per minute and compromising the heart's pumping ability.

Though most heart rhythm abnormalities are harmless—and surprisingly common—several types are quite serious and can lead to cardiac arrest and death.

First, we will look at benign arrhythmias—the normal speeding up and slowing down of the heart rate and the garden-variety palpitations that affect most of us at one time or another. Then, we will examine more serious heart rhythm disturbances, known as *supraventricular tachycardias* and *ventricular tachycardias*. Finally, we will explore the varying degrees and consequences of heart block and take a look at *sick sinus syndrome*, one of the most common indications for pacemaker implantation in older people.

Benign Arrhythmias

Just about everyone has felt his or her heart skip a beat or suddenly race in situations of anger or fear. These occasional and brief deviations from the heart's normal rhythm are harmless and common. Moreover, as part of its normal functioning, the heart speeds up to accommodate the demands of physical exertion or emotional stress and slows down during rest and sleep, when demands on it are low.

Tachycardia—*tachy* (fast) *cardia* (heart)—is the term used to describe a heart rate above 100 beats per minute. *Bradycardia*—*brady* (slow) *cardia* (heart)—refers to a heart rate that is slower than the norm—less than 50 beats per minute. (However, highly trained—and healthy—athletes often have heart rates below 60 beats per minute when they are at rest.)

Doctors call the normal speeding up and slowing down of the heart rate in response to everyday demands *sinus tachycardia* and *sinus bradycardia*. In sinus tachycardia and sinus bradycardia, the SA node—the heart's main pacemaker—is simply doing its job, boosting heart rate when necessary and dampening it when demand is low.

Two other types of usually harmless tachycardia involve premature contractions of the atria (known as *premature atrial complexes*) or the ventricles (called *premature ventricular complexes*). These feel like a skipped beat or palpitation and often are precipitated by external factors, such as smoking, drinking too much coffee, or taking decongestants or other stimulants. Premature ventricular complexes are common. Just about everyone experiences them occasionally. These early ventricular beats also accompany coronary artery disease.

Although premature ventricular complexes may not be harmful, people who regularly experience these too-early contractions run a higher than average risk of developing more serious ventricular arrhythmias. Moreover, in susceptible individuals, an episode of these irregular contractions can trigger a more dangerous type of arrhythmia.

In general, occasional skipped heartbeats are nothing to worry about. But if they occur frequently or last for more than a few seconds, have your doctor check them out. As with all odd sensations involving the heart, the prudent approach is to err on the side of caution.

Supraventricular Tachycardias

Sustained tachycardias—rapid and irregular heartbeats that are relatively long-lasting—are more serious and should always be evaluated by a physician. When the heart beats too rapidly, the ventricles do not have time to fill completely—and that can compromise the heart's pumping ability. These irregularities are classified according to where they originate in the heart. Site of origin is important: it will determine whether treatment is needed. It will also influence what type of treatment is chosen and help predict the long-term outcome of the patient. Supraventricular tachycardias arise in the area above the ventricles (the prefix *supra* means "above")—either in the atria or atrioventricular (AV) node. Ventricular tachycardias originate in the ventricles and are potentially more serious.

Supraventricular tachycardias may be associated with coexisting heart or lung disease, and they may arise after a heart attack or surgery for various cardiac or pulmonary disorders. These arrhythmias generally are not life threatening unless the heart is seriously compromised in other ways. Some types may require drug therapy or another form of treatment. Others require no treatment at all and represent little more than a nuisance.

Nonetheless, all persistent irregular heartbeats need to be carefully evaluated.

Supraventricular tachycardias are frequently occurring arrhythmias and encompass numerous subtypes. Those characterized as paroxysmal (of unpredictable onset, cessation, or duration) are frequently encountered and include atrioventricular reciprocating tachycardia and atrioventricular nodal reentrant tachycardia. They are called paroxysmal atrial tachycardias (PATs). These are generally benign unless cardiac function is compromised. The attacks may be disturbing or frightening to the patient. Rest and cautious, gentle massage of the carotid artery area in the neck, along with use of a beta-blocker such as atenolol, are useful. These arrhythmias are maintained by the atrioventricular junction, which is the area at the apex of the heart's center-dividing septum. These tachycardias are usually not associated with underlying cardiac disease.

One type of these paroxysmal tachycardias is Wolff–Parkinson–White syndrome, which is characterized by the ventricle's being electrically excited to action prematurely. Conduction goes awry usually—but not always—because connections exist outside the normal conducting tissue, linking atrium and ventricle. Generally, these occur congenitally and may be detected early, but tachycardia can occur at any age. The syndrome may be diagnosed with electrocardiography (not all cases can be picked up).

Because Wolff–Parkinson–White syndrome has been shown to be generated by an accessory pathway that can be anatomically identified and treated, its cure rates are now quite high. Both Wolff–Parkinson–White syndrome and supraventricular tachycardias in general can be treated by catheter ablation. Catheter ablation is being used as a primary or first-line therapy for some patients with these rapid heartbeats.

Another type of supraventricular tachycardia is atrial tachycardia. This type, along with atrial fibrillation and atrial flutter, is often associated with underlying cardiac disease, such as previous heart attack or valvular disease. Patients may have underlying metabolic disturbances (excess caffeine or alcohol intake, often paired with tobacco use) and be physically fatigued or overworked. These episodes require evaluation by a physician, ideally while they are in progress. A doctor can help patients understand the mechanisms causing the tachycardia, help them cope, and suggest and implement appropriate therapy.

Atrial flutter refers to the rapidly "fluttering" P waves this condition produces on an electrocardiogram. During atrial flutter, the atria may contract 250 to 400 times per minute. The ventricles, unable to keep pace, contract once for every two to four atrial beats. The heart's pumping efficiency declines, often leaving the person feeling weak or faint.

Atrial fibrillation, one of the most common cardiac arrhythmias, can occur in people with underlying heart, lung, or metabolic disorders, or it may arise in otherwise healthy individuals. Coronary artery disease, rheumatic heart disease, mitral valve dysfunction, and thyroid problems are common triggers. Atrial fibrillation becomes more common with advancing age, affecting about 10 percent of people older than age 75.

During atrial fibrillation, the upper chambers of the heart contract in an uncoordinated—and often rapid—manner. As a result, electrical impulses transmitted through the AV node get out of sync, producing erratic and inefficient contractions in the ventricles. People experiencing atrial fibrillation often report one or more of several symptoms, including heart palpitations or skipped beats, light-headedness, feeling faint or fainting, chest pain, or anxiety.

The chaotic and often rapid contractions in atrial fibrillation can lead to heart failure, a condition in which the heart fails to pump enough blood to sustain normal functioning. Moreover, atrial fibrillation poses serious risk for stroke. When the atria contract irregularly and inefficiently, they do not empty properly, allowing blood to pool within the chambers. This can set the stage for formation of a *thrombus*—or clot—that can later travel to the brain, choking off the blood supply and causing a stroke.

Most people with recurrent atrial fibrillation are placed on anticoagulant therapy—medications that inhibit blood coagulation and, therefore, clot formation. Without this therapy, a number of people who regularly experience atrial fibrillation would go on to have a stroke at some point in their lives. Anticoagulant therapy, however, is by no means benign. Although prescribed with therapeutic intent, it can have significant, even life-threatening, side effects, and it has a number of contraindications. New approaches to therapy involve ablating (removing by cutting or vaporizing) the AV node, which reduces the effect on the ventricles, and then implanting a pacemaker. This therapy has been used successfully in more than 20,000 cases in the last few years. Therapy for atrial fibrillation is also discussed on pp. 165–166 and pp. 445–446. The main forms of therapy remain digitalis preparations, quinidine, and cardioversion; ablation has been used in resistant cases.

Ventricular Tachycardias

Ventricular arrhythmias are the most serious type of heart rhythm disturbance. These heartbeat irregularities originate in the myocardium of the ventricles. Because the ventricles bear the major responsibility for propelling blood into the circulation, any significant dysfunction can have dire consequences.

The two primary types of ventricular arrhythmia—ventricular tachycardia and *ventricular fibrillation*—demand immediate medical attention. Ventricular fibrillation is a life-threatening emergency that requires cardiopulmonary resuscitation (CPR) and special medical equipment to prevent sudden death. These are different from the premature ventricular complexes, the early ventricular beats discussed above. *Nonsustained* ventricular tachycardias are several consecutive beats of ventricular origin. They are transitory but may be life threatening, and they often portend development of *sustained* ventricular tachycardia.

Ventricular tachycardia resembles a sustained run of premature ventricular complexes. This type of arrhythmia is strongly associated with coexisting heart disease, especially coronary artery disease, heart attack, and mitral valve dysfunction. In fact, ventricular tachycardia may develop in the days following heart surgery or a heart attack, as a result of either scarring or abnormal impulse conduction in the area involved. In addition, a host of other medical conditions, including infections, inflammatory disorders, and cancers that spread to the heart, can set the stage for ventricular tachycardia.

This type of arrhythmia can cause palpitations, breathlessness, fainting, light-head-edness, or a pounding sensation in the neck. Sustained ventricular tachycardia may lead to dangerously low blood pressure, difficulty in breathing, and heart failure. Untreated, ventricular tachycardia can degenerate into ventricular fibrillation.

In ventricular fibrillation, muscles in the ventricles are reduced to rapid, erratic quivering and twitching. In this chaotic state, the ventricles lose their ability to pump blood out of the heart. Without immediate intervention, blood flow to the brain stops, and sudden cardiac death follows. CPR may be able to sustain a reduced level of cardiac output during ventricular fibrillation, but a device called a defibrillator will be needed to "shock" the heart into a normal rhythm and prevent death. In the last few years, permanent pacemakerlike devices with defibrillating ability have been implanted in patients with arrhythmias.

Heart Block

In heart block, communication between the atria and the ventricles breaks down. The electrical impulses that originate in the SA node get delayed in the AV node or bundle of His, disrupting the coordinated rhythm of the heart. Some forms of heart block are well tolerated; others can cause bradycardia, the extremely slow heart rate that can lead to loss of consciousness or, in some instances, death.

A number of medical conditions can cause heart block. These include coronary artery disease and heart attack; such inflammatory diseases as rheumatoid arthritis; metabolic imbalances; infections; surgical interruption of the conduction pathways; and scarring. Some cardiac medications can cause or aggravate heart block, including beta-blockers, calcium channel blockers, and drugs used to correct other arrhythmias.

Despite the ominous-sounding name, not all cases of heart block pose a serious threat. Doctors designate three degrees of heart block, beginning with the least serious: *first-degree, second-degree,* and *third-degree (complete) heart block.* Symptoms range from none in the mildest form, to palpitations, extreme breathlessness, fatigue, weakness, threat of fainting, and finally, loss of consciousness and convulsions in the most serious cases.

In first-degree heart block, impulse transmission through the AV node is delayed. This mildest form of the disorder usually causes no symptoms (and often is detected only on an electrocardiogram). First-degree heart block usually requires no therapy other than attempting to identify and correct the factors that caused it, such as electrolyte imbalances, medications, or coexisting heart problems. However, first-degree heart block is noteworthy because it may be a person's first indication that he or she has underlying heart disease. Moreover, heart block can further compromise heart function in patients with heart failure.

In second-degree heart block, some of the electrical impulses passing from the atria get through to the ventricles, but others do not. The normal relation between atrial and ventricular contractions begins to unravel, resulting in uncoordinated and inefficient pumping of blood from the ventricles. Doctors further classify second-degree heart block into *Mobitz type I* (in which conduction delays precede conduction blockage) and *Mobitz type II* (in which conduction blockage occurs without a delay).

A Mobitz type I heart block usually originates just above the AV node and often is benign. Mobitz type II is more ominous. It usually occurs in the His–Purkinje system and often precedes development of complete heart block.

In third-degree heart block, communication between the atria and ventricles breaks down completely. The block can occur in the AV node, His bundle, or in the outer reaches of the Purkinje fibers. With no electrical impulses getting through to the ventricles, backup pacemaker cells in these lower chambers begin firing independently—but too slowly. Heart rate drops to dangerous levels, and blood flow to the brain dwindles, resulting in loss of consciousness and even death.

Sick Sinus Syndrome

Sick sinus syndrome is the name given to a generalized dysfunction of the sinus, or SA, node. The term encompasses a number of abnormalities, including delayed, erratic, or blocked impulse transmission from the SA node, and combinations of SA node and AV node conduction disturbances. A number of factors can contribute to sick sinus syndrome. These include damage to the SA node itself, inflammation or degeneration of the nerves surrounding the node, disease-related changes in the wall of the atrium, fat accumulation, and fibrosis. Degenerative changes in the SA node become more common with age.

A person with sick sinus syndrome may experience more than one type of rhythm abnormality. The heart may race on one occasion but beat too slowly on another (thus, the name of a subset of the syndrome: *tachycardia–bradycardia syndrome*). Some people may experience persistent bradycardia or intermittent sinus block or arrest. An episode of tachycardia may be followed by a long pause before normal sinus rhythm is reestablished.

Symptoms are dependent on the predominant rhythm abnormalities. But the most common ones are dizziness, mental confusion, fatigue, and fainting (or near-fainting spells called *grayouts*). In severe cases, loss of consciousness may occur.

Treatment for sick sinus syndrome almost always involves implantation of an artificial pacemaker. Arrhythmia medications may be added if necessary.

Treatment

Heart rhythm disturbances are among the most challenging heart problems to treat. Some, such as occasional premature beats, require no treatment at all and are more of an annoyance than a serious health problem. Others can be life-threatening emergencies. A careful diagnostic workup is essential to distinguish between benign arrhythmias and those that are potentially lethal.

In general, heartbeat irregularities arising in or involving the upper areas of the heart—*supraventricular arrhythmias*—are less serious and often respond well to medications. *Ventricular arrhythmias*—those originating in the lower chambers of the heart—can be quite serious and often require more complex interventions.

Treatment of heart rhythm disturbances can be complex. Sometimes more than one mechanism contributes to the irregular rhythm, and a two- or three-pronged therapy will be needed to address all the factors involved. Sometimes the medication given to correct one type of arrhythmia will trigger another type of irregularity. As is true for many other heart problems, successful treatment is a delicate balancing act.

The first step toward correcting an abnormal rhythm is to trace its origins in the heart and then try to identify which internal or external factors might be triggering the disturbance.

Diagnostic Foundation

Because arrhythmias may not always occur when the doctor is there to observe them, the patient's report of what happened can be crucial. If you experience an arrhythmia and seek medical attention, try to provide the physician with as much detail as possible. The more information you can provide, the better.

- What were you doing at the time— lying down, watching a basketball game, pushing the lawnmower, arguing with a coworker?
- What do the irregular heartbeats feel like? Does your heart race? Flutter? Skip a beat?
- When does the arrhythmia occur, and how long does it usually last?
- Do these abnormal heartbeats arise several times a day or just once in a while?
- Do they come and go suddenly or gradually?
- How do you feel during an episode? Does your chest hurt? Is it hard to catch your breath? Do you black out or feel as if you are going to faint?

These details can be important pieces of the diagnostic puzzle.

Your doctor also will review your medical history for clues. Coexisting cardiovascular diseases—and even some of the medications used to treat them—are common causes of arrhythmias. Noncardiac conditions—such as thyroid disorders, inflammatory diseases, endocrine problems, or infections—also may be to blame.

The doctor will obtain a medical history and do a full physical examination and may order blood tests to check for an overactive thyroid or electrolyte imbalances—low levels of potassium or magnesium, for example. Because a variety of substances can touch off arrhythmias, your doctor will ask about your use of caffeine, alcohol, cigarettes, decongestants (such as those containing pseudoephedrine), diet aids, and recreational drugs. If the arrhythmia is still in progress, he or she may perform what are called *vagal maneuvers.* These are indirect physical manipulations of the vagus nerves, which help regulate heart rate. By gently massaging the carotid sinus, a dilated area in the carotid arteries in the neck, the doctor may be able to slow your heart rate. Your heart's response to these maneuvers can provide important diagnostic information.

Electrocardiograms

The electrocardiogram (ECG or EKG) is the cornerstone of arrhythmia diagnosis. Like fingerprints found at a crime scene,

ECG tracings are important pieces of physical evidence.

The various phases of the ECG tracing—P wave, PR segment, QRS complex, and T wave—correspond to the different stages of electrical activity associated with a cycle of a heartbeat. An abnormal wave signals a problem in a particular area or function of the heart and may, in some instances, provide enough information to establish the diagnosis. In other cases, 24-hour ambulatory (Holter) ECG monitoring or electrophysiologic studies (discussed below) will be needed to determine conclusively the cause of the arrhythmia. (For a description of ECG tracings, see pp. 29–31.)

As part of the initial diagnostic workup, you also may be monitored by one or more variations of the standard ECG. Your doctor may want an *exercise ECG*, recorded while you walk on a treadmill or pedal a stationary bike, to observe your heart's activity during strenuous exertion.

You may be asked to undergo ambulatory ECG monitoring—an around-the-clock recording of your heart rhythm as you perform your usual activities. In ambulatory monitoring, you will wear a portable ECG monitor (sometimes called a *Holter monitor*) 24 hours a day and may be asked to record each of your activities—eating, sleeping, walking the dog, watching television—along with the time of day and any symptoms you experienced during the activity. That way the doctor can correlate any rhythm irregularities with the type of activity that may have triggered them.

Ambulatory monitoring is a very important diagnostic test. It may provide one of the few noninvasive ways for your doctor to observe and record your heartbeat abnormality as it occurs. If the arrhythmia remains elusive, an *event recorder* may be used. With one of these devices in place, you can call in to a main computer as soon as you feel the irregular rhythm, and your ECG will be transmitted over the phone line.

Electrophysiologic Studies

If the origin of an apparently serious arrhythmia remains a mystery, or if the doctor needs more specific information before selecting a treatment, you may be asked to undergo electrophysiologic testing. Electrophysiologic studies are an important diagnostic and therapeutic tool. These invasive, in-hospital procedures can be used to "map" the heart's electrical conduction system, to provoke an abnormal rhythm (for diagnostic purposes), to test the effects of various drugs, and to guide a treatment called *catheter ablation* (see "Catheter Ablation" below in this chapter).

In electrophysiologic testing, specialists pass electrode-tipped catheters through blood vessels into the heart. Typically, the catheters are inserted through the veins and into the right atrium and right ventricle. The electrodes record electrical impulses within the heart and allow doctors to trace the heart's conduction pathways. Following the impulses through the heart allows physicians to pinpoint the area where the system breaks down and an arrhythmia starts.

In addition to sensing electrical activity within the heart, the electrodes are able to deliver low-level electrical current to heart muscle, much as a pacemaker does. This capability to stimulate the heart allows the specialists to reproduce the rhythm abnormality in the controlled setting of the electrophysiology laboratory.

There, too, doctors can test the effects of various medications with a relative degree of safety. Typically, the electrophysiology specialists will provoke the arrhythmia and then give the patient a selected drug. Afterward, if they are unable to provoke the abnormal rhythm while the patient is medicated, the drug has a high likelihood of preventing the problem under everyday circumstances.

Electrophysiologic testing is conducted in a catheterization or electrophysiology laboratory. The lab will be equipped with recording and stimulating devices, imaging equipment to check placement of the electrodes, machines to monitor vital functions, and defibrillating devices in case complications arise. A cardiologist specially trained in the technique and an assistant will perform the testing, with the help of a nurse anesthetist and one or more other technicians.

The procedure can take as long as two or three hours, depending on what the cardiologist finds and how many medications are tested. Less complex cases may be completed in under an hour. As with other procedures involving catheterization, the patient usually remains awake but mildly sedated during the testing.

Local anesthetic will be injected at the catheter insertion sites. Typically, two or three tiny catheters will be passed through the femoral vein in the groin, and one may be passed through the jugular vein on the right side of the neck. (These catheters have extremely small diameters and can easily fit into the femoral or jugular vein.) The catheters are then advanced along the vein until they reach the superior or inferior vena cava, and then are introduced into the right side of the heart through the upper chamber (right atrium).

You probably will not feel the electrical current as the doctor stimulates your heart. When an arrhythmia is triggered, however, you may experience the same sensations you have when the out-of-sync rhythm occurs naturally. You may feel anxious (although the sedative will help), unable to catch your breath, or faint, and you may even black out. But it is important to remember that you are surrounded by specialists trained to revive you quickly and to restore a normal heart rhythm with the use of sophisticated equipment.

When testing is complete, the catheters are removed and the insertion sites are cleaned and checked for bleeding. Bruising may occur at the sites, but trauma to the area usually is minimal. Complications from electrophysiologic studies are rare—occurring less than 1 percent of the time. Potential problems at the insertion site include bleeding, development of a blood clot, or infection. More serious—but again rare—complications include damage to blood vessels or the heart, stroke, ventricular fibrillation, and death.

A cardioversion/defibrillation device is always on standby during electrophysiologic testing. These devices can convert a sustained tachycardia into a normal sinus rhythm (*cardioversion*) or terminate ventricular fibrillation (*defibrillation*) by delivering an electrical shock to the heart. The electrical current stimulates all or most of the myocardium at once, briefly suspending all heart activity. This provides an opportunity for the heart's natural pacemakers to regain control of heart rhythm and for natural electrical impulses to resume. (Electrical cardioversion also may be used in nonemergency situations to restore normal heart rhythm in patients with sustained tachycardia.)

Drug Therapies

Many cardiac arrhythmias can be managed with medication, although finding the most effective drug or best dosage often requires experimentation and perseverance. With some types of arrhythmias, electrophysiologic testing can simplify the process considerably. Electrophysiologic studies, however, are invasive, expensive, and not without risks. For simpler, less serious heart rhythm disturbances, a doctor may prescribe an appropriate medication and monitor the patient's response on ambulatory ECG.

The initial doses of some antiarrhythmia medications may need to be given in the hospital, where the patient's response can be carefully monitored. Some of the drugs used to treat arrhythmias can trigger arrhythmias or worsen preexisting arrhythmias, through a process called *proarrhythmia*. A number of medication-induced heartbeat abnormalities are known to exist. Moreover, because some of these medications are effective only when given in amounts that approach a toxic level, it is often safer to adjust dosage in the security of the hospital setting.

A wide array of medications are used to suppress heartbeat irregularities. These include beta-blockers, calcium channel blockers, quinidine, digitalis preparations, and procainamide. Other, more potent medications may be used, especially to treat ventricular arrhythmias. Many of these medications have desensitizing or anesthetic effects that make heart muscle less reactive to stimuli, and can slow conduction of impulses through the heart. Because of their numerous side effects—including the potential to trigger other arrhythmias—these powerful drugs are reserved for people whose risk of sudden death is high enough to justify the risks of the medication.

An antiarrhythmia medication may be given intravenously in an acute situation—to suppress an arrhythmia in progress or to convert the heart to a normal sinus rhythm (called *pharmacologic cardioversion*). That drug may or may not be continued in oral form afterward.

All medications used to treat cardiac arrhythmias have side effects. These range from the generally mild side effects associated with beta-blockers and calcium channel blockers, to the more serious problems that may arise with the desensitizing medications. A doctor will weigh the potential benefits of drug therapy against the possible risks. Unfortunately, these risks and benefits are not always clearly defined—and that has made drug therapy for certain types of arrhythmia controversial. In recent years, for example, cardiologists have learned that a medication's ability to suppress potentially lethal ventricular arrhythmias in certain patients does not necessarily translate into improved survival.

Landmark studies called the Cardiac Arrhythmia Suppression Trials (CAST) examined the effects of suppressing serious ventricular arrhythmias in heart attack survivors with significant left ventricular dysfunction. When the trials were extended to patients with less serious arrhythmias, the researchers found that the patients treated with any of three antiarrhythmia medications had a higher risk for sudden death than did untreated patients. The results of these and other studies underscore the complex nature of heart rhythm disturbances. Researchers continue to try to define the risks and benefits of various drug therapies and to identify which subgroups of patients are more likely to have improved outcomes with medication.

In the meantime, nondrug therapies—such as catheter ablation and implantable cardioverter/defibrillators—increasingly are being used to prevent or interrupt serious heart rhythm disturbances.

Invasive Interventions

Invasive approaches to arrhythmia management involve the expense, discomfort, and risks associated with any surgery or catheterization. In many instances, though, they can provide a permanent solution to a bothersome or dangerous rhythm disturbance.

For some arrhythmias, implantation of a pacemaker or defibrillator is the treatment of choice. In other instances, the patient may prefer an invasive procedure to a lifetime of taking multiple medications that may be only partially protective or fraught with side effects.

Whatever the circumstances, nondrug therapies for arrhythmias have come a long way and offer excellent solutions to many rhythm abnormalities.

Pacemakers

Artificial pacemakers have become so commonplace that it is easy to forget how revolutionary the first ones really were. Dramatically smaller, "smarter," and considered almost routine today, pacemakers are lifesaving devices that allow tens of thousands of people to go about their usual activities each day, with little thought

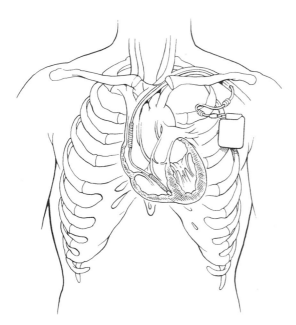

Figure 9.1. Placement of the defibrillator is usually in the pectoral region (left chest, as shown, or right).

given to their once-debilitating rhythm abnormalities.

Pacemakers are used most often to correct bradycardia, a heart rate that is dangerously low; however, they may also be implanted after surgical or catheter ablation has been used to intentionally destroy a malfunctioning AV node or other arrhythmia-provoking tissue. (For more on pacemakers and the implantation procedure, see Chapter 10.)

Implantable Cardioverter/Defibrillators

Before the advent of implantable defibrillating devices, most people unlucky enough to experience ventricular fibrillation far away from a hospital or without the immediate response of a well-equipped emergency team died of cardiac arrest within minutes. When the ventricles' steady rhythm degenerates into the rapid, chaotic quivering and twitching of fibrillation, an electrical shock is needed to suspend heart activity—and then allow it to initiate a normal rhythm.

Today, patients can "carry" their own personal defibrillators, usually within their chest wall (Figure 9.1). The most recent ones can be implanted in the pectoral muscle in an upper quadrant of the chest, and they utilize a structure known as an "active can." Called *implantable cardioverter/defibrillators,* these highly sophisticated devices can sense an abnormal rhythm and then automatically deliver one or more lifesaving jolts of energy to shock the heart out of its chaos. In doing so, they can rescue patients from the grip of ventricular tachycardia and ventricular fibrillation.

Implantable cardioverter/defibrillators essentially are minicomputers connected to the heart. With the introduction of transvenous leads, it is no longer necessary to open the chest to implant them. The devices have become smaller and smaller (weighing less than 10 ounces) and increasingly versatile. The more sophisticated ones can be programmed for varying sensitivity to abnormal rhythms and for production of a range of energy—from low-energy bursts for converting heart rhythm, to high-energy bursts for defibrillation.

With those cardioverter/defibrillators capable of being implanted without major surgery (without thoracotomy—that is, surgical opening of the chest), the active "can" is placed in the pectoral region and a lead goes through a vein into the heart. Once the device is in place, the cardiologist or cardiothoracic surgeon will conduct numerous tests of its sensing and defibrillating functions. The device will be tested again before the patient is discharged from the hospital and anytime thereafter when arrhythmia medications are changed for any reason. (More than half of patients who have implantable defibrillators require drug therapy, but usually the number of drugs or the dosages are reduced.)

Newer implantable defibrillators typically last seven or eight years, depending on how frequently they are called upon to perform their lifesaving task. The implantation surgery is associated with a variety of potential complications, including *pericarditis* (inflammation of the pericardium), heart attack, congestive heart failure, postoperative stroke, and infection, among others. One to three percent of patients die during or after thoracotomy, usually because of serious arrhythmias that resist correction or because of other heart or lung problems. Fortunately, the traditional open-chest implantation surgery is obsolete now, since almost all of the current defibrillator leads are implanted transvenously and connected to the pulse generator that is placed in the pectoral area. Implantation below the skin in the pectoral muscle without thoracotomy has meant a reduction in the number of patients who experience serious complications or die. One study reported that the risk for death around the time of implantation was less than 1 percent, a rate similar to that for pacemaker implantation. Cost also falls because of shortened hospitalization. Some researchers propose using it for appropriate patients as a frontline, or initial, therapy, which they believe would improve patient care and reduce costs overall.

Implantation of a defibrillator may have a number of psychological side effects as well. Because the devices rescue patients after the life-threatening episodes are under way—rather than prevent the arrhythmias—the painful shocks are a stark reminder of the seriousness of their condition. Psychological counseling may help patients overcome the fear, anxiety, and depression that can complicate life with an implantable defibrillator.

Although this form of treatment certainly is not without risks or potential complications, the people who require an implantable defibrillator already have a

high risk for sudden death. Studies suggest that without an implantable defibrillator 20 percent of these high-risk individuals would die within two years. Having a defibrillating device in place reduces the five-year risk to 5 percent.

Catheter Ablation

Sometimes the best way to treat an arrhythmia is to destroy the tissue where it originates. In certain heartbeat irregularities, a group of cells begins firing electrical impulses independently, throwing heart rhythm into disarray. Other times, electrical impulses get hung up in a re-entry loop—a "short circuit" in the heart. Although medication is used to suppress many of these arrhythmias, incomplete response, side effects, or other considerations may make other options more attractive.

Deactivating the tissue responsible for the arrhythmia may be accomplished by a technique called *ablation*. This can be accomplished directly with surgery, or through a catheter (Figure 9.2). Success rates are generally high. Depending on the type of abnormality being treated, most patients will achieve a complete cure. Others will gain better control of their condition, either with or without continuing medication. For a small percentage, the procedure brings no improvement.

Catheter ablation (*ablate* means "to remove"; *ablation* means "removal") was a

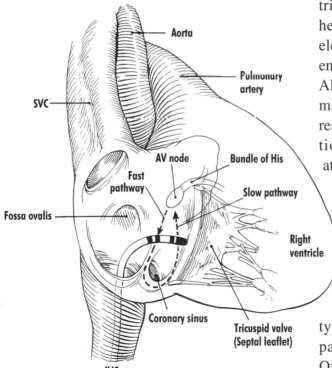

Figure 9.2. Catheter ablation. The ablation catheter enters the right atrium through the inferior vena cava (IVC). This procedure is meant to modify the atrioventricular (AV) nodal slow pathway in a patient with AV nodal reentrant tachycardia, a common type of supraventricular tachycardia. The superior vena cava (SVC) extends above the atrium.

natural outgrowth of electrophysiologic mapping studies. Once cardiologists could identify and stimulate target areas in the heart's conduction system, they began trying to adapt the catheters to a treatment modality.

The first adaptations delivered direct-current electricity to the heart muscle. Although effective in destroying the target tissue, the powerful direct current was associated with a high degree of "overkill," damaging healthy tissue in the surrounding area. Today, most catheter ablations use radiofrequency energy to destroy target tissue. Radiofrequency ablations accomplish their task (Figure 9.3) through controlled heat production. This newer procedure causes minimal pain, does not cause other muscles in the body to contract, and requires that the patient undergo only local anesthesia.

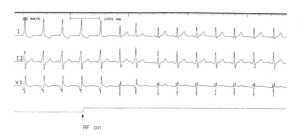

Figure 9.3. This electrocardiogram tracing shows how after radiofrequency (RF) catheter ablation the accessory pathway conduction is eliminated within less than one second. This patient had Wolff–Parkinson–White syndrome.

Summary

Our understanding of cardiac arrhythmias has evolved considerably in recent years. Today physicians have sophisticated ways to map the heart's conduction system and identify underlying abnormalities. Refinements in drug regimens and the diagnostic and therapeutic applications of medical technology have extended the lives of patients with extremely serious heart rhythm disturbances. Development of new arrhythmia medications, advances in pacemaker technology, the advent of implantable defibrillating devices, and progress in ablative techniques have led to more effective treatments for many heart rhythm disturbances.

CHAPTER TEN

Controlling Arrhythmias: Pacemakers, Ablation, and Surgery

BY JAMES B. YOUNG, M.D.

Overview of Pacemaker Systems

Understanding the electrical conduction system of the heart is important. Indeed, insight into the electrical control of cardiac rhythm, with subsequent development of devices that can capture and regulate this activity, has been a major triumph. Particularly fascinating has been the manufacture of sophisticated electrical components (particularly transistors) that has made possible extraordinary miniaturization of complex cardiac pacing and arrhythmia control devices. Cardiac pacing systems have evolved from large tabletop, vacuum tube–laden boxes resembling radios from the 1930s or 1940s, to sleek, metal-sheathed electronic wizardry slightly larger than a 50-cent piece. Two principal factors enabled the current sophistication of electronic cardiac pacing and arrhythmia control. First was understanding the electrical nature of myocyte contraction and cardiac impulse propagation. Second was the great advances made in electronics in general during the first half of the twentieth century.

It is estimated that well over 2 million patients, worldwide, have received a permanent cardiac pacemaker of one sort or another. This does not include the vast number of patients who have benefited from temporary pacemakers, with removal of these devices when the acute difficulty has resolved. Pacemaker research has led to highly sophisticated devices that can stimulate multiple cardiac chambers using heart rate–responsive systems designed to detect increasing demands placed on the cardiovascular system by exercise, for example. Systems today can even be programmed into different modes by transmitting magnetic field signals through the skin. Telemetry interrogation of many devices is also possible, and this provides insight into dysrhythmias over time. Microprocessor-based electronic circuitry

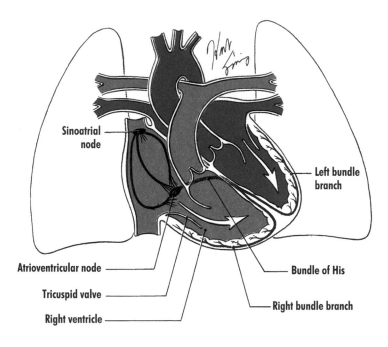

Sinoatrial node

Left bundle branch

Atrioventricular node

Tricuspid valve

Right ventricle

Bundle of His

Right bundle branch

Figure 10.1. Electrical conduction system of normal heart.

has allowed incredible miniaturization and set the stage for long-life power systems. Newer lead designs have greater energy delivery efficacy with vastly improved electrical control of potentially life-threatening cardiac rhythms. Reliability of the devices has improved dramatically as integrated circuitry and power sources have evolved.

The Heart's Electrical Conduction System

Before pacemaker devices are reviewed in more detail, it is important to understand the relation of the heart's cardiac conduction system and properties of electrical

propagation to heartbeat and cardiac rhythm (Figure 10.1). An important characteristic of the myocyte is its ability to shorten regularly and rhythmically, and when cells are linked synergistically, produce a contracting mass that translates power into discharge of a mechanical load. In the case of the heart, this represents forward blood flow through the right and left sides of the heart, past the tricuspid, pulmonic, mitral, and aortic valves, into the pulmonary and systemic vascular circuits. The inherent contractility of the myocyte is regulated by charged or ionic salts passing back and forth across the cell membrane. These particles such as sodium, potassium, calcium, and chloride, among others, create electrical gradients that ultimately trigger contractile machinery and also precipitate propagation of electrical impulses throughout the heart.

Directing this harmonious process is the sinoatrial node anatomically located at the junction of the right atrium and superior vena cava. Electrical impulses generally originate from this point and pass through the myocardial fibers of the right and left atria, subsequently activating the atrioventricular node, which is located at the four-corner junction of the two atria and ventricles. Cardiac nodal tissue is a distinct type of non-contractile cardiac cell that spontaneously depolarizes and produces rhythmic electrical discharge and conduction. From the atrioventricular node, electrical activity spreads rapidly through a specialized collection of conduction fibers called the "bundle of His." This is located in the muscular septum separating the right and left ventricles and divides as it courses distally into the right and left bundle branches, which then fan out over the left and right ventricular muscle.

The electrical conduction system of the heart has many analogies to wiring systems in any structure. As the electrical impulse from the sinus node passes through the atrial tissue, contraction of these chambers is induced. This forces blood from the atrial chambers across the atrioventricular valves (the tricuspid and mitral valves) and into the right and left ventricles. Atrial contractility is synchronized to occur in cardiac diastole. After coursing through the ventricular conduction system, the impulse reaches ventricular fibers, subsequently causing integrated contraction of these tissues as well. This results in configurational change of ventricular shape and volume ejection.

Interference with the conduction system at one or more locations can produce a variety of difficulties, such as a first-degree, second-degree, or third-degree "heart block." Pacemakers are sometimes indicated when heart block occurs, since this disorder can slow heart rates, which then produce inadequate circulation and symptoms, such as syncope. Intrinsic abnormalities of the sinus node can also cause slow heart rates or actual cessation of heartbeat, which also will obviously produce symptoms. So that one can understand why and when some artificial pacemakers are useful, a review of the various types of slow heartbeats (bradycardia) or heart block is necessary. *First-degree atrioventricular block* simply represents a delay in the transmission of electrical impulses from the atrium to the ventricle. Electrical conduction activity is slowed. Because all impulses generated by the sinus node are transmitted, there is little or no decrease in heart rate or change in its regularity. It appears as an abnormality on electrocardiogenic recordings.

First-degree atrioventricular block can be caused by fibrosis of the conduction system, or by certain medications given patients with heart disease. It is not usually an indication for the insertion of a pacemaker device.

Second-degree atrioventricular block is subcategorized into two forms. Type I is characterized by a progressive delay in the electrical transmission of impulses, with fatigue of conduction occurring such that ultimately the electrical impulse is blocked from entering the ventricle, and a normal heartbeat is dropped. This creates a situation in which the atria may beat three times while the ventricle beats only twice. Dropped heartbeats can be noted on an electrocardiogram; this form of heart block is usually reversible and generally benign. It often is associated with acute myocardial infarction but can also be due to certain medications such as digitalis. It is sometimes referred to as *Wenckebach phenomenon* after the gentleman first describing the arrhythmia.

Type II second-degree atrioventricular block has a different pattern and a more ominous prognosis. In this form of heart block the impulse may be transmitted from the atria without delay one time but may not pass through the atrioventricular node into the ventricles at all during the next heartbeat. This form of second-degree heart block is often unstable and may suddenly progress to third-degree, or complete heart block. It is a frequent indication for permanent pacemaker insertion.

Third-degree atrioventricular block is also sometimes referred to as "complete heart block" or "complete atrioventricular dissociation." It generally is an extremely serious condition. As indicated, one characteristic of myocardial tissue is that it will depolarize or contract spontaneously, without extrinsic electrical stimulation, but the rates of these spontaneous contractions are variable and generally much slower than the rate dictated by sinus node impulse formation. In complete heart block, the heart may cease contracting entirely, an event that is referred to as *asystole.* The electrical activity that then does trigger contraction begins in ventricular muscle cells themselves; the rate is thus slow and unstable, and sometimes no contraction whatsoever occurs.

When atrial and ventricular contraction is occurring independently and unrelated, the difficulty is termed *atrioventricular dissociation.* Contractions of the atria and the contractions of the ventricle are occurring as dissociated patterns and, generally, at two completely different rates, with the atrial rate being higher than the ventricular rate.

When complete heart block occurs suddenly, it generally causes loss of consciousness and fainting. In these arrhythmias, patients rarely have any premonitory symptoms or signs, and suddenly have what is often referred to as a "drop attack." These fainting spells are also labeled *Stokes-Adams attacks* after the physicians who first described the relation between sudden syncope and cardiac rhythm disturbance. Unfortunately, the life expectancy of a patient with acquired complete heart block is usually significantly decreased. Pacemakers may attenuate this diminution, but life expectancy is also determined by the underlying conditions that led to the difficulty in the first place. When complete heart block occurs as a consequence of myocardial infarction, the prognosis is worse than when it occurs spontaneously secondary to fibrosis developing in the conduction system. Sometimes complete heart block can develop from drug administration (drugs such as beta blockers, digitalis, or certain calcium channel blockers such as Verapamil or Diltiazem can cause the problem). Complete heart block can also occur in inflammatory heart disease or myocarditis. When the condition is due to drug therapy or diseases that can spontaneously resolve, permanent pacemaker therapy may not be necessary. Rather, temporary pacing units might be inserted. In any case, pacemaker insertion improves quality of life in these patients and allows maintenance of adequate circulation in a setting of very slow or no spontaneous heartbeat activity.

Historical Aspects of Cardiac Pacing

It was the growth of radio and its associated industry that stimulated production of small electrical components and batteries in the late 1920s and 1930s that were critical to development of today's implantable pacemaker devices. The creation of a semiconductor transistor in 1948 by William Schockley, John Bardeen, and Walter Brattain, who subsequently won the Nobel Prize, coupled with more potent and long-lasting batteries, led to modern microprocessor pacemakers. The use of electricity to stimulate the heart is relatively new. Though a variety of attempts at resuscitation of asystolic hearts, some successful, were reported in early medical publications, it was Albert S. Hyman, a physician working at the Beth David Hospital in New York City, who is credited as the originator of the artificial cardiac pacemaker. In 1932, Hyman described an effective method of stimulating hearts in ventricular standstill. Indeed, he was able to resuscitate several patients with transthoracic needle electrodes placed so that they came in contact with the right atrium. The original pacemaker was a large spring-driven magneto-like device that had to be hand-cranked every few minutes to maintain its charge. It was Hyman who first referred to a device of this sort as an "artificial pacemaker." Though the original device was crude, our current pacemakers operate theoretically in the same fashion. Interestingly, Hyman noted that the device was "small enough to fit into a doctor's bag," and could operate on "a common flashlight battery" as its energy current source. Hyman's report referred to several previous attempts at electrostimulation of asystolic hearts in animals and, in particular, an Australian named Lidwill, who had reported the case of a stillborn infant who was resuscitated by electrical stimulation of the heart in 1929. Lidwill actually suggested that cardiac "revival" using electrical stimulation could be applicable in ". . . cardiac failure during anesthesia, cases of drowning if combined with intratracheal insufflation, certain types of gas poisoning, sudden death during the incidence of acute diseases such as diphtheria, and possibly, sudden death during cardiac disease." The link to modern cardiopulmonary resuscitation (CPR) is obvious.

The concepts of Lidwill and Hyman remained fallow for over two decades. Virtually no work was done on the development of pacemaker devices because of the unavailability of sophisticated electronic equipment and lack of knowledge regarding appropriate surgical approaches. It was not until 1952 that P. M. Zoll demonstrated that a high-voltage external pacemaker device, utilizing plate electrodes strapped to the chest wall, could resuscitate the heart in ventricular standstill. This was obviously a difficult and painful procedure. Subsequently, however, by using small epicardial leads placed directly into the myocardium at the time of cardiac surgery, Lillehei demonstrated that patients in whom heart block developed could be paced at better rates for some time. This observation, coupled with disenchantment with Zoll's transthoracic pacing device, spurred S. Furman and J. B. Schwedel to develop an endocardial electrode designed for long-term use that could be placed transvenously. This would allow more chronic pacing of the heart, though still in "temporary" fashion, because only external pacemaker generators were available.

With the evolution of transistors in the late 1950s, a stage was set for implantable, battery-operated, electrical pulse generators to be coupled with endocardial and epicardial electrodes to pace the heart. The first device implanted used a rechargeable power source. Senning and Elmquist performed the procedure in Sweden in 1958. A year later, Greatbach developed the first self-contained implantable pulse generator that relied on a zinc-mercury battery. The Greatbach device contained 10 zinc-mercury cells that provided the power source, and the pacemaker components (battery and circuit transistors) were enclosed in an opaque epoxy resin with an outer coating of silicone rubber.

Early devices were solely "asynchronous," meaning that periodic stimuli were delivered to the ventricles regardless of the underlying ventricular rhythm at any given moment. Large bipolar electrodes were attached to the surface of the heart, and one obvious disadvantage was that the procedure required thoracotomy. Also, the rather large pacemaker system made subcutaneous implantation difficult, if not impossible. Still, experience began to accumulate with this method of long-term treatment for Stokes-Adams syncopal attacks. During the subsequent decade, improvements in electronic circuitry allowed electrocardiographic QRS sensing techniques to be developed, and "demand" pacemaker systems emerged. These units were remarkable for sensing periods of asystole long enough to produce difficulties, and only then would there be subsequent activation of the pacemaker. The result was to restore reasonable underlying rhythms only when necessary. This obviously decreased battery drain and improved overall patient function and satisfaction.

As can be imagined, a reliable power source for these sophisticated electronic devices was problematic in the early 1960s. Battery life was short, and a search began for alternatives with more reliable voltage-generating systems. This led to the proposal that "nuclear" batteries or power sources be used since estimated pacer life could be extended to 25 or 30 years with these systems. The first nuclear, power-source-containing pacemaker was implanted in France in 1970, and although these devices demonstrated the longest cumulative pacemaker survival rate, possible radiation injury to both the patient and to others, with contamination of the environment if the pacemaker case should rupture, led to abandonment of these devices quickly. Lithium-based battery cells have been used more recently, and since 1972 have provided the basic power source for these units.

With advances in lead and electrode development and miniaturization of the pacemaker system itself, the necessity for a major thoracotomy operation to use them could be avoided. By pacing the leads into a large central vein (subclavian or internal jugular vein) and burying the leads and connecting pacemaker "box" subcutaneously, the surgeon could spare the major surgical procedure with general anesthesia. Difficulties can still be encountered, however, with wound infection; lead and electrode perforation of the heart; dislodgement of electrodes lead; wire fracture; and inadvertent muscle or diaphragmatic stimulation complications, seen more commonly with the percutaneous transvenous pacemaker approach. Fortunately, further improvement of electrodes, insulation materials, and pacing circuitry led to diminution of these problems. Lead durability has increased considerably with multifilar and carbon filament leads and replacement of silicone as a lead insulator with polyurethane. Also, development of leads with tips that can be screwed into the endocardial surface of the heart, or elute steroids to decrease contact point inflammation and fibrosis, has been helpful.

The electrodes of transvenous intracardiac pacemakers are positioned in the right ventricle by passing them into a peripheral vein and then manipulating the lead and contact electrodes into appropriate position within the right ventricle. Multiple-lead systems can be placed and two or three leads can be attached to various places in the right atrium, coronary sinus, and right ventricle. The pacing device itself containing its power source is then tucked under the skin below the clavicle (collar bone) with direct connection between the pacemaker lead and the device being made. The current average pacemaker weighs but a few ounces, and the size is that of a large coin (Figure 10.2).

Indications for Permanent Cardiac Pacing

At first, the only indication for permanent cardiac pacing was severely symptomatic Stokes-Adams attacks. Patients without a

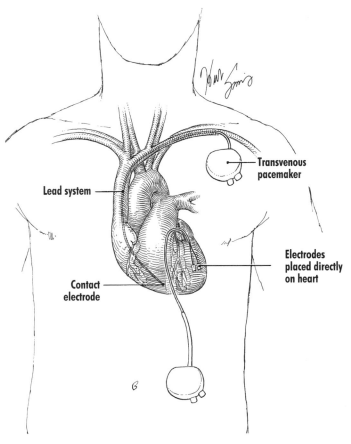

Figure 10.2. Schematic diagram of two general types of pacemakers used, those surgically implanted and connected to electrodes placed in epicardial fashion, and those implanted superficially in the infraclavicular region using transvenous leads and electrodes.

pacemaker placed for this syndrome had a high incidence of sudden cardiac death syndrome and generally substantive congestive heart failure. Furthermore, syncopal episodes characterizing this syndrome were unanticipated, frightening, and terribly debilitating. With the improvement in pacing systems, and, particularly, development of pacemakers that could regulate a variety of cardiac chambers and provide programmable modes, less serious bradycardias (slow heartbeats) could be effectively treated by pacemakers. Indeed, today's range of pacemaker options and pacing modalities has allowed matching a wide variety of clinical conditions to varying pacemaker types. Symptomatic second-degree atrioventricular block has, therefore, become an indication for permanent pacemaker insertion. Basically, any cardiac rhythm that produces an inappropriately slow heart rate that is associated with symptoms and is otherwise not amenable to treatment, might benefit from pacing therapeutics.

Implantable Pacemaker System

The implantable pacemaker system as a whole is comprised of the pacemaker pulse generator, which includes the power source and the generator circuitry. Original zinc-mercury pacers remained standard for more than 15 years but had unpredictable failure patterns and an average life span of only two to four years. Rechargeable nickel-cadmium batteries were more reliable, but patients frequently had to recharge their power source. Lithium anode batteries have become the mainstay of

pacemakers today, with greater reliability of pulse generation and longer life spans. The pulse generator circuitry is what controls the pacing discharge rates and types, native heart electrocardiographic sensing circuits, and various electronic accessories that allow programmability, telemetry, memory, dual chamber, and rate responsive sensor controls. A variety of switching devices are used to control these pacemaker activities.

The pacemaker lead and contact electrode delivers the electrical charge generated by the pulse generator to the myocardium and transmits electrocardiographic potentials back to the sensing circuitry in the pacemaker. Though epicardial leads were used initially, the requirement for thoracotomy to insert these wires stimulated development of transvenous endomyocardial lead systems (inserting the lead wires through a peripheral vein to the heart), which are the overwhelming choice today. Two major types of lead systems are used; one is the so-called unipolar lead with only one electrode on the lead itself (the cathode, or active, positive pole). In unipolar systems, the anode (or negative pole of the system) is located on the metal casing of the pacemaker pulse generator. Current flows from the pacing generator through the pacemaker lead and cardiac electrode, returning to the anode to complete the circuit. In contrast, a bipolar lead has both the anode and the cathode poles on the lead itself, but stationed a variable distance from each other. Both electrodes are positioned within the heart, and the circuit is completed at this level rather than transthoracically (through the chest wall).

Originally, bipolar leads were large and difficult to use. Modern pacing systems with coaxial bipolar leads and low profile connecting hubs are used more frequently today. Unipolar pacing has the disadvantage of oversensing. This enhanced sensing capability makes such systems more likely to detect electrical potentials arising from skeletal muscle rather than cardiac muscle contraction. Another disadvantage of single polar pacing is the proximity of skeletal muscle to the pacemaker box anode lead. This might induce skeletal muscle contraction when the current is returning to the anode after myocardial stimulation. This difficulty is usually addressed by having the anode facing the subcutaneous tissue rather than the muscle tissue.

The cardiac electrode is the actual myocardial contact and stimulating part of the pacemaker lead and is responsible for delivering the electrical charge to the heart muscle itself. Systems today have high impedance, low-stimulation threshold, and energy-efficient cathode tips. Several systems that screw into the endocardium make them less likely to become displaced over time.

Pacing Modes

The ability to use a spectrum of pacing modes has been one of the more important advances in the field of pacemaker therapy. The initial pacemaker devices were not synchronized with intrinsic cardiac electromechanical action (they were asynchronous) and were therefore limited in their application. In 1962, the first atrioventricular synchronous pacemaker was implanted in a patient. This pacemaker was the first to create more physiologic paced rhythms. Initial impulses were delivered to the right atrium, with atrial contraction followed by ventricular contraction after impulse delivery to this chamber had been delayed for an appropriate interval. Various adjustments in the atrioventricular electromechanical coupling delay could be introduced with programmable forms of this pacemaker. Pacemakers also evolved so that ventricular contraction could be synchronized to the heart's intrinsic atrial P-wave activity.

Improvement in leads and pacemaker circuitry ultimately led to the development of dual-chamber pacemakers that could sense both atrial and ventricular activity and deliver impulses to both of these chambers based on a variety of electrophysiologic situations. Pacemakers could be easily designed so that impulses were delivered synchronously with electrocar-

Table 10.1. Pacemaker Codes

I Chamber Paced	II Chamber Sensed	III Response to Sensing	IV Functions and Modulations	V Functions
V Ventricle	**V** Ventricle	**T** Triggers pacing	**P** Programmable rate and/or output	**P** Antitachycardia
A Atrium	**A** Atrium	**I** Inhibits pacing	**M** Multiprogrammability of rate, output, sensitivity, etc.	**S** Shock
D Double	**D** Double	**D** Triggers and inhibits pacing	**C** Communicating (telemetric)	**D** Dual (P + S)
O None	**O** None	**O** None	**R** Rate modulation	**O** None
			O None	

SOURCE: Data from the North American Society of Pacing and Electrophysiology and the British Pacing and Electrophysiology Group.

NOTE: Positions I through III are for antibradycardia functions; position V is for antitachycardia functions. In position II, sometimes manufacturers append an S to atrium or ventricle to indicate a single chamber.

diographic R-wave generation, or pacemaking firing could be inhibited by the presence of a native cardiac R-wave complex. Interestingly, a variety of physiologic responsive pacing systems have emerged. Sensors can be placed that detect metabolic changes associated with exercise. These sensors are linked to rate- responsive circuitry that increase or decrease the frequency of electrical pulse generation so that metabolic demands associated with exercise can be more appropriately handled by the heart and artificial pacemaker.

Because of the vast array of mode combinations that can be programmed into pacing devices, a standardized code and reference system has been developed. This allows physicians to communicate with specificity when describing the type of pacing system implanted, as well as the mode of pacing planned and programmed. Patients are usually informed of the device programs as well.

Table 10.1 summarizes these codes. A series of letters is designated and placed in sequential position (there are five positions given I through V Roman numeral sequencing status). The first position delineates the chamber paced; the second position is the chamber sensed; the third position is the chamber responding to sensing signaling; the fourth position is the programmable functions of the pacemaker; and the fifth position is the antitachycardia management functions (to be discussed). Not all options are available in every pacemaker. The chamber paced can either be the ventricle (V), the atrium (A), or both the atria and the ventricle (D for Double). Position II uses the same abbreviations and refers to the cardiac chamber sensed. Position III indicates the response to sensing with (T) standing for "triggers" pacing, (I) meaning "inhibits" pacing, and (D) indicating that the system both triggers and inhibits pacing. Therefore, a dual-sensing chamber, atrioventricular sequential pacing mode pacemaker would be described as a DDD system. The fourth position in the sequence refers to programmable functions and, specifically, rate modulation capabilities. (P) indicates that the pacemaker has a programmable rate or output characteristic. (M) suggests multi-programmability capabilities (rate, output, sensitivity, etc.); (C) suggests the pacemaker has telemetry or communicating functions; and (R) indicates rate modulation abilities. The fifth position refers to antitachycardia functions of pacemakers, with (P) indicating a tachycardia characteristic present, (S) indicating shock-delivery capabilities, and (D) indicating for both antitachycardia and shock capabilities being present. These latter func-

tions will be addressed subsequently. Patients with permanent pacemaker systems implanted are always given a record of one sort or another, documenting the type of system placed and which pacing mode has been programmed. The sequence of capital letters on the card refers to these different options.

The most common system implanted currently is VVI, or a ventricular inhibited pacing system. In this format, spontaneous electrocardiographic QRS potentials are sensed by the pacemaker in the ventricle (V), and if noted to be appropriately timed and present, the subsequent ventricular (V) pacing stimulus is inhibited (I). A pacing stimulus will occur when the pacemaker rate is set above the native heart rate, as determined by the time interval between QRS complexes. A DDD pacemaker system is a fully automatic atrial and ventricular pacing device whereby both the atria and ventricle are sensed and paced. Ventricular pacing, as a result of either atrial pacing or atrial sensing, will occur with an atrial inhibited and a ventricular inhibited response to activity noted in any of the respective chambers.

Pacemakers that are fully automatic must have highly complex programmable features. Pacemakers are programmed by predetermined magnetic pulses passed through the chest wall with devices held directly over the pacing unit designed to trigger a menu of responses within the system. Telemetry is a noninvasive function linked to pacemaker programmability whereby the status of the generator can be determined by information transmitted to the pacemaker programmer during electromagnetic interrogation of the device. Information, such as identification of pulsing state parameters and pulse generator type, battery life status, lead characteristics, electrocardiographic events, and arrhythmia documentation, are examples of features that can be transmitted externally for review from the pacemaker system.

Because pacemaker devices are generating electromagnetic fields and responses, as well as programmable functions induced by magnetic fields, the potential for altering pacemaker activity exists when electrical field charges are encountered (microwave ovens, for example). With the development of more sophisticated, better integrated and insulated, and more reliable pacemaker devices, this difficulty is unlikely to occur today. Still, however, one will see signs warning pacemaker patients to stand clear of powerful microwave emitting transmitters. Although being close to more ordinary household electrical products is not likely to generate interference with these devices, common sense dictates that care should be exercised with respect to potentially powerful magnetic fields. Concern about the possibility that electrical equipment can cause pacemaker

dysfunction has probably been overexaggerated. Each person with a permanent pacemaker should discuss his particular activities with his physician, understanding the exact type of device implanted.

Pacing Systems for Treatment of Tachycardias

Pacemaker systems have been used in two distinct fashions for treatment of tachycardias, or rapid heartbeat arrhythmias. These complex automated antitachycardia devices are not used much now because of the great success of catheter-based ablative techniques and surgical approaches to treat certain tachycardias. In the past, these antitachycardia pacemaker devices were often used in patients with disabling tachycardias resistant to or intolerant of drug therapy. Proof of physiologic efficacy with regard to tachycardia interruption by pacing methods is, obviously, required before these devices are inserted. By and large, the tachycardias treated with pacing systems are supraventricular (atrial) in origin. Ventricular tachycardias, however, can also be treated with these pacing systems sometimes. The pacing system is required to first recognize the noxious tachycardia, and then capture the appropriate cardiac chamber with the heart at a rapid burst of pacing energy. The arrhythmia should terminate when the burst capture dissipates. Obviously, the pacing device must first diagnose the rhythm disturbance and then deliver an appropriate burst stimulus to capture the desired cardiac chamber.

Another device now available for arrhythmia treatment is the implantable cardiac defibrillator. Again, this is a self-contained diagnostic and therapeutic device that provides automatic detection of malignant ventricular tachycardias with delivery of electrical countershock in the hopes that the arrhythmia will be terminated. Because many instances of sudden cardiac death in the face of coronary heart disease or cardiomyopathy appear due to derangement in the heart's electrical stability, devices having this capability or both the capability of treating potentially lethal bradycardias as well as ventricular tachycardia and fibrillation, can be lifesaving. Because ventricular fibrillation will not respond to ventricular pacing, this arrhythmia must be aborted by delivery of a potent electrical countershock. Ventricular tachycardia, on the other hand, that responds to rapid ventricular pacing, could be treated with the rapid ventricular pacing mode.

Countershock techniques are dramatic and have been proved effective in animal models with ventricular tachycardia and fibrillation since Zoll demonstrated in 1954 the ability to defibrillate the heart with externally applied electrical discharge. Furthermore, "synchronized"

cardioversion has been used since 1961 to terminate atrial fibrillation. The transthoracic shock was timed to the electrocardiographic R-wave that prevented the direct current shock from precipitating ventricular fibrillation when trying to convert a supraventricular arrhythmia.

Internalizing these concepts has been challenging. More than a decade of research went into the creation of the first automatic implantable cardiac defibrillator. The objective of the device was to sense ventricular fibrillation and rapidly deliver an electrical countershock to restore normal sinus rhythm. Second-generation and improved devices could discern both ventricular fibrillation and tachycardia from the other cardiac dysrhythmias. Obviously, it is extraordinarily important to differentiate one arrhythmia type from another, since the devices must employ different strategies for different arrhythmias.

The first automatic implantable cardiac defibrillator was placed in a patient in 1980. To date, more than 25,000 such devices have been implanted with third-generation systems incorporating additional improvements such as programmability, back-up pacemaker capabilities, antitachycardia pacing options, improved sensing and arrhythmia discrimination, and the ability to deliver programmed electrical stimulation to study ventricular arrhythmias from an electrophysiologic perspective. Figure 10.3 demonstrates one

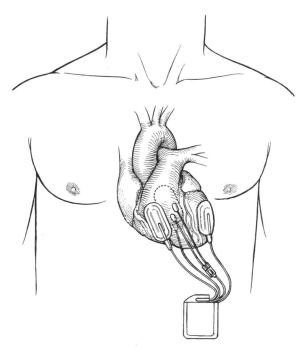

Figure 10.3. An example of modern, multiple-task, integrated pacemaker system with multiple pacing, cardioverting, and defibrillating leads that are placed in epicardial fashion.

lation or syncopal or hypotensive ventricular tachycardia that is not associated with acute myocardial infarction, and not due to remedial cause (such as drug toxicity, electrolyte derangement, or active cardiac ischemia). The arrhythmia should be neither controlled by acceptable drug therapy after appropriate testing nor amenable to definitive therapy with surgical ablation. Implantation of these devices may also be indicated after spontaneously occurring, but noninducible, documented syncopal or hypotensive ventricular tachycardia not due to one of the foregoing difficulties. These devices might also be indicated after ventricular tachycardia/ventricular fibrillation cardiac arrest or after an operation for ventricular tachycardia or ventricular fibrillation if the ventricular arrhythmia remains inducible.

multidimensional system that includes pacemaker, cardioverting, and defibrillating capabilities. The device shown is configured for epicardial patch and electrode placement and requires thoracotomy for implantation.

These devices have served patients with life-threatening ventricular arrhythmias well, sometimes in combination with more traditional antiarrhythmic drug therapy. Currently, indications for implanting cardioverting and defibrillating devices are one or more episodes of spontaneously occurring and inducible ventricular fibril-

Ablation Techniques to Control Cardiac Arrhythmias

From an electrophysiologic standpoint, "ablation" refers to the use of physical agents or catheters to modify or destroy cardiac conduction tissue in specific regions of the heart felt responsible for tachycardias. Tissue ablation techniques work best when a discrete and anatomic foci of arrhythmia can be identified. A diffuse substrate for the arrhythmia, such as the atrium in atrial fibrillation, would be difficult to treat with an ablation technique. Atrioventricular block, however, can be created in atrial fibrillation patients by ablation of the atrioventricular node. Because cardiac conduction will be impaired and atrial fibrillation–directed impulses diminished in number across the atrioventricular node, back-up pacing after ablation is required and allows more control of the ventricular rate in this setting. More discrete arrhythmias, such as supraventricular tachycardia due to abnormal conduction paths (as occur in Wolff-Parkinson-White syndrome), can be treated with ablation catheters if the location of these conduction pathways can be precisely mapped out during electrophysiologic study. Direct ablative procedures can be done at the time of thoracotomy and cardiotomy with incisions made directly into the heart at the pathway focus or by use of devices to induce thermal or electrical injury. Percutaneous ablation techniques most often have radiofrequency energy sources. Catheter ablative techniques have rapidly progressed and dramatically changed the approach to treatment of patients with, in particular, supraventricular tachycardia. If specific arrhythmia foci can be identified, ablative procedures often are curative. In some situations, tachycardias can be corrected by ablation of atrioventricular conduction pathways with subsequent pacemaker

insertion in a fashion similar to the described approach for atrial fibrillation. Indeed, complete atrioventricular junctional node ablation is the procedure of choice for many patients with atrial arrhythmias refractory to drug therapy. Although some patients with ventricular arrhythmias may benefit from these catheter ablative techniques, most are better treated with drugs, implantable cardiac defibrillating devices, or direct surgical procedures.

Surgical Treatment of Cardiac Arrhythmias

Fueled by progressive insight into the anatomic and electrophysiologic abnormalities responsible for supraventricular tachycardias, cardiac arrhythmia surgical procedures evolved during the past two decades. The ability to map atrial and ventricular pathways responsible for conduction in the heart using sophisticated electrophysiologic mapping systems made it possible to surgically sever the bypass tracts responsible for tachycardia. Patients with syndromes, such as the Wolff-Parkinson-White syndrome, atrioventricular nodal reentry tachycardia, automatic atrial tachycardia, and ischemic and nonischemic ventricular tachycardias, have all been treated by electrophysiologically guided surgical resection of the abnormal conduction pathways.

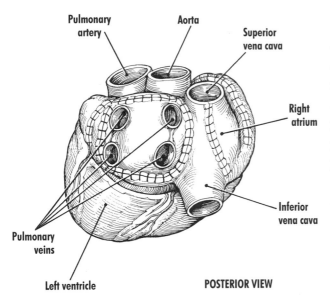

Pulmonary artery

Aorta

Superior vena cava

Right atrium

Inferior vena cava

Pulmonary veins

Left ventricle

POSTERIOR VIEW

Figure 10.4. Depiction from the posterior and superior views of the incisions used for performing the maze procedure to treat atrial fibrillation.

Interestingly, parallel development of the previously described antitachycardia pacing devices and demonstrated utility of implantable cardioverter defibrillator devices has decreased the indications for surgical intervention for refractory ventricular tachycardia. Still, some surgical advances have been recently made with respect to arrhythmia surgical treatment. The recent development of a technique for the treatment of atrial fibrillation whereby multiple incisions are made throughout the atrium (the maze procedure for atrial fibrillation) is an example of this (Figure 10.4). The multiple incisions in the atrium alter conduction dynamics of this chamber and sometimes improve atrioventricular mechanical transport in some patients with atrial fibrillation. A variety of endocardial resection techniques in patients with ischemia-induced ventricular tachycardia have also been utilized to decrease the incidence of these hemodynamically unstable rhythms. These operations are often combined with drug therapy and pacemaker or arrhythmia-terminating device insertion, and the multiple therapeutic methods available should dictate strategy in a highly individualized and specific fashion.

Summary

Pacemaker therapy, arrhythmia ablation, and surgical intervention to control cardiac arrhythmias provide clinicians with a broad-spectrum armamentarium designed to treat patients with rapid and unstable heart rhythms, as well as bradycardias, as effectively as possible. Each approach has a variety of advantages and disadvantages. However, the sophisticated newer devices, particularly with their incredible miniaturization, make them a profoundly important arm of antiarrhythmic therapy.

CHAPTER ELEVEN

Hypertension

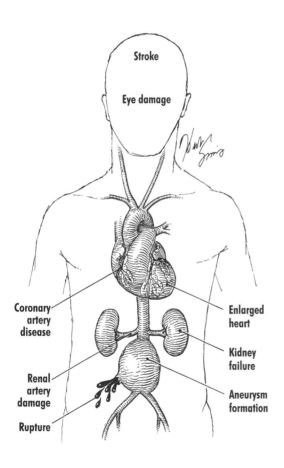

Figure 11.1. The consequences of hypertension encompass threats to the coronary and renal arteries, risk for kidney failure, the possibility of aneurysm formation and rupture, and the burdens of illness caused by an enlarged heart. Stroke and eye damage are also risks.

The Silent Killer

The dramatic phrase—"the silent killer"—is used frequently to describe high blood pressure, or *hypertension*. Hypertension earned this name by having no noticeable symptoms: a person can have high blood pressure for years without knowing it. But if hypertension is ignored and goes undiagnosed and untreated, it can have serious, even deadly, consequences (Figure 11.1). Uncontrolled hypertension can cause a stroke, enlarge the heart, and damage the kidneys. It can cause aneurysms to form, large arteries to rupture, and the heart or kidneys to fail. Hypertension may also result in damage to the retina and loss of eyesight. A major risk factor for cardiovascular disease, hypertension is also the leading chronic adult illness in the United States today, affecting more than 50 million Americans.

Although hypertension is a highly serious medical condition, it is also highly treatable. Once hypertension is diagnosed, it can be managed through a program of lifestyle changes and medications tailored to the individual. Controlling mild hypertension can help prevent more serious complications, and lifestyle changes can help prevent hypertension in many people who are free of the disease but at risk for developing it.

Blood Pressure and Its Measurement

When the heart beats, it pumps blood to other parts of the body through arteries. Arteries are so named because the ancients believed these vessels carried air. Blood pressure is a measure of the force that blood exerts against the arterial walls as it is pumped throughout the body. The heart muscle contracts to push blood through the arteries, much as an engine forces water through a fire hose. The force of water rushing through the fire hose is water pressure; the force of blood pumping through vessels is blood pressure. Arteries are flexible, able to expand or contract in response to the force against their inner walls. Blood pressure is one of life's necessities. Without it, blood could not circulate throughout the body, and the body's vital organs would be deprived of the oxygen and nutrients essential to continued functioning.

Arterial blood pressure is most often measured using a stethoscope and a sphygmomanometer, a device that consists of an inflatable cuff, a bulb to inflate it, a control to deflate it, and a tube of mercury marked off in millimeters (mm Hg). (*Sphygmo-* is from Greek, meaning "throb" and "pulse"; a *manometer* is any instrument for measuring pressure of gases or vapors.) The measurement is the level of pressure at which the artery opens and blood begins to flow through it again. To measure blood pressure, a physician or nurse wraps the cuff around the arm and inflates the cuff to stop blood flow in the main artery (the cuff is inflated to the point at which the pressure exceeds that in the artery and the artery is collapsed). Then the cuff is slowly deflated (see Figure 3.9). The first sound heard is the systolic pressure, created as the heart contracts or beats. The person measuring blood pressure checks to see what the mercury level is at that moment, and this number becomes the top number in a blood pressure reading, or the systolic pressure (normally about 110 to 140 mm Hg in an adult). The cuff is then deflated until no further sounds are heard; this is the diastolic pressure, the pressure between heartbeats (normally about 70 to 90 mm Hg). This measure becomes the second number in a blood pressure reading.

Low Blood Pressure

Low blood pressure (hypotension) can be a chronic condition or one that develops suddenly. Chronic hypotension is not unusual and ordinarily is not a serious health problem. It can result from taking high blood pressure medications or from diabetes, arteriosclerosis, pregnancy, malnutrition, excessive weight loss, or other conditions. A loss of blood caused by hemorrhage or shock or infections, fever, or other disorders can initiate a sudden drop in blood pressure to dangerously low levels.

A temporary condition called *postural hypotension* affects some people, typically older adults. Individuals who have postural hypotension will feel dizzy or lightheaded when they stand up from a seated or reclining position because their blood pressure has fallen and blood flow to the brain is temporarily decreased. If you experience this light-headedness, stand up slowly before starting to walk. This action should relieve the problem. If it does not, or if frequent dizziness or fainting spells occur, discuss the problem with a physician.

High Blood Pressure

Blood pressure is regulated by arterioles, which are small branches of the arteries. If the arterioles become narrowed, the heart struggles to pump blood, and both systolic and diastolic pressures will increase. Blood pressure guidelines classify blood pressure in stages: optimal, normal, high normal, and high blood pressure. High blood pressure, in turn, has four stages, ranging from mild to very severe (Table 11.1). There is no single ideal blood pressure reading; rather, acceptable blood pressure falls within a range.

Table 11.1. Categories of Adult Blood Pressure

Category	Blood Pressure (mm Hg)	
	Systolic	Diastolic
Optimal°	Below 120	Below 80
Normal	Below 130	Below 85
High normal	130 to 139	85 to 89
High blood pressure		
Mild	140 to 159	90 to 99
Moderate	160 to 179	100 to 109
Severe	180 to 209	110 to 119
Very severe	210 or higher	120 or higher

SOURCE: Data from *Fifth Report of the Joint National Committee on Detection, Evaluation, and Treatment of High Blood Pressure* (Bethesda, Md.: National Heart, Lung, and Blood Institute, 1992).
° Readings that are unusually low require evaluation by a physician.

Blood pressure can vary widely, not only from day to day but also within the same day, and even the same hour. Blood pressure can be affected by a variety of factors, such as the stress of being at the doctor's office (often called *office* or *white coat high blood pressure*), excitement, recent exercise, or some illnesses and medications. These changes in blood pressure are perfectly normal.

For most adults, blood pressure is considered to be high when systolic pressure is greater than 139 mm Hg or diastolic pressure is greater than 89 mm Hg for an extended time period. You should not assume that you have high blood pressure based on one reading alone. To confirm a diagnosis of hypertension, your physician will measure blood pressure over multiple office visits, preferably over a period of several weeks. You also may be asked to monitor your blood pressure at home using portable manual or semiautomatic devices.

Risks of Hypertension

Unfortunately, high blood pressure often has no symptoms, so a person can have hypertension for years and be unaware of it. Severely high blood pressure may cause headaches and bleeding into the blood vessels of the eye. High blood pressure can cause the heart to become enlarged and the arteries to become scarred and less elastic. Hardened and narrowed arteries are less able to carry the amount of blood needed by the body's organs and tissues. The longer blood pressure remains high, the greater the risk for damage to body organs. Narrowed arteries also can lead to the formation of blood clots, which can cause heart attacks and strokes.

Types of Hypertension

There are two types of high blood pressure: *secondary* and *essential,* or *primary,* hypertension. Secondary hypertension results from the presence of a specific disease or medical condition, such as kidney disease, adrenal tumor (primary hyperaldosteronism), renal artery stenosis, coarctation, Cushing's disease, hyperthyroidism, or pregnancy. Once the disease or condition is identified and resolved or corrected, the high blood pressure usually will disappear as well. Secondary hypertension represents only a small percentage of all hypertension cases.

A common and very curable cause of secondary hypertension is renal artery stenosis (narrowing of the renal arteries). When the arteries serving the kidney narrow, it is usually because of atherosclerosis (about 66 percent of cases). Fibrous dysplasia, which accounts for most of the remainder of these cases, can also narrow a renal artery and result in hypertension, causing a type of hypertension most common in women younger than 35. Complete obstruction of the artery is uncommon with atherosclerotic stenosis and unobserved with fibrous dysplasia.

Cases of renovascular hypertension represent only about 3 percent of all instances of hypertension. The most telling indication of renal artery stenosis is the sudden appearance of uncontrollable hypertension in patients for whom high blood pressure was never a problem or in patients whose hypertension was well controlled. Patients with renovascular hypertension, in comparison with patients with essential hypertension, are less likely to be black and less likely to be obese.

Surgical therapy is the usual response to renal artery stenosis, although drug therapy is likely to be used in mild cases. Percutaneous angioplasty has been increasingly used with success in cases caused by fibrous dysplasia, but in about one third of patients the arteries narrow again, especially in atherosclerotic cases.

Essential, or primary, hypertension is by far the more common form of high blood pressure. Essential hypertension is hypertension in which there is no known underlying cause. It occurs when the vessels are excessively contracted or contain excess fluid. Essential high blood pressure is responsible for 90 to 95 percent of all hypertension cases. Important to understand is that essential hypertension cannot be cured, but with lifestyle changes and medication, it can be controlled.

Risk Factors for Essential Hypertension

While the exact cause of essential hypertension cannot be pinpointed, there are specific, often interrelated risk factors that seem to play important roles in its development.

Uncontrollable Risk Factors

Some risk factors for hypertension, such as heredity, age, sex, and race, cannot be controlled.

- *Heredity.* An individual who has a parent or other close blood relative with hypertension is more likely to develop it eventually than an individual with no family history of hypertension. Individuals who have close family members who either have hypertension or have suffered strokes or heart attacks at a young age should be especially vigilant about regularly monitoring their own blood pressure.
- *Age.* Blood pressure increases with age, and high blood pressure occurs more often after age 30.
- *Sex.* High blood pressure is more common in men than in women until early middle age, but this situation reverses in early middle age, when hypertension becomes more common in women than in men.

(See pp. 409–410 for more information on women and hypertension.)

- *Race.* High blood pressure occurs at a younger age and occurs twice as frequently in black people compared with white people.

Controllable Risk Factors

Other important risk factors for hypertension, such as obesity, a sedentary lifestyle, heavy alcohol consumption, and high sodium in the diet, can be modified (Table 11.2).

Obesity

Obesity (see Table 7.8, page 102) is closely linked with hypertension. Obesity causes the heart to struggle to supply excess tissue with blood. Controlling weight is an important factor in preventing and treating high blood pressure, and blood pressure has been found to decrease in proportion to weight loss. Weight loss also has been found to improve the effectiveness of blood pressure medications.

Sedentary Lifestyle

People who are sedentary, or *couch potatoes* in popular jargon, have been found to be 50 percent more likely to develop hypertension than those who are active. Regular aerobic physical activity can lower systolic blood pressure by approximately 10 mm Hg in hypertensive patients. Taking part in physical activity every day is more likely to lower blood pressure than is exercising only a few times per week. Low- to moderate-intensity aerobic exercise is as helpful in reducing mild to moderate high blood pressure as is high-intensity aerobic exercise. All individuals should check with their physicians before beginning an exercise program.

Alcohol Consumption

Excessive alcohol consumption can raise blood pressure and can cause resistance to high blood pressure medications. Reducing alcohol consumption has been found to lower blood pressure in those people with normal blood pressure levels,

Table 11.2. Lifestyle Changes to Reduce Risk for High Blood Pressure

Factor	Goal
Weight	Achieve a desirable body weight and maintain it.
Activity level	Participate in physical activities regularly.
Alcohol intake	Limit daily alcohol intake to no more than 2 drinks daily (see Table 11.3)
Sodium	Keep daily sodium intake below 2,400 mg.

Table 11.3. One Alcoholic Drink: Equivalents

Alcohol	Amount (fluid ounces)
Regular or light beer	12
Table wine	5
Fortified wine (sherry, port, marsala, or Madeira)	3
Liquor	
80-proof	$1\frac{1}{2}$
100-proof	1

NOTE: Limiting intake to no more than 2 drinks per day is recommended.

in those with high blood pressure, and in alcoholics as well as nonalcoholics. Lowering alcohol intake also may help prevent the development of high blood pressure. People with hypertension who choose to drink alcoholic beverages should do so only in moderation. Moderate alcohol intake is defined as no more than 2 ounces of 100-proof whiskey, 10 ounces of table wine, or 24 ounces of beer daily (Table 11.3). Research has yet to determine conclusively whether consuming alcohol below these levels increases risk for hypertension.

Sodium

A strong link binds sodium consumption to blood pressure. Sodium causes the body to retain extra fluid. This puts an additional burden on the heart and narrows blood vessels, which, in turn, raises blood pressure. A diet that is high in sodium also decreases the effectiveness of medications used to treat high blood pressure. Sodium is obtained primarily from sodium chloride, or common table salt, although it also is found in large amounts in such substances as baking powder, monosodium glutamate (MSG), and soy sauce. The National High Blood Pressure Education Program recommends that healthy adults consume no more than 2,400 mg of sodium per day (about $1\frac{1}{8}$ teaspoons of salt). American adults typically consume an average of 4,000 to 5,800 mg per day—more sodium than their bodies need. Some recent research has suggested that not all people are susceptible to sodium's induction of high blood pressure. However, this finding is controversial, and recommendations for patients have not been changed. (More detailed information on sodium in the diet can be found in *The New Living Heart Diet.*)

175

Other Dietary Issues

Scientists have learned that some nutrients, in particular, potassium and calcium, have a beneficial effect on blood pressure levels. A high intake of potassium can offer protection against developing high blood pressure, and a low intake can increase blood pressure. Potassium also seems to strengthen the advantages of lowering sodium intake. Potassium is found in significant amounts in many fresh fruits and vegetables. Foods high in potassium and low in sodium include bananas, potatoes, beans, cantaloupes, and yogurt. (*The New Living Heart Diet* lists the potassium content of selected foods.)

It has been reported that calcium deficiency is linked with a greater incidence of high blood pressure and that a high calcium intake may help decrease blood pressure, although some authorities have questioned this relation. Most people do not need to take large doses of calcium to gain its blood pressure benefits; the recommended daily allowance (RDA) appears to be sufficient. (The RDA for calcium is 1,200 mg for people ages 11 to 24 years, and 800 mg for younger children and for adults age 25 and above.) The best sources of calcium are dairy products; smaller amounts of calcium are found in dark green leafy vegetables and some fish and shellfish.

Other Lifestyle Issues

The word hypertension sometimes makes people think that this condition is caused by stress or emotional tension. Individuals who have hypertension are not necessarily more anxious or nervous than other people, although stressful situations or a stressful environment can raise blood pressure. While some evidence does point to stress as a factor in the development of hypertension, research has not actually found that practicing stress management techniques can prevent or control high blood pressure. But controlling and managing stress in a positive way is known to improve overall well-being.

Cigarette smoking, while not directly linked to the development of hypertension, is a major heart disease risk factor and the greatest single preventable cause of death in the United States.

Special Hypertension Issues for Women

Hypertension has been found to be more common in women who have taken oral contraceptives for five years or longer than in those women who have not taken oral contraceptives. The risk appears to increase with age, with length of oral contraceptive use, and perhaps with weight. Women age 35 and older who take oral contraceptives and smoke cigarettes are at greatest risk. If they continue to smoke, they should consider discontinuing the use of oral contraceptives. Most cardiovascular deaths linked to oral contraceptive use have occurred in women who smoked cigarettes.

Hypertension also can develop in women during the last three months of pregnancy. If left untreated, this condition can be dangerous to both the mother and the baby. Hypertension that develops during pregnancy usually disappears after delivery. If it does not, it should be medically treated and controlled in the same way as other types of hypertension. A woman who already has hypertension when she becomes pregnant should be carefully monitored by a physician. Pregnancy may or may not make hypertension more severe, but with careful treatment, a woman should be able to have a normal pregnancy and a normal baby.

Controlling Hypertension

While essential hypertension cannot at present be cured, it usually can be managed. The effects of hypertension can be prevented or reduced if the condition is treated early and kept under control. Anyone with hypertension, even hypertension that is categorized as mild, is at increased risk for additional medical complications.

If you have been diagnosed with hypertension, or believe you have hypertension, you should be under a physician's care. The physician should take a complete medical history to assess your risk factors for hypertension, such as high sodium intake, excessive alcohol usage, and family history of the disease. The physician may also perform a physical examination and ask you to undergo various laboratory tests and diagnostic procedures, including a complete blood count; a urinalysis; electrocardiography; and blood glucose and lipid measures. Results from these tests will help determine the possible causes of your hypertension, the extent of any organ damage, and overall estimated risk for cardiovascular disease.

The physician should explain your condition, set a blood pressure goal for you, and outline ways to meet that goal that are tailored to your needs and your medical history.

There are two basic approaches to lowering blood pressure levels: lifestyle modification alone (see Chapter 26 for general lifestyle measures to improve cardiovascular health) or lifestyle modification in combination with medication.

Unless there is an immediate need for medication because of severe hypertension or other medical complications, most patients will be advised to try to lower their blood pressure levels by making lifestyle changes. For many who have mild hypertension, lifestyle modifications will lower their blood pressure to a normal level.

Hypertension Medications

If lifestyle changes are not effective in lowering blood pressure after a three- to six-month period, physicians may then prescribe medication to control high blood pressure. Physicians prescribe medications in addition to lifestyle changes, not instead of them. Making lifestyle modifications can cause hypertension medications to work more effectively and may permit a reduction in medication.

Hypertension can be treated by several different types of medications. Patients react differently to medications, and some may experience side effects. Side effects often can be moderated or eliminated by lowering dosage or by substituting another medication. A physician frequently will prescribe various types of hypertension medications in combination with one another to maximize their effectiveness and to allow individual medications to be taken in smaller dosages, thus lowering the possibility of dose-dependent side effects. Medicines prescribed for hypertension include diuretics, beta-blockers, and other drugs.

Diuretics

Diuretics are often the first type of medication prescribed for treatment of hypertension. Diuretics eliminate excess fluid and salt that accumulate in the tissues surrounding the arteries and thus lower blood pressure. Side effects sometimes associated with diuretics include harmful effects on the blood lipid profile (although these effects are modest and transient with the thiazide diuretics), weakness, and loss of potassium.

Beta-blockers

If diuretics are not effective in lowering blood pressure, a beta-adrenergic blocker, called beta-blocker for short, may be prescribed in combination with a diuretic. Beta-blockers have a complicated mechanism that involves decreasing heart rate and force of contraction and altering plasma volume. Side effects that have been linked with beta-blockers include fatigue, insomnia, and aggravation of congestive heart failure. Some beta-blockers can increase triglyceride and decrease high-density lipoprotein (HDL) cholesterol levels (that is, they have adverse lipid effects); others can decrease triglyceride and increase HDL-cholesterol levels (that is, they have beneficial lipid effects).

Other Types of Medications

Other types of hypertension medications, including adrenergic inhibitors, angiotensin-converting enzyme (ACE) inhibitors, calcium antagonists, and vasodilators, work by opening constricted blood vessels. ACE inhibitors may interfere with kidney function and cause coughs and rashes. Calcium antagonists may cause headaches and dizziness. Vasodilators may cause headaches, tachycardia, and fluid retention. Most of these agents are neutral in their effect on blood lipids.

If your physician prescribes antihypertension medicine for you, be sure to report any new or unusual symptoms that occur after you begin taking it. Determining the medication or combination of medications that will most effectively lower your blood pressure with the fewest side effects may take time.

Maximizing the Effectiveness of Medication

You can maximize the effectiveness of high blood pressure treatment by keeping all appointments with your physician, following medical recommendations for making lifestyle modifications (such as losing weight, getting regular exercise, and moderating alcohol intake), and taking all medications as directed.

If a physician prescribes hypertension medications for you, it is very important that you continue taking them, even if you are feeling good, or, at the opposite end, if you are experiencing side effects. Discuss side effects with your physician. Medication can control hypertension, but it cannot cure it. Taking the blood pressure medication in the amounts and at the times your physician prescribed is important in achieving success with your therapy. If your physician prescribes medication, be sure you understand the correct dosage (amount of drug and number of times per day), the preferred method of taking it (with food or without), and the side effects you may experience.

Make your medication a part of your daily routine. Some people find it helpful to have a pillbox with compartments for each day of the week; others put a check mark on the calendar every time they take a pill. Always be sure to refill your prescription before you run out of pills so that you will not miss a dose. Carry a day's supply of current medications with you at all times, and if you are traveling, always carry your medications on your person (not in your luggage).

Even if you feel better, or if you experience side effects, never decide on your own to change your dosage or to stop taking your medications. Do not stop taking your medication if your blood pressure is normal when you have it checked, for it is probably the medication that is causing your blood pressure to be normal. Always keep your appointments with your physician to have your blood pressure checked.

The Patient's Responsibility

Successful blood pressure treatment involves a team approach, with the patient and supportive family members or friends working in partnership with the physician and other health care professionals. The patient should maintain regular contact with the physician. The patient's condition and needs may change over time, and the physician may need to modify medications.

It is crucial that the patient realize that, while essential hypertension can be controlled, it cannot be cured. Hypertension requires lifetime management, but the severity of this condition can be lessened with careful compliance with the prescribed treatment regimen.

CHAPTER TWELVE

Diseases of the Veins

In contrast to the arterial system, in which arteriosclerosis or atherosclerosis is a common cause of disease, the venous system is rarely attacked by arteriosclerosis. In general, diseases of the veins are nonatherosclerotic. To be sure, patients may have severe arteriosclerotic arterial disease with relatively normal veins, and on the other hand, patients may have severe disease of the veins with a relatively normal arterial system. It is also possible for a patient to have both arteriosclerotic arterial disease and venous disease not caused by arteriosclerosis.

Although blood flow in the arterial system is propelled by the heart and takes place under high pressure, the pressure in the venous system is ordinarily quite low. Blood is returned to the heart through the low-pressure venous system by external compression from muscular movements that propel the flow from the peripheries through unidirectional valves. Under pathologic conditions, the level of venous pressure may be greatly increased. For example, in the patient with pulmonary hypertension, the pulmonary veins are subjected to a high pressure, and severe atherosclerotic changes may develop. Thus, it is probable that it is the relatively low pressure that protects the venous system from the development of atherosclerosis.

Varicose Veins

The most common problem affecting the venous system is varicose veins. The varicosities occur mainly in the network of saphenous veins in the legs. They are caused by incompetence of the valves, which permits backflow or leakage, or by occlusion in the deep system of veins within the legs. This condition occurs predominantly in females in a ratio of 5 to 1, often with onset after pregnancy. A family history can usually be obtained. Varicosities are generally classified as primary or secondary. The primary form is considered an isolated disorder involving the superficial veins (the saphenous system) of the legs. The secondary varicosities are considered to be the consequence of deep venous insufficiency often associated with stasis dermatitis, edema, and ulceration. It is important to distinguish between these two forms, since both prognosis and treatment are different. In addition to pregnancy, this condition is accelerated by conditions that require prolonged standing or immobility.

Symptoms of primary varicosities are somewhat variable. Most patients complain of the cosmetic effect of the visibly distended veins. They may also complain of a heavy or fatigued sensation on prolonged standing. Occasionally, usually from trauma, bleeding may occur. Treatment of primary varicosities is less complicated if the disease is located primarily within the saphenous system itself, and the deep veins are uninvolved. It is, therefore, important to confirm the patency and competency of the deep venous system. This can be done by the simple Trendelenburg test, which consists in elevating the leg to observe emptying of the veins, or by applying a well-fitted elastic stocking, following which the patient feels improved.

Conservative treatment includes avoiding prolonged standing or crossing the legs. Fitted elastic support stockings may be useful. If indicated, weight loss should be encouraged as well as exercise by walking. In patients with more severe and symptomatic involvement, two forms of treatment may be used, namely injection sclerotherapy or excision. Sclerotherapy is indicated in well-localized varicosities of short length and in spider varicosities. In the more extensive varicosities, ligation and stripping are preferable. There is sufficient collateral circulation so that the ligated, excised, or sclerosed segment of the vein will not lead to venous congestion in the leg. If the venous disease progresses to the point that ulceration develops, skin grafting may be required. A much more serious situation occurs when the patient has thrombosis of the deep veins of the leg. More than 125 years ago, Virchow originally presented a hypothesis of venous thromboembolism. He thought that venous thrombosis resulted from damage to the wall of the vein, due to changes in the blood and sluggishness of circulation, which promoted coagulation.

An embolus is a portion of a thrombus or clot that breaks off and is carried to a distant part of the circulation, where it lodges in another blood vessel. An embolus from the legs usually lodges in the lungs and is referred to as a pulmonary embolism. Even today, the precise causes have not been defined. Thrombosis of the deep veins of the leg tends to develop in patients who are immobilized for periods of time, have stasis of blood due to varicosities or congestive heart failure, are pregnant, have trauma to the legs, or have an increased number of red blood cells and various types of malignant diseases. An inflammatory phase associated with thrombosis is referred to as *phlebitis* or *thrombophlebitis*. The thrombosis and inflammation may be primarily superficial, deep, or both. The clinical manifestations may be mild to severe, and pulmonary embolism can be a dangerous complication. On rare occasions there may be a massive reaction in the leg, progressing to severe edema and inflammation termed *phlegmasia cerulea dolens*. This occurs with thrombosis of the iliofemoral vein because of its anatomic location. The patient in such cases is acutely ill, and death may ensue or the leg may be lost. Long-term complications include venous insufficiency of the leg and recurrent bouts of thrombophlebitis.

Patients with thrombophlebitis of the superficial or deep venous system should be treated with bed rest, elevation and wrapping of the legs, and anticoagulation with the drug heparin. It may be desirable in some patients to use thrombolytic therapy. This requires the intravenous injection of a substance such as urokinase, streptokinase, or tissue plasminogen activator to dissolve the thrombus. In some instances, venous thrombectomy, that is, the direct removal of the venous thrombosis, may be required. Such surgical treatment should be performed as soon as possible for severe forms of phlegmasia cerulea dolens.

The treatment of pulmonary emboli requires special consideration aimed at preventing recurrence. Fortunately, most of these emboli are small. Treatment of the acute attack consists in bed rest, elevation and wrapping of the legs, and anticoagulation. Anticoagulant treatment is continued after the acute period. If the patient has a further pulmonary embolus while on anticoagulants, or if for some reason these drugs cannot be used, it may then become necessary to interrupt the venous system at the level of the inferior vena cava to prevent recurrence of embolization. This is performed preferably by the placement of a caval filter or "umbrella" in the inferior vena cava. It can be simply inserted by a catheter through the vein in the groin.

Occasionally, in the patient with a massive acute pulmonary embolism with hypertension or shock and evidence of right ventricular failure, it may be necessary to perform *embolectomy* as an emergency life-saving measure. This procedure was originally suggested in 1908 by Friedrich Trendelenburg and first performed successfully by Martin Kirschner in Germany in 1924. The first successful operation for acute massive pulmonary embolism by embolectomy with use of temporary cardiopulmonary bypass was performed at the Cardiovascular Center of the Methodist Hospital in 1961. This approach allows enough time to permit clearing of the emboli from the pulmonary artery and has subsequently been successfully used on a number of patients.

Chronic Venous Insufficiency

Chronic venous insufficiency, sometimes referred to as a *postphlebitic syndrome,* is caused by obstruction to the venous return from the legs, owing to obstruction or incompetence of the deep venous system, usually from the thrombosis. Usually there is a history of thrombophlebitis. There may also be a history of trauma or fracture. The condition is classified by progressive edema, a reddish brown hyperpigmented appearance in the lower leg just above the ankle, recurrent skin ulceration, and poor wound healing.

Treatment should begin with conservative measures, including particularly the use of compressive elastic stockings, elevation of the leg at least one foot above heart level during the night while sleeping, meticulous skin care, and avoidance of injury to the leg. In patients with ulceration, the Unna boot may be used. This consists in an absorbent dressing applied

to the ulcer with a semirigid compressive dressing wrapped around the lower part of the leg from the foot to the knee, kept in place for about one week, and reapplied until the ulcer heals. Antibiotic therapy may also be required.

More aggressive surgical treatment may be considered for patients with multiple recurrences, despite adequate conservative therapy, who experience considerable incapacitation. These procedures require careful and precise evaluation preoperatively of both the superficial and deep venous systems as well as the perforating veins. It is also essential to have this performed by an experienced surgeon in this field.

It is important that patients understand the chronic, relapsing, and intractable nature of the postphlebitic syndrome as well as the limitations of complete curative therapy—medical or surgical. Unfortunately, the highly successful surgical techniques that have been used in the treatment of arterial disease have not been found useful in the treatment of the venous diseases. Further research directed toward this objective should be encouraged.

CHAPTER THIRTEEN

Atherosclerosis

When arteries are healthy, they have strong, flexible walls and a smooth inside lining that allow them to transport blood freely to all parts of the body, much as a garden hose carries water. But the inner lining of an artery can become laden with

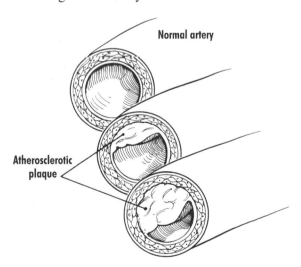

Figure 13.1. In the progression of atherosclerosis, the inner lining of an artery becomes filled with a build-up called *plaque,* which ultimately causes the artery to become clogged, stiff, and hardened. This series of drawings illustrates the build-up of plaque, which eventually can reduce or totally stop blood flow, increasing risk for heart attack, stroke, kidney failure, and other clinical events.

fatty substances such as cholesterol (lipids), calcium, and other materials. This build-up is called *atherosclerosis,* a name first proposed by the pathologist Felix Marchand in 1904 and constructed from the Greek roots *athero,* which means "gruel" or "porridge," and *sclerosis,* which means "hardening." Atherosclerosis is appropriately named: it involves accumulation of soft, fatty deposits that can look like porridge, and the build-up ultimately causes the artery to become hardened and stiff. The lesions, often called *plaque,* clog the artery much in the way that rust, grease, and scale block the pipes in a kitchen sink (Figure 13.1).

Atherosclerosis refers specifically to a disease of the intima, or the innermost layer, of the arterial wall. *Arteriosclerosis* is a broader term and includes conditions such as calcification of the media, or middle layer, of the arterial wall, which occurs in many elderly individuals.

Many people in modern industrialized societies have lifestyles that contribute to atherosclerotic disease, eating diets that are high in saturated fat, getting little or no exercise, and smoking cigarettes. But atherosclerosis is not exclusively a "modern" disease. The disease existed even in ancient times. Evidence of atherosclerosis has been found in Egyptian mummies from the third millennium B.C. and in Peruvian remains from the first millennium B.C.

Consequences of Atherosclerosis

Atherosclerosis can be found in many different arteries. If atherosclerosis develops in the coronary arteries, which run along the heart and supply blood to the heart muscle itself, the result is coronary heart disease, also called *coronary artery disease.* Atherosclerosis does its damage insidiously, usually progressing silently in the body for many years. The first symptom of coronary atherosclerosis may be chest pain (angina pectoris) or a heart attack (myocardial infarction). A heart attack occurs because a coronary artery has become totally blocked and can no longer supply blood to the heart, which causes part of the heart muscle to die. As many as 10 percent of heart attacks may be silent—that is, individuals have them without being aware of them. Unfortunately, in a significant proportion, the first indication of coronary

disease is sudden cardiac death. Whether or not there is a blood clot, in such cases the patient develops ventricular fibrillation, which is a fatal cardiac arrhythmia. Unless resuscitative measures are immediately instituted or unless the patient has an implantable defibrillator or is in a hospital setting where a defibrillator is available, the result invariably will be death. Whether sudden cardiac death occurs as a complication of a heart attack or is independent of a heart attack, underlying coronary atherosclerotic disease typically is present. (Coronary artery disease is discussed further in Chapter 17.)

Atherosclerosis can also develop in the aorta, the large vessel that carries blood away from the heart. And atherosclerosis can form in the cerebral, carotid, renal, femoral, and brachial arteries (that is, the arteries of the brain, neck, kidneys, thighs, and arms, respectively). If an artery that supplies blood to brain tissue becomes blocked by a clot, a stroke may result. If a vessel that provides blood to the kidney is blocked, hypertension failure may occur; if the blocked vessel is one providing blood to a leg or arm, damage to the leg or arm may ensue.

A blood vessel may become completely blocked because a blood clot, or thrombus, has formed at the surface of the atherosclerotic lesion, or because there has been bleeding into the lesion. In either case, a

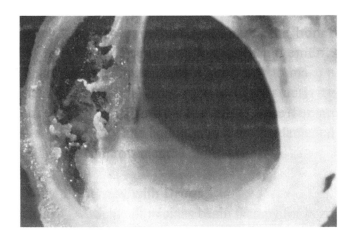

Figure 13.2. These 3 photographs show atherosclerotic lesions of the coronary arteries. Researchers now believe that lesions such as the one pictured at the top may be responsible for most heart attacks. Notice its soft, pulpy, lipid-rich contents and the thin cap separating the contents from the vessel's interior. Such lesions, which may be called *unstable*, *vulnerable*, or *culprit lesions*, are prone to rupture and to initiate the body's blood-clotting mechanism. The results of this process are pictured in the middle photograph. In contrast, some lesions (bottom) lack a soft lipid core and may be more stable, although a lesion of this size would be a candidate for a procedure such as bypass grafting or balloon angioplasty because it leaves little room for blood flow through the vessel. Heart attacks typically occur when a blood clot causes complete blockage of a coronary artery, cutting off blood supply to heart muscle and causing the muscle to die. Thus, severe narrowing of a vessel's opening by atherosclerosis is not required for a heart attack, and mild or moderate lesions usually far outnumber severe lesions. It may be possible, however, to stabilize lipid-rich culprit lesions through lifestyle changes and drug therapy designed to decrease blood cholesterol concentrations (photographs courtesy of Dr. M. J. Davies).

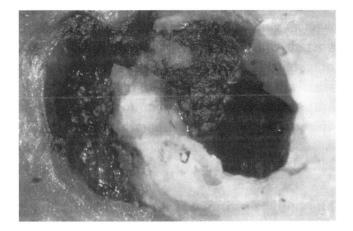

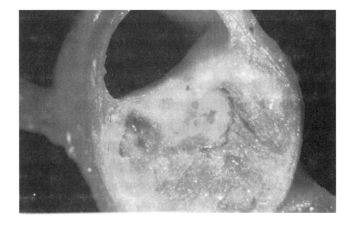

vital organ is deprived of the oxygen and other nutrients that are transported in the blood.

Researchers previously thought that the lesions most likely to form blood clots and lead to heart attacks were those causing 70 to 90 percent narrowing (stenosis) of a vessel. Based on information obtained from recent angiographic studies, it is now believed that the "culprit lesion," or the lesion that is most likely to have a blood clot, is one with a lipid-rich core and usually a thin, rather than thick, cap. The degree of vessel narrowing may be only 30 to 50 percent. Such a lesion is shown in Figure 13.2. Fissuring, or cracking, occurs around the edge of the lesion and leads to bleeding into the wall of the artery and a blood clot that totally blocks the blood flow through the damaged vessel. An individual with atherosclerosis usually has many more of these lesions causing less severe narrowing than lesions causing severe narrowing. The lesions with a lipid-rich core and a thin cap may be more unstable (rather like a jelly doughnut as opposed to a crusty hard roll). This new knowledge underlines why it is important to adhere to interventions—for example, dietary changes and use of lipid-lowering drugs—that can slow the atherosclerotic process throughout the vascular system.

Angiography is the radiologic technique usually used to visualize vessel narrowing in the living body. (Many examples of arteriograms of vessels are included in Chapter 19 as well as other chapters of this book.) It is currently the only radiologic method for reliable visualization of the coronary arteries. Some arteries, such as those in the neck and thighs, may also be assessed by ultrasound. Some researchers are using techniques such as ultrafast computed tomography (CT, or CAT, scanning) to detect calcium build-up in blood vessels, and positron-emission tomography (PET scanning) may be used to determine if tissue is well supplied with blood.

Mechanisms of Atherosclerosis Development

The leading hypothesis about how atherosclerosis develops is that it begins as a response to injury. The hypothesis states that when the endothelium (the layer of cells that lines the cavity of the blood vessel) sustains some type of injury or damage, platelets, fibrin (a clotting material in the blood), cellular debris, and calcium become deposited in the arterial wall. The blood vessel can become injured for a variety of reasons, including elevated blood lipid levels, high blood pressure, and cigarette smoking, or perhaps, as some speculate, a viral or bacterial infection. Heredity undoubtedly also plays a role in the development of atherosclerotic plaque. (Risk factors for atherosclerotic disease are discussed in detail in Chapter 7, which begins on page 79.)

As a result of the injury to the endothelial cells, the wall of the artery may become more easily permeated by low-density lipoprotein (LDL) particles. That is, the injury to the endothelial layer of the blood vessel may speed up the process by which LDL-cholesterol, or "bad" cholesterol, leaves the blood and enters the intima, the innermost layer of the arterial wall. Once within the arterial wall, the LDL may become oxidized or chemically modified. This modified LDL may incite a reaction that is similar to an inflammatory reaction.

The original response-to-injury hypothesis holds that various factors, including platelet-derived growth factor, cause a change in the characteristics of the smooth muscle cells, transforming them from a resting state to an active state and resulting in their proliferation, as well as their migration from the media to the intima of the arterial wall. This is still believed to be an important factor in early lesion development and certainly is important in the arterial wall that is subjected to percutaneous

transluminal coronary angioplasty (PTCA) (see below).

Oxidized or otherwise modified LDL is able to induce endothelial cells to secrete a substance that promotes the migration of macrophages or monocytes (which are types of white blood cells) from the bloodstream into the arterial wall. This is believed to be a key step in atherosclerosis formation. Some of the smooth muscle cells that have migrated into the intima may also be transformed into macrophages. The macrophages produce various substances that contribute to a type of inflammatory reaction. The "culprit lesion" described above has many of the characteristics of an acute inflammation.

As an atherosclerotic lesion progresses, a lipid core accumulates, which damages the arterial wall and increases the likelihood of blood clot formation. What is seen is a lipid core with an accumulation of activated macrophages and T lymphocytes (another form of white blood cell), characteristic of an acute inflammatory reaction near the surface of the lesion. It has been postulated that activated macrophages release enzymes called *matrix metalloproteinases* (MMPs), which then cause the breakdown of connective tissue and lead to a destabilization of the lesions. This is a complex reaction, and the details are not well understood.

Interestingly, the culprit lesion that is about to undergo formation of a blood clot contains very few smooth muscle cells. Whether these are somehow damaged or just why they disappear is not yet understood. The dramatic reductions in rates of clinical events—for example, in heart attacks and coronary heart disease deaths— observed in relatively short periods of time with vigorous lipid-lowering therapy are thought to be related to stabilization of atherosclerotic lesions, which is perhaps induced by decreasing lipid core contents. This is still an active area of investigation, but the above scheme provides a rational way of viewing and explaining the pronounced benefits of aggressive lipid lowering, and in particular, LDL-cholesterol lowering, in patients with established coronary heart disease.

The earliest lesions of atherosclerosis appear to be fatty streaks, which contain lipid-filled macrophages. Fatty streaks are small, flat, yellowish patches. They are believed to originate in childhood, and, in fact, have been found in children as young as 1 year of age. Not all fatty streaks turn into the more advanced lesions of atherosclerosis, but at least some fatty streaks eventually do become more mature lesions (Figure 13.3).

A subsequent stage of atherosclerosis is the fibrous plaque, in which the lesion becomes filled with calcium, fibrous tissue,

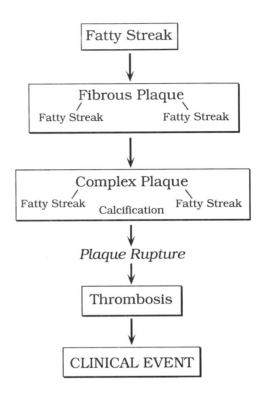

Figure 13.3. One scheme of the progression of atherosclerosis.

and connective tissue debris and begins to protrude into the opening (lumen) of the artery. Advanced plaques, which also are called complicated lesions or complex plaque, eventually may develop. Advanced plaques contain even larger accumulations of fatty substances and cellular debris and occur with greater frequency as a person ages.

As noted above, some researchers are investigating whether an infection could contribute to the vascular injury thought to occur in the development of atherosclerosis. While at first this idea might seem a little far-fetched, there is interesting evidence from a bird model of atherosclerosis and from studies in human tissues. Chickens infected with Marek's disease virus, a member of the chicken herpesvirus family, can develop massive atherosclerosis. The disease in chickens is different from that in humans in that the lipid-filled cells in the artery wall are derived mostly from smooth muscle cells rather than from macrophages. While an infectious virus cannot be isolated from the chicken's atherosclerotic lesions, viral proteins and the genetic material of the virus are present in the cells of the lesion.

In humans, a number of studies were conducted in the mid-1990s to evaluate the association of a cytomegalovirus (CMV), a human herpesvirus, with atherosclerosis. (The herpesvirus family is a large one and in humans includes, for example, herpes simplex virus 1, which causes cold sores; herpes simplex virus 2, which usually causes genital lesions; herpesvirus 3, or varicella-zoster virus, which causes chickenpox; herpesvirus 4, which is Epstein–Barr virus; and herpesvirus 5, which is CMV.) In one such study, conducted at Baylor College of Medicine, the genetic material for CMV was found in 90 percent of the tissue samples from 135 patients undergoing surgery to correct vascular disease. Both the atherosclerotic plaque

and uninvolved aortic tissue samples from these patients gave similar results. In addition, 86 percent of the patients who had positive tissue samples also had serum antibodies to the CMV. As with the Marek's disease virus, no infectious CMV particles have been found in patient arterial tissue in any study. Thus, it would appear that latent CMV infection of arterial tissues is quite common in patients with atherosclerosis. It has also been observed that patients who undergo heart transplantation, who can develop active CMV infections, experience accelerated atherosclerosis in transplanted vessels.

Other data have suggested that *Chlamydia pneumoniae* (a bacterium that causes a mild form of pneumonia in humans), *Helicobacter pylori* (a bacterium that causes gastritis and ulcers in humans), and herpes simplex virus may be associated with the development of atherosclerosis. Research in progress in a number of laboratories should provide, over the next few years, a better understanding of how infectious agents might contribute to the atherogenic process.

Regression of Atherosclerosis

Until very recently, atherosclerosis was thought to be a relentless process. Now, however, research has shown that the progress of atherosclerosis can be delayed, stopped, and occasionally even reversed. In a number of clinical trials, aggressively lowering LDL-cholesterol by the use of dietary changes and/or lipid-lowering drugs led to a decrease of plaque in a small percentage of patients with coronary heart disease. In many additional patients, the progression of plaque in the coronary arteries was either stopped or delayed. In contrast, atherosclerosis continued to progress in the groups of patients randomly assigned to usual care or placebo in these trials. Also, cholesterol-lowering therapy in these trials led to greater-than-expected reductions in rates of coronary events, such as heart attacks, sudden cardiac death, and need for bypass grafting or balloon angioplasty. New research suggests that the use of cholesterol-lowering therapy can shrink the soft, lipid-rich atherosclerotic lesions that are more likely to rupture, and some scientists believe there may be additional beneficial effects, such as endothelial healing.

In these trials looking at the effects of therapy on the coronary arteries, angiography was used to image the arteries. The researchers measured on the angiograms whether the vessel diameters were larger, smaller, or the same at the end of the trial, without knowing which patients received treatment and which did not. In the preponderance of the trials, these measurements were made using computerized systems. The trials typically lasted between one and three years. Other cholesterol-lowering trials have used angiography or ultrasound to visualize the arteries in the neck or thighs and found similar results of slowed atherosclerotic lesion progression and occasional regression. All told, the results of the cholesterol-lowering "regression trials" support the lower LDL-cholesterol goal of less than 100 mg/dl set by the National Cholesterol Education Program for adults with atherosclerotic disease (see pp. 90–93).

Lesion-prone Areas and Individual Differences

One of the interesting aspects of atherosclerosis is that it tends to occur at specific sites where arteries branch or curve. As in a river or brook, these are sites where fluid flow patterns may be complex. Some investigators believe that variations in the circulation's shear stress at such points may result in chronic minimal injury to the endothelium, an injury that can be worsened by such factors as an elevated cholesterol level, high blood pressure, tobacco smoking, or a viral infection. Atherosclerotic lesions may tend to occur at sites of low or oscillating shear stress. Laboratory experiments have shown, for example, that low shear rates encourage proliferation of smooth muscle cells, an important component of the formation of athero-sclerotic lesions. A vicious circle may develop, since injury to the vessel wall can impair the vessel's ability to adapt its diameter to control shear stress. Healthy arteries have the ability to sense shear stress and to remodel themselves to keep shear stress within a narrow range (the "biosensor" may be the endothelial cell); in some cases, a vessel may have an inher-ently impaired ability to remodel itself because of a genetic abnormality. Hemodynamic shear stress may also be important in understanding plaque progression (often a slow process) or plaque rupture and thrombosis (typically abrupt changes). Dr. Stefan Jost and colleagues found progression of coronary heart disease to be most frequent in arte-rial segments with larger diameters; they speculated that the result may reflect lower shear stress in those segments.

Other theories about why atheroscle-rosis preferentially occurs at curves and branch points include high pressure, low pressure, and turbulence at those locations. Studies of fluid dynamics and "geometric" risk factors (for example, a small branch angle may be a geometric risk factor in some coronary arteries) in the develop-ment of atherosclerosis may help us under-stand the complex riddle of why and where atherosclerotic disease occurs. It involves dynamic interactions among a variety of cellular, biochemical, and bio-physical factors.

Studies of populations have shown that atherosclerotic lesions occur earliest and most extensively in the aorta. They develop later and are less extensive in the coronary and cerebral (brain) arteries, as well as the renal (kidney) arteries. The pulmonary (lung) arteries are less suscep-tible to atherosclerosis. In an individual, the severity of disease in one artery does not predict the severity of disease in another artery. It needs to be remembered that in individual patients, findings may fall well outside of generalizations.

Dr. DeBakey and some colleagues studied the records of almost 14,000 men and women who, over the course of 35 years, were admitted to The Methodist Hospital in Houston because of atheroscle-rotic disease causing severe arterial blockage. It was found that the disease tends to assume characteristic patterns that may be classified by predominant site or distribution (Figure 13.4) into five major categories: (1) the coronary arteries, (2) the major branches of the aortic arch (including the carotid, or neck, arteries), (3) the visceral arterial branches of the abdominal aorta (including the renal arteries), (4) the terminal, or lower, abdominal aorta and its major branches (including the femoral, or thigh, arteries), and (5) a combination of any of these simultaneously. The fourth category included the highest proportion of patients (about two-fifths of patients), and the first category included the second highest proportion (almost one-third). The third category included the lowest proportion of patients (only 3 percent). Patients in the first and third categories were significantly younger than those in the other categories.

Atherosclerosis also varies among individuals in how quickly it progresses, or builds up. In some patients, the disease

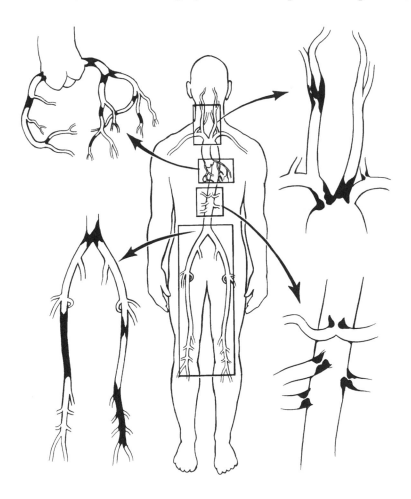

Figure 13.4. Predominant anatomic locations of atherosclerotic occlusive disease: coronary arteries (top left), major branches of the aortic arch (top right), major visceral branches of the aorta (bottom right), and major branches of the terminal aorta (bottom left).

remains relatively stable over a period of years. In others, it progresses rapidly, and in yet others, lesions progress at an intermediate rate. The younger the individual at the time clinical disease is indicated (for example, symptoms such as angina pectoris develop), the more rapid the progression. Averaged across groups of untreated patients—for example, the control patients or placebo recipients in angiographically monitored cholesterol-lowering trials—coronary atherosclerosis has been found to progress at a fairly constant rate. With cholesterol-lowering therapy, progression can be retarded, as is discussed above. Besides elevated blood cholesterol, factors such as diabetes or cigarette smoking may be associated with a more rapid rate of lesion progression. Also, there is undoubtedly a strong genetic influence, since rapid lesion progression has been observed in some families with relatively mild abnormalities in known risk factors. Still, the most important concept to be remembered in discussing variable susceptibility to atherosclerosis at different arterial locations or among individuals is that researchers believe that the key factor determining differences in the extent of atherosclerotic disease among populations is, as emphasized in this book, lifestyle factors—for example, the amount of saturated fat in the diet and smoking habits.

Accelerated Atherosclerosis

In contrast to spontaneous, or native, atherosclerosis, as described in the preceding section, which may occur prematurely in individuals with risk factors such as elevated blood cholesterol, smoking, diabetes, or a family history of premature atherosclerotic disease, researchers have described what is termed *accelerated atherosclerosis*. This occurs in some patients after heart transplantation or PTCA (percutaneous transluminal coronary angioplasty). It also occurs, uncommonly, after coronary artery bypass grafting using vein grafts (CABG is an acronym you may hear pronounced as "cabbage"). The development of these forms of atherosclerosis appears to have much in common with spontaneous atherosclerosis—notably, occurrence as a response to injury—but also some unique aspects. However, much more research is needed, in particular regarding how to prevent accelerated atherosclerosis. As in spontaneous atherosclerosis, the development of each kind of accelerated atherosclerosis is very complex.

Atherosclerosis in the Transplanted Heart

The principal cause of death in heart transplant recipients who survive the first year after surgery is premature coronary atherosclerosis. Although these patients usually receive healthy hearts, atherosclerosis can develop rapidly after surgery, and about half of heart transplant recipients who survive five years are found to have coronary atherosclerosis. Posttransplantation atherosclerosis often causes a characteristic concentric narrowing of coronary arteries. It is possible that injury to the vessel leading to atherosclerosis results from immune-mediated chronic rejection or infection with CMV (see above). Elevated blood lipids may contribute to posttransplantation arterial disease, since elevated levels occur in a large proportion of heart transplantation recipients. In a study of 100 patients at our institution conducted by Dr. Gotto, Dr. Christie Ballantyne, Dr. John Farmer, and other colleagues, average total cholesterol increased from 168 mg/dl before heart transplantation, to 234 mg/dl three months after surgery. Increases in blood lipid levels may result in part from the use of immunosuppressive drugs such as cyclosporine, and heart transplant recipients may have had artificially low lipid levels because of heart failure before transplantation. Lipid deposition in the vessel wall may occur after chronic immune injury. In a randomized study, cholesterol-lowering therapy using a drug called an HMG-CoA reductase inhibitor (or statin) increased

the one-year survival rate and decreased accelerated atherosclerosis and the incidence of rejection causing hemodynamic compromise in patients who had undergone heart transplantation.

Atherosclerosis after PTCA

Accelerated atherosclerosis is the key factor limiting the success of balloon angioplasty. In this case, the accelerated atherosclerosis occurs in the blood vessel that has been treated by angioplasty for atherosclerosis: the vessel's opening narrows again—restenosis occurs. Within three to six months of angioplasty, as many as one-fourth to one-third of patients have restenosis. The initial injury that causes proliferation of smooth muscle cells appears to involve the angioplasty itself, and the response is viewed by some as an effort by the vessel to heal itself. The risk conferred by restenosis is typically recurrence of symptoms (angina), and CABG or repeat angioplasty may be required: the patient may become an "old customer." Initial presentation of restenosis as a heart attack or sudden death is uncommon.

Increased risk for restenosis appears to exist if there is angina, residual stenosis, or a positive perfusion scan soon after angioplasty. Among other risk factors for which there is some evidence are elevated lipoprotein[a] (see pp. 96–97), a low HDL-cholesterol level, total occlusion, previous restenosis, diabetes, and angioplasty performed in the left anterior descending artery. Lifestyle and drug interventions to decrease restenosis have proved disappointing: the risk factor control that has proved so successful against native atherosclerosis has not proved effective against restenosis. Still, it is important for patients who have undergone angioplasty to adhere strictly to atherosclerosis risk reduction measures such as those designed to lower blood cholesterol or blood pressure, since the impact of these measures against the development or progression of lesions at other locations is by no means diminished. The problem of restenosis likely will be solved after a better understanding of the basic biologic and molecular phenomena underlying it is achieved. The area is one of intensive research.

Atherosclerosis in Vein Grafts

When possible, grafts from the internal mammary artery rather than vein grafts are used in coronary bypass surgery (see pp. 277–279). Ten years after surgery, 90 or 95 percent of mammary grafts remain patent (that is, widely open, so that they can fully supply blood to the heart), compared with only about 50 percent of saphenous vein grafts. (Saphenous veins are veins in the legs.) Patients who have received mammary artery grafts survive longer and have fewer cardiac complications than patients who have received only saphenous vein grafts. Most of the saphenous vein grafts that close up do so because of atherosclerosis. Aspirin given from the time of surgery onward can decrease the frequency of vein graft occlusion, and attention to modifiable coronary heart disease risk factors (discussed in Chapters 7 and 26) can also help keep grafts open for as long as possible. In the Cholesterol Lowering Atherosclerosis Study, conducted in middle-aged men who had undergone CABG, aggressive lowering of LDL-cholesterol using the drugs colestipol and nicotinic acid resulted in a significant reduction in the formation of new atherosclerotic lesions in vein grafts. Results from the large Post-CABG trial also indicate that lowering LDL-cholesterol can significantly reduce the risk for progression of atherosclerotic lesions in saphenous vein grafts.

Why accelerated atherosclerosis occurs in vein grafts is poorly understood. Occlusion that occurs soon after surgery appears to be related to the formation of clots (thrombosis). Vein grafts are subject to mechanical injury during harvesting and handling; this injury may lead to thrombosis, but in most cases the vessel wall heals quickly. Later atherosclerosis in vein grafts represents proliferation of smooth muscle cells and superimposed additional atherosclerotic changes.

The excellent long-term results with mammary artery transplantation have helped make CABG one of the most commonly performed and successful operations in improving quality of life for patients with angina. The results have encouraged surgeons to investigate performing CABG using other arteries taken from the patient's own body (that is, other autologous arterial grafts, *auto* meaning "self," as in *autobiography*), since mammary artery transplantation is not always possible. An example is transplanting to the heart the gastroepiploic artery of the greater curve of the stomach. Using vessels from sources other than the patient's own body (that is, using nonautologous sources) is also being investigated.

CHAPTER FOURTEEN

Therapeutic Procedures

Moving blood through its chambers and out through the arteries, the heart works to deliver life-giving oxygen and nutrients throughout the body. The heart keeps the blood moving and making all of its regularly scheduled deliveries. However, like any transportation system, this one occasionally encounters obstacles.

In an ideal system, the heart would be like an airport control tower on a clear day, sending passengers and goods into a barrier-free space, with few external factors affecting its on-time service. Oxygen and nutrients would have only to stay on course. But in reality, the heart is more like a railroad station, sending its passengers and freight out on predetermined tracks, with countless unpredictable hazards along the way. As the tracks age, are damaged, and fail to be maintained, they pose threats to safe transport. When might track damage or debris endanger a fast-moving train? These tracks, part of a labyrinthine system, allow the train to bring its cargo to countless places along the route and to carry it back again to the station when all sites have been served.

But what if the train encounters obstacles on the tracks, and it has to come to a halt until the blockage is moved? Or what if the train has difficulty getting back to the station because it does not have the power it needs for the round-trip?

These problems are like those caused by coronary blockages and a slowed heartbeat. A response is required when a clot or fatty deposits in the blood vessels obstruct blood flow or a slow heartbeat fails to regulate blood flow properly. Physicians have responded with such procedures as percutaneous transluminal coronary angioplasty (PTCA), stents, atherectomy, thrombolytic therapy, and pacemaker placement. These highly technical, modern medical solutions, once out of reach, have been transformed by time and experience into remedies practiced around the globe.

Percutaneous Transluminal Coronary Angioplasty

Although its development goes back to the 1920s, when a physician first inserted a catheter into his own vein as an experiment, and to the 1960s, when physicians first attempted to obliterate atherosclerosis with coaxial dilators, percutaneous angioplastic dilation of a coronary artery was first performed in 1977. Now used worldwide, this technique enlarges a blood vessel's passageway by applying pressure from the inside out. Under carefully controlled conditions, a cardiologist or surgeon positions a very slender tube (a catheter) in a constricted vessel, and by exposing and inflating a balloon carried along within this tube, the physician is able to compress and split the plaque obstructing the vessel and simultaneously stretch the vessel wall, widening the passageway. This pressure clears the way for freer transport of circulating blood.

Patients who need to undergo this procedure have a coronary artery blocked by fatty deposits around the inside of the vessel that make it difficult or impossible for the blood to flow through the passageway freely. This condition is known as atherosclerosis (see Chapter 13). Chest pain (angina) may result when the atherosclerotic blockage significantly reduces the flow of blood to the heart and the supply of oxygen to the heart muscle. When it

affects the flow to the brain, dizziness, temporary loss of speech, or overwhelming weakness may occur. When atherosclerosis leads to total occlusion of an artery supplying the heart or brain, a heart attack or stroke results.

After being diagnosed as having significant atherosclerosis of a coronary artery, a patient may undergo PTCA. In this procedure, a physician, typically a cardiologist, performs the catheterization; nurses assist the physician and ensure the proper supplies are at hand; a radiologic technician makes sure that the radiology equipment provides the best visualization of the vessels; and another technician monitors the patient's heartbeat and breathing. A cardiovascular team should be available to perform surgery if necessary. If the patient has many sites that are narrowed, the cardiologist may recommend coronary artery bypass grafting instead.

In PTCA, the physician inserts what is called a *guiding catheter* through the femoral artery, a major blood vessel in the thigh, to the opening (ostium) of the coronary artery to be dilated. Using a fluoroscope to visualize the vessels, and administering some drugs to help the heart and vessels undergo the procedure without problems, the physician then inserts a dilation catheter, which carriers an uninflated balloon (Figure 14.1). By injecting contrast material that will be visible on the fluoroscope, the physician can carefully monitor

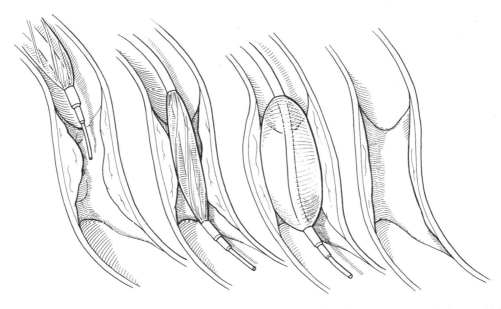

Figure 14.1. Clogged vessels may be reopened with percutaneous transluminal coronary angioplasty, which is also called balloon angioplasty. A tiny, specially designed balloon, uninflated and inside a catheter, is inserted through the femoral artery. The catheter is threaded to an area within the vessel where blood passage is difficult, usually because of atherosclerosis. Once there, the balloon is positioned at the narrowest portion and inflated, widening the channel.

the catheter's progress into the artery. Once the balloon at the tip of the dilation catheter is placed across the area of the most serious narrowing and its position is confirmed by fluoroscopy, it can be inflated. The physician opens and closes the balloon, sometimes several times. (If he or she believes the vessel is likely to close again after the procedure, a stent may be placed in it. See below.) After the artery has been successfully dilated, the physician administers more drugs, monitors the patient for stability, and withdraws the dilation catheter. Then arteriograms are made, and the guiding catheter is removed if all is well.

After angioplasty, the patient is watched in observation before being taken to a regular hospital room. Nurses monitor the patient closely. A patient can expect to be discharged in about 48 hours.

Complications occur in only 2 to 5 percent of patients. The most serious complication is the sudden closing of an artery. Doctors may use drugs, a flexible guide wire, angioplasty, a stent, or surgery to open the vessel again. Among other possible complications are coronary artery rupture, vessel perforation, arrhythmias, and embolism, but these are all uncommon.

Initial success rates are high—the interior diameter of the vessel is enlarged; the

What's in a Name?
Percutaneous Transluminal Coronary Angioplasty

Although the name of the procedure is long, each word in its name is straightforward. *Percutaneous* means "through the skin" (*cutis* is Latin for skin, and is also the root in *cuticle*). *Transluminal* means "through the lumen" (the lumen is the channel within a blood vessel). *Coronary* refers to the heart vessels, and *angioplasty* is plastic surgery of a vessel (compare it with *rhinoplasty,* which refers to plastic surgery of the nose). The combining word *angio* comes from the Greek word *angos,* which means "vessel." Thus, as described by the four words, the physician inserts the catheter *through the skin* and threads it *through blood vessels* that serve the heart, enabling him or her to undertake the needed surgical repair of the vessel without having to make a long incision in the chest to expose the heart. At the tip of the dilation catheter is a small balloon used to widen the vessel lumen, which has given the procedure the nickname *balloon angioplasty.*

high local pressure on the vessel is reduced; symptoms associated with poor blood supply to the heart muscle (myocardial ischemia) are moderated or eliminated; and surgery is avoided. However, the vessel narrows again in a significant proportion of patients within three to six months.

Short-term success is marked by relief of angina, improved circulation, better ability to exercise, and better heart function, even at rest. Long-term studies show that about 30 to 40 percent of patients experience recurrence. In these cases, the angina returns, and a treadmill test usually reveals that the heart is not getting the blood it needs. Angioplasty can be repeated, and success rates with the repeat procedure can be as good or better than those of the first procedure, but often are not.

After angioplasty, the physician will institute a medication schedule that will incorporate several medicines. Nitrates and calcium antagonists will be on the list throughout the hospital stay, and they may be part of the daily medication regimen for the next three to six months. Aspirin (up to 650 mg/day in two 325-mg doses) will also be prescribed and may remain part of the drug plan for six months. Many physicians also order ticlopidine, an antiplatelet agent. Because these drugs affect the outcome of angioplasty—that is, they may help prevent the vessels from narrowing again—it is important to follow the doctor's orders.

If you undergo angioplasty, be sure to ask your doctor about when you can return to work, what kind of activities you can undertake, and when he or she will see you again. The answers you receive will help you know what to expect. The doctor may want to perform other tests, including a stress treadmill test, within about two weeks. The tests may also be scheduled on a regular basis over an extended period to monitor the success of the angioplasty.

Stent Implantation

The perplexing problems of the reclosing of the coronary artery experienced by patients three to six months after angioplasty or of the intraprocedure sudden collapse of the vessel requiring emergency surgery (this experienced by 5 to 7 percent of patients) prompted development of new technology to address them. The solution was the coronary stent, a less than 1-inch-long tube of wirelike stainless steel that is expanded within the artery and left in place to brace the walls of the vessel, much as supporting structures keep subway tunnel walls in place, ensuring free passage.

Stents can be lifesaving for patients whose arteries suddenly spasm or collapse and close during angioplasty, setting off a heart attack. They also help patients avoid coronary artery bypass surgery, or at least buy time for planning a future heart surgery while avoiding the risks of emergency surgery. Furthermore, with the stent in reserve, physicians can attempt more aggressive angioplasty and broaden options for patients who have problems that prevent them from being candidates for bypass surgery.

Patients who have already undergone coronary artery bypass grafting are also candidates for stenting when their saphenous vein grafts narrow with disease. Within 10 years of surgery, occlusive disease develops in about 50 percent of saphenous vein grafts. Stents offer a therapeutic alternative to these patients, who are at higher risk for death and complications with every repeated bypass procedure (and some have had up to four).

Often resembling a coil spring, stents are implanted after balloon angioplasty (Figure 14.2). Using the catheter system already in place, the cardiologist will mount the stent over a balloon catheter and, with the stent inside a sheath, return the catheter to the dilated vessel. There the sheath is retracted, the balloon inflated, and the stent thereby expanded and positioned. The balloon is deflated, withdrawn into the sheath, and removed. Arteries of the heart and those extending from the intestinal region into the thighs are candidates for stent buttressing. Stent size varies according to application, and physicians may use more than one in a series as needed. A study of one type of coronary artery stent performed by 19 cooperating medical institutions with almost 500 patients found it successful in 95 percent of patients.

Before the procedure, the cardiologist will prescribe *anticoagulants,* drugs to disengage in part the body's coagulation mechanisms in order to avoid *occlusion.* The patient may take some of these drugs before entering the hospital, and others may be administered intravenously before, during, and after the procedure. Drugs that may be part of this plan include aspirin, ticlopidine, warfarin, and heparin.

Whereas angioplasty alone usually requires a hospital stay of no more than two or three days, stent placement may require a stay of four to seven days. While in the hospital, the patient will be on complete bed rest for about 24 hours after the catheter's femoral sheath is removed. The physician may recommend a soft restraining device be used briefly for the leg where the sheath was inserted, in order to prevent any strain that would initiate bleeding. Patients should report any chest pain, shortness of breath, nausea, or profuse perspiration. These may be indications of reocclusion.

Patients are asked to drink a lot of liquids to flush the contrast solution out of their bodies. Diet recommendations will include limiting intake of vitamin K, which inhibits anticoagulation efforts. Patients should also advise their other physicians and their dentist that the stent has been placed. The cardiologist may also make other dietary or lifestyle recommen-

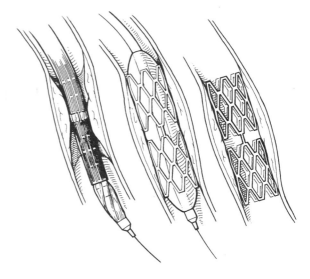

Figure 14.2. Stents are implanted using a catheter system. The stent is mounted over a balloon catheter, covered with a sheath, and placed within the vessel (left). The cardiologist retracts the sheath and inflates the balloon, thereby expanding and positioning the stent (center). With the stent in place, the balloon is deflated, withdrawn into the sheath, and removed. The stent remains (right). Some physicians use anticoagulants to coat stents as a way to reduce blood clot formation and to allow lower dosage of anticoagulation therapy.

dations to enhance the prospect of good cardiac health.

Some physicians have used heparin as a stent coating to lower doses of anticoagulation therapy and to reduce blood clot formation. Other cardiology researchers are working on similar refinements, including coatings meant to inhibit vascular tissue growth and thereby reduce the probability of restenosis. In the future, device enhancements are expected to lead to improved care. New techniques and devices based on the angioplasty approach, rather than supplanting others, are expected to find specific uses for which they are best suited and to offer physicians and patients a broader spectrum of therapies.

Atherectomy

Atherectomy is the excision and physical removal of obstructing atherosclerotic plaque from coronary arteries. Used in place of or as an adjunct to balloon angioplasty, atherectomy widens the vessel by tissue (plaque) removal and by balloon inflation and direct mechanical dilation. As with other procedures, freer passage afterward is thought to be partially due to vessel wall and plaque stretching. Success is achieved in about 95 percent of patients, but 20 to 30 percent experience restenosis. Acute occlusion occurs in less than 5 percent of patients.

One type of device used for this procedure has a cylindrical cutting blade, an atheroma collection chamber, and a balloon as essential elements. The device is advanced through the atheromatous lesion. The balloon is then inflated, pressing a cutting edge against the obstruction. Next, the cylindrical rotary cutter moves forward and shaves away vessel wall deposits. The debris is pushed into the specially designed collection chamber, and afterward the balloon is deflated. The device is reposi-

tioned and the process is repeated until the physician is satisfied by angiographic results that the job is completed. When the device is withdrawn, the tissue debris comes with it.

The device is better suited for some types of atherosclerotic lesions (for example, those of proximal large vessels) than others, and the technique requires advanced skills in angioplasty. Other types of atherectomy devices are, like the one described above, under study.

Thrombolytic Therapy

Although still considered investigational in the 1980s, thrombolytic therapy is now approved by the U.S. Food and Drug Administration and has become a full-fledged member of the array of procedures used to stop a heart attack. Thrombolytic therapy employs drugs to dissolve a blood clot (thrombus) that is obstructing the blood's path to the heart and preventing it from receiving oxygen and nutrients. Known commonly as "clot-busting" therapy, this method reinstates blood flow in 60 to 90 percent of patients.

When such blood components as platelets and fibrin collect on an atherosclerotic plaque, cells are entrapped and a blood clot may totally obstruct the vessel (Figure 14.3). Chest pain (angina) results, indicating the threat of a heart attack—

what doctors call a *myocardial infarction.* The sooner any blockage is treated, the better. Studies have shown that thrombolytic therapy can reduce the number of deaths resulting from coronary artery blockage.

If you experience pain in the center of the chest that radiates to the shoulders, neck, or arms, and you feel faint or nauseated, or experience shortness of breath or sudden sweating, you should go immediately to a hospital with 24-hour emergency cardiac care. Getting the help you need as fast as you can get it will decrease your chance of dying and the chance of doing serious damage to your heart. You can't choose where you will have a heart attack, but knowing where to go if it happens when you are at home or work can save time. Don't wait until you need this kind of help to learn where to find it. Contact the hospitals near your home and near your office to identify which ones provide 24-hour emergency cardiac care, including thrombolytic therapy.

The physician performing the thrombolytic therapy will work quickly to restore the flow of blood to the heart. Angiograms can be used to delineate the thrombus and its location. After an initial injection of a thrombolytic agent into the blocked coronary artery, the physician will continue therapy with an intravenous (IV) drip containing a clot-dissolving drug. Heparin, a blood thinner, will also be given. An

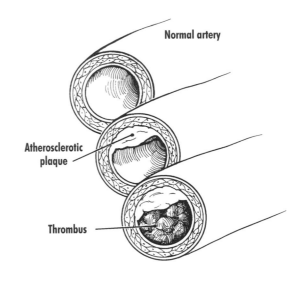

Figure 14.3. The normal coronary artery has 3 layers, and blood flows through the channel, or lumen, in its center (top). After atherosclerotic plaque forms within the channel, blood flow is restricted (middle). With the addition of a thrombus, the vessel is blocked (bottom).

alternative approach is to use IV administration only, basing administration on clinical symptoms such as chest pain and on electrocardiographic indications of acute myocardial infarction. (Electrocardiography will be used to monitor the heartbeat throughout the procedure.) If blood flow is not restored within established time limits, the physician may increase the dose of the thrombolytic agent or use other techniques that will help the thrombolytic drugs do their job better. Even after the vessel has reopened, the physicians will continue to infuse the drug for a while to ensure that the threat of the clot has been eliminated.

What's in a Name? Thrombolytic Therapy

Therapy, we know, means "treatment." But what kind of treatment is *thrombolytic treatment?*

It is a therapy that lyses thrombi. Still confused? These are not words we use in everyday conversation. Except, think of *electrolysis*—it is a procedure that destroys or kills (lyses) hair roots with an electrical current (*electro* is a combining word referring to electricity). *Thrombo* refers to a thrombus, a blood clot that remains at its point of origin (whereas an embolus travels). *Thrombolytic therapy,* then, means "thrombus-destroying treatment."

Within 24 hours, up to 85 percent of the blood flow through the vessel can be reestablished. Afterward, the patient may need to take medicines to keep the vessels open and to prevent the blood from coagulating inappropriately.

Complications occur in a small percentage of patients undergoing thrombolytic therapy. Some patients have fever, and some experience bleeding, usually at a puncture site. If the bleeding becomes significant, the physician will apply pressure to the site, stop the thrombolytic therapy, and begin to infuse blood products and perhaps other drugs to reduce bleeding. Because bleeding sometimes occurs internally, doctors will use drugs beforehand to try and prevent it. Unfortunately, about 20 percent of patients have

been known to experience the shutting down of the vessel a second time and the recurrence of heart attack. In these cases, treatment must be on a case-by-case basis, and physicians will choose from instituting long-term drug therapy to prevent coagulation, performing coronary angioplasty, or performing revascularization surgery.

Well-known examples of thrombolytic agents are tissue plasminogen activator (t-PA) and streptokinase.

Pacemaker Implantation

What follows below is a brief overview of pacemaker implantation, including what the patient can expect before and after implantation. For a full look at the history of pacemakers, their variations and uses, and their abilities, see Chapter 10.

Things have changed greatly since the late 1950s, when the implantation of the first cardiac pacemaker was performed in Stockholm. Found to improve greatly the life of elderly patients with bradycardia (a condition of a slow-beating heart), pacemakers, one of the highest achievements of modern medicine, have come a long way since they used to set off passenger surveillance equipment at airports.

Not simple metronomelike devices keeping a steady beat, many pacemakers today can respond to changes in physiologic requirements, follow programming, and communicate. Some know when you are at rest or quiet (for example, watching TV), and they know when you're active or excited (for example, rushing to get to work, jogging to catch the bus, or running along the sidewalk to make an appointment on time). Various pacemakers can sense physical movement, body temperature, and breathing rate. Pacemakers respond to changes in these factors with changes in the heart rate to meet the needs they sense. Pacemakers send electrical impulses to the atrium, the ventricle, or both, ensuring that the heart beats fast enough and regularly enough for proper functioning.

A pacemaker may be temporary or permanent. Those patients most likely to need one have slow heart action that can fall to life-threateningly low rates. Drug therapy may prove ineffective. These patients are subject to the symptoms of debilitating fatigue, chronic exercise intolerance, and frightening episodes of loss of consciousness due to insufficient blood flow to the brain. Pacemakers can meet their needs.

A pacemaker has a pulse generator, which is often a circular device, slightly larger in diameter than a quarter, that houses electronic circuitry and lithium batteries. Both lie within a titanium or stainless steel case that is hermetically sealed. Attached to it are one or two leads, which are insulated electrical conductors that convey the electrical pulses from the generator to the tips of the leads positioned in the heart's chambers.

Pacemakers with internal leads but an external pulse generator may be placed temporarily when patients need rate regulation immediately. These patients may be recovering from a heart attack, and their heartbeat may be abnormal. Not knowing whether the abnormality will disappear as the heart heals or whether it will persist, the physician will use a temporary system. Fluoroscopy will be used to guide the cardiologist in positioning the leads properly. These pacemakers may stay in place for only a few days or for several weeks. They are replaced by a permanent pacing system if one is required as soon as the patient is strong enough to undergo the procedure. Complications include risk for infection and cardiac perforation.

Surgeons and cardiologists have recommendations from a task force composed of representatives from the American Heart Association and the American College of Cardiology to guide them in properly selecting patients for permanent pacemaker implantation.

Patients are asked not to eat anything for six or eight hours before the procedure, but aside from routine tests, patients will not be asked to meet any other preoperative requirements. Only local anesthesia is given, and a mild sedative will be administered before the procedure.

If your job or favorite sport requires repetitive use of one of your hands, the physician will probably place the pacemaker generator on the opposite side. During the procedure, the leads are guided through a vein underneath the collarbone, and their tips are positioned in the ventricle, atrium, or both. The physician attaches the leads to the pulse generator and then tests the pacemaker twice to make sure the pacing is right for the patient and the sensing function is working properly. Sensing devices are in the tips of the leads. The pacemaker is placed in a "pocket" (a naturally occurring depression) just above the pectoral muscle, and it is rechecked before the physician closes the pocket with sutures. (The pectoral muscles extend from the breastbone over to the arm and shoulder, at the top of the chest on each side.)

Patients remain in the postoperative recovery room until they are mostly free of the effects of the sedation and stable enough to be moved. The heart will continue to be monitored around the clock by electrocardiography. A chest x-ray will indicate whether the leads have been placed correctly and provide a check that no air or gas has accumulated in the pleural cavity. Within a day or two the patient will be able to leave the hospital.

Results of a study of more than 1,000 patients who had temporary pacemakers inserted indicated that complications occurred in 14 percent of patients. There were no fatalities, but complications included blood or air in the pleural cavity and inflammation of a vein in relation to a blood clot. Complications in permanent pacemaker placement may represent failure of the device to work properly—failure of the electrical impulse to make the ventricle contract, failure of the sensors to sense changes in the heart's needs accurately, and failure of the pacemaker to pace the beats of the heart. Common placement problems include damage to the lead as it is passed beneath the collarbone, and loss of sensitivity on the tip of the lead because of a chemical reaction (involving oxygen) or scarring around the tip of the lead (which can be decreased by using steroid-coated leads). Other complications include a fast-beating heart, infection, injury to the heart during a procedure, thrombosis, and embolism.

After pacemaker implantation, the physician will monitor the pacemaker's performance, make adjustments to ensure effectiveness, and take preventive measures against infection. Activities that require moving the elbow above the shoulder—driving, playing basketball, firing a rifle, swimming, for example—may have to be discontinued until the tenderness at the incision resolves. Although operation of the new pacemaker models is unlikely to be jeopardized by being near microwave ovens, powerful electromagnetic fields may affect their functioning. Patients need to ask their physician what precautions to take. Patients with cardiac pacemakers are restricted from magnetic resonance imaging (MRI). Do *not* have an MRI scan if you have a pacemaker.

The pacemaker's performance will be monitored during visits to the physician's office and also through calls that may be made to an office able to receive special signals from the pacemaker and to produce an electrocardiogram. This monitoring office will be able to advise you and your physician about the need for replacement. Pacemakers are driven by batteries with a life of up to 15 years, and the devices will emit signals indicating that the time to replace them is nearing. Unlike a watch, the pacemaker cannot simply have its batteries replaced and go back to work. Because its case cannot be opened and reclosed and remain airtight, the old generator must be replaced with a new one containing a new battery supply.

Summary

These solutions for cardiac problems offer dramatic treatment improvements for patients. In scarcely a generation, coronary artery angioplasty has become a mainstay in treatment strategy, and thrombolytic therapy has emerged from experimental status to recognition as standard practice. With experience, physicians are advancing the art even further, tackling more complex cases.

CHAPTER FIFTEEN

Developments in Cardiovascular Surgery

Few medical specialties have shown the phenomenal progress that cardiovascular surgery has made during the past half century. A number of factors are responsible for this momentous advancement. Among the most important are: 1) development of relatively safe, readily applicable angiographic techniques, which permit precise delineation of the location, nature, and extent of disease in the heart and arterial system; 2) development of highly successful surgical procedures of vascular replacement (with restoration of normal circulation or replacement of the excised diseased segment with an arterial substitute); and 3) a tremendous surge of interest and intensification of investigative endeavors, undoubtedly a result of the stimulating initially successful surgical procedures for some cardiovascular problems that had long seemed hopeless.

Although the era of modern cardiovascular surgery may be considered to encompass the past four or five decades, certain developments preceding this period are not only of historical interest but are helpful in providing a better appreciation of subsequent events. The idea of suturing blood vessels was conceived more than two centuries ago by an Englishman named Lambert, who suggested the method to his colleague, Mr. Hallowell. On June 15, 1759, Hallowell successfully applied it to an artery in a patient's arm, which had been punctured for therapeutic bleeding—a popular treatment for various illnesses at that time. Further work on suturing blood vessels was soon discouraged because of the unsuccessful experiments of Conrad Asman of Groningen in the Netherlands in 1773, and the procedure was abandoned for more than a century. Additional factors that may have contributed to the decline of work along these lines were the prestige accorded the Hunterian ligature after its development in 1785 and the dominant concepts of Antonio Scarpa regarding the healing of aneurysms. John Hunter (1728 1793) was one of the great English surgeons and investigators who devised the principle of treating aneurysms (widening or dilatation) of the arteries of the limb by a single ligature (tying off of a blood vessel) applied to the healthy part of the artery well above the aneurysm. Of historical interest is the observation that in describing his procedure, Hunter made no reference to the fact that Antyllus, a contemporary of Galen in the second century, described ligation of the artery above and below an aneurysm (in the extremities only), and that Aetius of Amida, a Byzantine surgeon during the seventh century, described the same procedure without referring to Antyllus. Antonio Scarpa (1752–1832), a great and influential Italian surgeon and anatomist who lived in the late eighteenth and early nineteenth centuries and whose teachings had great influence, stated that ". . . a complete and radical cure of aneurysm cannot be obtained . . . unless the ulcerated, lacerated, or wounded artery from which the aneurysm is derived is, by the assistance or of nature combined with art, obliterated and converted into a perfectly solid ligamentous substance . . . ."

Toward the latter part of the nineteenth century, interest in vascular suturing was revived, probably because of the impetus given to experimental surgery by the Listerian doctrine, which, by providing an aseptic environment, greatly reduced the incidence of infection, a previously grave complication. Further interest in vascular suturing was stimulated in 1881 by its successful application in a patient with an injured jugular vein by Vincenz Czerny of Germany and by P. Postempski in Italy, five years later, in a lateral wound of the femoral artery. The development of endoaneurysmorrhaphy (obliteration of the lumen of an aneurysm by suturing together the inner wall and all openings to it) in 1888 by Rudolph Matas, one of the great American pioneers in vascular surgery, was a tremendous impetus to the revival of interest in the suturing of blood vessels. It provided the first successful challenge to the "law laid down by Scarpa" more than 100 years earlier. In 1889, Alexander Jassinowsky of Germany performed a series of experiments demonstrating the successful suturing of blood vessels.

The next few decades witnessed intense investigative activity in the field, both in America and abroad, distinguished by the work of a number of surgeons.[1] At the turn of the century several investigators, including particularly Alexis Carrel and C. C. Guthrie, had clearly demonstrated experimentally the feasibility of excising arterial segments and restoring continuity by end-

---

[1] Nikolai Eck, J. B. Murphy, Julius Dörfler, Erwin Payr, Alexis Carrel, C. C. Guthrie, E. Bode, E. Fabian, and Alexander Jassinowsky

to-end anastomosis or by use of arterial grafts, as well as by organ transplantation, such as the kidney and heart. A few patients with aneurysms or injuries of peripheral arteries had been treated by these methods with some success. In 1896, John Benjamin Murphy of Chicago, after establishing the success of the procedure in a series of experiments, resected about one-half inch of a patient's femoral artery that had been lacerated by a bullet and sutured the ends together. In 1906, D. José Goyanes of Spain reported the successful excision of an aneurysm of the popliteal artery with restoration of continuity by grafting a vein. The following year Professor E. Lexer, in Germany, reported a similar successful operation in the axillary artery.

Except for the individual efforts of a few surgeons at that time, little consideration was given to the application of these principles in the treatment of aortic disease. In 1902, for example, Professor Marin Théodore Tuffier of Paris reported an unsuccessful case of ligation of the neck, or opening of the aneurysm, in a patient with a sacciform (a saclike bulge from the arterial wall) aneurysm of the ascending aorta, but this experience convinced him of the feasibility of excisional therapy with lateral repair by suture. The foresight of some of these early scientists is further illustrated by another pioneering French surgeon, Professor René Leriche, who predicted in 1923 that

the ideal treatment for occlusive disease of the abdominal aorta (since termed Leriche's syndrome) would be excision of the diseased segment and its replacement with an aortic graft.

About 50 years were to elapse before Tuffier's recommendation was put into practice, and 30 years before Leriche's prediction became a reality. A number of factors contributed to this delay. For one thing, certain ancillary surgical measures, particularly induction of anesthesia, blood transfusions, chemotherapy, and antibiotic therapy, had not developed adequately to support extensive vascular procedures. For another, the specialty of surgery had not matured sufficiently to accept this more rigorous and aggressive approach to complex surgical problems. Finally, arteriography, an important diagnostic procedure for identifying the type and location of arterial disease, had not yet been developed.

The interest in vascular surgery was probably revived initially in 1944 by successful treatment of coarctation of the aorta (by excision and repair with end-to-end anastomosis) by Clarence Crafoord in Sweden and Robert Gross in Boston. A few years later, Robert Gross and Charles Hufnagel reported the successful repair, with aortic homografts (removed from a cadaver), of the defect in the aorta, resulting from excision of coarctation when the ends could not be approximated. Considerable impetus was thus given to further development of these approaches to treatment of arterial disease; this led to renewed interest in using homografts to bridge excised segments and thereby permitted broader application of this method to other aortic lesions. In 1951, J. Oudot in Paris reported the first case of occlusive disease on the lower abdominal aorta treated by excision and replacement with homograft, as originally recommended by René Leriche almost 30 years before. In the next year, Charles Dubost of Paris, and shortly afterwards, Michael E. DeBakey successfully performed the procedure for aneurysm of the abdominal aorta (Figure 15.1). In 1953, DeBakey also performed the first successful case of resection of fusiform aneurysm of the descending thoracic aorta with restoration

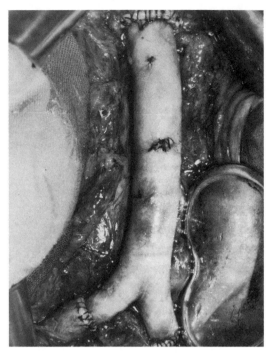

Figure 15.1. Photograph taken at operation showing aortic bifurcation homograft used to replace defect following resection of an aneurysm of the abdominal aorta (1952).

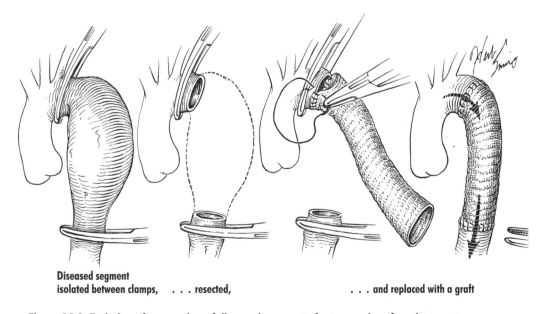

Diseased segment isolated between clamps,   . . . resected,   . . . and replaced with a graft

Figure 15.2. Technique for resection of diseased segment of artery and graft replacement.

of continuity by an aortic homograft (Figure 15.2), and in the following year, he did the first successful resection and graft replacement of an aneurysm of the descending thoracic aorta. During the next few years this method of surgical excision and graft replacement was also successfully used by DeBakey in the treatment of aneurysms of the ascending aorta, the thoracoabdominal segment, and the entire aortic arch, as well as in dissection and dissecting aneurysms of the aorta. Thus, within a decade, excisional therapy of aortic lesions

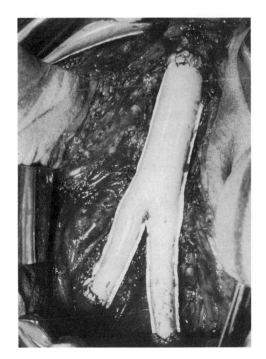

Figure 15.3. Photograph taken at operation showing Dacron® bifurcation graft made of two sheets of Dacron® cloth, with the edges sewn together on a sewing machine, used to replace the defect after resection of an aneurysm of the abdominal aorta on September 2, 1954.

had become a reality, and the centuries-old challenge had been successfully met.

During this early period, aortic and arterial homografts (removed from cadavers) were used to replace the excised diseased segments, and although they functioned satisfactorily, they had a number of disadvantages, the most important being their limited availability and the inconvenience of their procurement, sterilization, and preservation. Later studies also indicated that the tissue elements of the graft gradually deteriorated and led to complications. For these reasons, in 1950 DeBakey, as well as a number of other investigators, directed efforts toward development of an arterial substitute that had none of these disadvantages. Stimulated by the experimental observations of A. B. Voorhees, Jr., showing that a fabric woven of Vinyon "N" thread (a plastic) could function as an aortic substitute, DeBakey tried to obtain some similar plastic fabric, such as nylon, at a department store. He was informed by the store clerk that they had run out of nylon but had just received some new plastic fabric called Dacron.® DeBakey purchased a yard of this material and fabricated a tube-like structure of the Dacron® fabric by cutting two strips of appropriate width and sewing the edges on each side using his wife's sewing machine. These were then implanted in experimental animals to determine their safety and function.

Although other materials such as nylon, Orlon, and Teflon were subsequently studied experimentally in a similar manner, Dacron® was found to be the most satisfactory and is considered by DeBakey to be the best material even today. On the basis of these early experiments, DeBakey used such a Dacron® graft, made on his wife's sewing machine, for the first time to replace the defect after resection of an aneurysm of the abdominal aorta in a 54-year-old man on September 2, 1954 (Figure 15.3). The patient remained well for 10 years and then died suddenly of a heart attack.

With the assistance of Thomas Edman of Philadelphia, Professor and a textile expert, a new knitting machine was designed and built to produce seamless knitted Dacron® tubes in different sizes and in the form of bifurcations (Figure 15.4). An important feature of this Dacron® arterial substitute is its porosity, which permits the blood to seep through its wall until sufficient clotting has occurred in the interstices of the fabric to seal it and thus prevent further leakage of blood. This porosity also permits subsequent ingrowth of tissue to produce firm attachment of the new intima lining the inner surface. In other words, the body builds its own new tissue around the Dacron® fabric and thus creates a new artery.

Our experience with these Dacron® grafts as arterial substitutes for a variety of

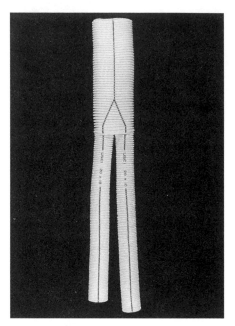

Figure 15.4. Dacron® bifurcation vascular graft.

aortic and arterial diseases in more than 50,000 patients has been extremely gratifying. Follow-up studies extending over a period of more than four decades have shown that the long-term function of these grafts is excellent. We have many patients with functioning grafts after 30 years. There is every reason to believe that these grafts should last the entire lifetime of the patient. Late failure of the graft may occur, but this is usually due to exacerbation of the disease in the artery distal to the anastomosis. The resulting decrease in blood flow through the graft may be sufficient to precipitate clotting in much the same way as when this occurs in the diseased artery.

During the early 1970s, DeBakey designed a new type of Dacron® graft, which was a result of his experimental work on the artificial heart. Efforts to find a better lining for these heart pumps led to the development of a velour fabric, which had the advantage of providing firm adherence of the new inner lining. This observation led us to experiment with velour as an arterial substitute. The Dacron® velour fabric is warp-knitted in such a way that loops of yarn are extended almost perpendicular to the fabric surface (Figure 15.5). This produces the velvety appearance that one sees on the inner surface of the graft. The fibrin and circulating cells become trapped and firmly attached to these loops. The ingrowth of tissue is better and more adherent to this velour surface. After laboratory experiments had demonstrated these advantages, we used the graft in patients, and experience now with thousands of cases has proved to be a further improve-

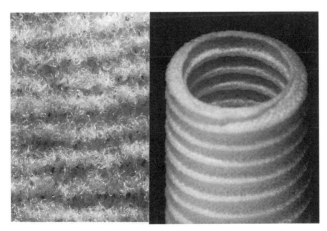

Figure 15.5. Magnified view (left) of velour fabric used to line interior. It is also used in some Dacron® vascular grafts for the exterior surface (right).

ment of previously used Dacron® grafts. More recently, DeBakey made an additional contribution by coating the Dacron® graft with albumin to seal the interstices of the graft, and thereby the need was obviated to use the patient's blood to clot and seal the graft. This is particularly important in patients whose clotting mechanism is temporarily blocked by heparin, which is necessary when the patient requires the use of the heart-lung machine. Experimental studies have shown that the albumin is absorbed in about six weeks, and healing around the graft takes place as it does in the absence of albumin.

In devising *endarterectomy* in 1947, Professor J. Cid dos Santos of Lisbon, Portugal, whose father performed the first abdominal aortography, made another important contribution to vascular surgery. After observing that certain forms of atherosclerosis could be easily peeled away from the remaining arterial wall (which he discovered by serendipity during an attempt to remove a clot in the femoral artery), he reasoned that this might constitute the basis for surgical treatment. In certain forms of atherosclerosis, the plaque-like lesion is well localized, with normal artery above and below it. This can be determined precisely by arteriography (radiographic visualization of the lumen of the artery after injection of radiopaque material).

The procedure of endarterectomy consists in applying occluding clamps to

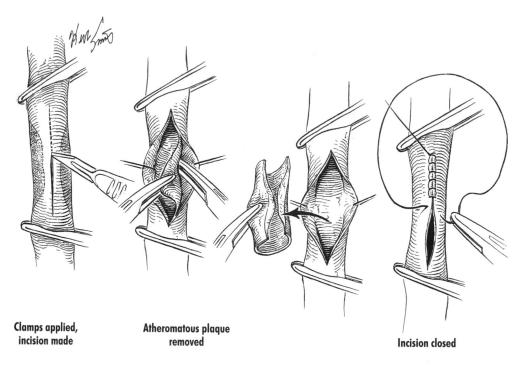

Clamps applied,
incision made

Atheromatous plaque
removed

Incision closed

Figure 15.6. Technique for removing atherosclerotic lesion by endarterectomy.

the artery above and below the lesion and then making a longitudinal incision through the arterial wall and the occluding lesion into the normal arterial wall immediately above and below the lesion (Figure 15.6). A proper cleavage plane is then found at the base of the lesion, usually between the media and intima, and it is carefully separated and peeled away from the remaining arterial wall with a blunt-ended instrument in much the same way as one would peel the skin of an orange. After the atheromatous plaque has been completely removed, the edges of the remaining arterial wall are sewed together or by use of a patch graft, and blood flow

through this new lumen is restored by removal of the occluding clamps. The procedure was rapidly and widely adopted by vascular surgeons and has proved to be eminently successful when properly applied.

Another contribution in this connection was the development of *patch-graft angioplasty* by DeBakey. It was observed that after completion of endarterectomy, closure of the incision in the arterial wall sometimes necessitated use of some of the circumference of the arterial wall, and this caused narrowing of the resulting lumen. To overcome this, a patch of Dacron® fabric, or a small segment of vein that was

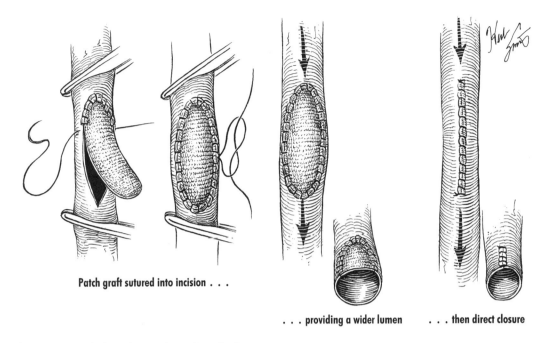

Patch graft sutured into incision . . .

. . . providing a wider lumen   . . . then direct closure

Figure 15.7. Technique for patch-graft angioplasty.

slit open, was inserted between the two edges of the artery and sutured into place (Figure 15.7). This provided an excellent method of repairing the opening in the artery without narrowing the lumen. We later found this method useful in certain types of arterial disease in which the lumen was narrowed, but in which endarterectomy was not indicated. The narrowed arterial segment could thus be widened by use of such a patch graft and blood flow restored through the normal lumen.

Still another important contribution to vascular surgery was made by Professor J. Kunlin of France, with whom DeBakey

had the good fortune to be associated as a foreign assistant working under Professor René Leriche at the University of Strasbourg. Professor Kunlin observed that certain forms of occlusive disease in the arteries of the leg were well localized and that beyond the diseased segment the artery was normal. Circulation to the leg beyond the obstructed segment was maintained through small collateral communications, which is nature's way of trying to overcome the decreased circulation produced by the obstructed arterial segment. Circulation through these small vessels may be adequate to maintain viability, but it is often not adequate to

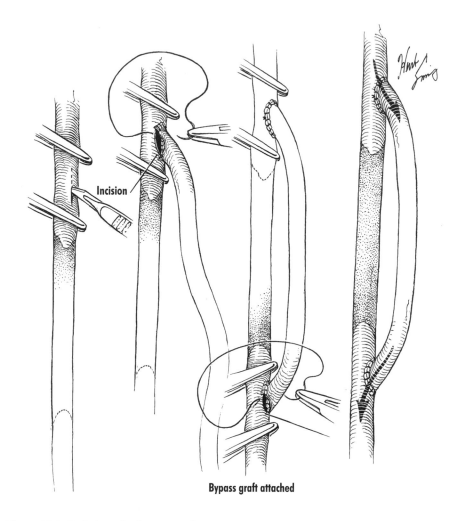

Incision

Bypass graft attached

Figure 15.8. Technique for bypass graft to shunt blood around diseased segment of artery.

maintain normal function. On this basis, Professor Kunlin reasoned that it should be possible to aid nature's efforts to restore circulation around the obstructed segment by attaching a graft (using a segment of the vein taken from the leg) to an opening in the side of the normal artery above the obstructed segment, and then in similar fashion, to the normal artery below the obstructed segment (Figure 15.8). In this way, blood would be shunted through the graft around the obstructed segment, and thus normal circulation would be restored. For this reason, the operation is referred to as a *bypass graft*.

In 1949, Professor J. Kunlin reported successful performance of this procedure on a patient suffering from circulatory problems in the leg due to occlusion of the femoral artery. Since then, this method has been widely used to restore circulation for various types of disease. It is of historical interest that Ernst Jeger, a young German surgeon, described and illustrated the concept of this bypass procedure in 1915 but never actually performed it. He died shortly thereafter while serving in the German army in World War I.

One of the most important contributions to cardiovascular surgery was the development of angiography, which provided the underlying basis for many brilliant achievements in the field. This diagnostic procedure made possible the radiographic visualization and precise delineation of diseases of the heart and blood vessels. It also established the fact that many arterial lesions are well localized to one segment, with relatively normal arteries above and below the lesion, and are therefore amenable to direct surgical treatment.

Radiographic visualization of the blood vessels became a reality shortly after the monumental discovery of x-rays by Wilhelm Konrad Roentgen of Germany in 1895. Within a month of this epochal discovery, scientists began experimenting with its potential clinical application for such ailments as bone fractures. In January 1896, E. von Haschek and O. T. Lindenthal of Germany injected a *radiopaque* substance into the blood vessels of an amputated hand, and thus first demonstrated the feasibility of radiographic visualization of blood vessels.

The potential diagnostic value of this procedure fired the imagination of a number of medical scientists. The major problem that limited the clinical application of the method was the need for an injectable, non-toxic, opaque substance. This problem proved difficult to resolve, and indeed, it was not until 1923 that the next major advance occurred. Two French scientists, J. A. Siccard and J. Forrestier, injected into a patient's femoral veins Lipiodol, an oil-iodine mixture that they had developed to visualize the bronchial tree on the x-ray, and watched it on the fluoroscope proceed to the heart and then to the lungs. In the same year two German scientists, J. Berberich and S. Hirsch, developed a bromide solution that they used to demonstrate arteriography and venography for the first time in a living man. The next year, Barney Brooks, an American surgeon, showed that injection of sodium iodide provided good visualization of the arteries of the legs, was useful in visualizing atheromatous disease of the arteries, and could indicate when amputation was necessary. It took nearly a half century of intensive investigation before finally developing a non-toxic, injectable, radiopaque substance for clinical use.

The early twentieth century was an exciting developmental period for angiography. Medical scientists from different parts of the world were eagerly pursuing the clinical objective of devising a unique and precise diagnostic procedure. The Portuguese medical scientists proved to be pioneers in this endeavor. Thus, Egas Moniz, a Portuguese neurosurgeon, devised the technique of carotid arteriography to visualize the arteries of the brain, and later, *angiopneumography,* to visualize the pulmonary vessels. R. dos Santos of Lisbon devised the technique of translumbar aortography, a method still used today but with much safer radiopaque solutions and simple use of percutaneous catheter insertion.

Although the technical feasibility and diagnostic value of arteriography had by then been demonstrated, the injectable solutions used were still not satisfactory; they were often irritating and produced other undesirable complications. A substance was needed that provided good radiographic visualization but produced no untoward reactions. An important breakthrough toward this objective came in 1929, when M. Swick of Germany reported the use of an organic iodide solution developed by two German scientists, A. Binz and C. Roth. This stimulated other workers to synthesize other radiopaque drugs that finally led to highly effective and safe injectable solutions as are used today.

Cardioangiography and cardiac catheterization were also major developments

that significantly influenced cardiac surgery. Studies in this regard began in 1928 with the experiments of Werner Forssmann of Germany, who became intrigued with the idea of cardiac catheterization as a means of injecting therapeutic drugs directly into the heart. Working on cadavers, he easily inserted a catheter into a vein in the arm and moved it to the right atrium. He did the first clinical experiment on himself despite the fact that his chief, after Forssmann informed him of his idea, forbade it. Using a fine catheter ordinarily used for urologic purposes and with the aid of an assistant, he inserted the catheter through a wide-bore needle into one of the veins in his arm. As the catheter approached his heart, his assistant became so fearful that he refused to continue, and the trial ended. But with the firm conviction of a dedicated scientist, Forssmann decided to proceed by himself a week later. After inserting the catheter through a vein in his arm and pushing it into his right atrium, he walked a distance, up stairs, to the x-ray room and radiographically confirmed the location of the catheter. Later, using this same technique, he injected a radiopaque substance through the catheter into the right atrium and obtained a roentgenogram of the cardiac chambers. The next day he thought he should tell his professor that he had performed the procedure, and by showing him the x-ray, his professor would be pleased. Unfortunately, his professor, the eminent Ernst Ferdinand Sauerbruch, reacted angrily and promptly fired him with the comment: "With such circus tricks you never can obtain a position in a decent German clinic." He later entered general practice and subsequently was correctly recognized by being awarded the Nobel Prize, along with A. Cournand and Dickinson W. Richards in 1956. During the next decade, several investigators[2] added further significant technical improvements and refinements and thus made it a versatile diagnostic method applicable to all forms of cardiovascular disease.

Medical history abounds with pioneering surgical developments stimulated by military or civilian injuries. This is particularly true of some of the early surgical procedures on the heart. In the early nineteenth century Baron Larrey, Napoleon's great military surgeon, successfully drained blood and fluid from the pericardial sac around the heart, and thus defied the erroneous prediction by a distinguished English surgeon, Stephen Paget, who had just previously written that ". . . surgery of the heart has probably reached the limits set by nature to all surgery. No new methods and no new discovery can overcome the natural difficulties that attend a wound of the heart." Another distinguished Professor of Surgery in Vienna, T. H. Billroth, expressed this rather prevailing pessimistic attitude by writing, in 1893, that "A surgeon who tries to suture a heart would lose the esteem of his colleagues." Yet only three years later, another German surgeon, Ludwig Rehn, successfully sutured a wound of the heart.

The first successful case of suture of the heart in the United States was performed by L. L. Hill, the father of the late distinguished Senator Lister Hill of Alabama. The operation was performed on September 14, 1902, on a 13-year-old boy who had been stabbed causing a wound in the left ventricle. The operation was performed on a table in the cabin of the boy's parents at one o'clock at night, about 8 hours after the stabbing, with two lamps to provide light for the surgeon. The patient recovered completely. In his report of this case, published in the *Medical Record* in 1902, Hill reviewed the medical publications on the subject and found 38 cases in addition to his own, with recovery in 12. He strongly recommended operation for this type of injury. In 1903, Professor Marin Théodore Tuffier, a famous French surgeon, removed a bullet that had lodged in the wall of the left atrium. During World

<hr>

[2] P. Rosthoi of Sweden, P. Ameuille of France, A. Castellanos of Cuba, and G. P. Robb, I. Steinberg, and F. M. Sones of the United States

War II, Dwight Harken, a distinguished American surgeon, demonstrated the feasibility of removing retained foreign bodies in the heart, and thus provided another illustration of how surgery of trauma inspired further advances.

The first cardiac operation, exclusive of traumatic cases, was performed by a French surgeon, Edmond Delorme, in 1898 for infection of the pericardium; the operation was also later done by the German surgeon, V. Schmieden. In 1902, Sir Thomas Lauder Brunton advocated surgical treatment for mitral stenosis, but more than two decades elapsed before his suggestion was followed. In the meantime, two French surgeons attempted to dilate stenosed heart valves. In 1913, Eugéne Doyen attempted to dilate a stenotic pulmonary valve, and one year later, Théodore Tuffier made a similar attempt on the aortic valve, but with little success. In 1923, Elliott Cutler and S. A. Levine of Boston devised a special valvulotome, which could be inserted into the chamber of the heart to cut the mitral valve. They performed this operation on a few patients with limited success. Two years later, Sir Henry S. Souttar, an English surgeon, inserted his left forefinger through an opening in the left atrium to feel the stenosed mitral valve, but found that it was already dilated, and he decided not to section the valve. Although convinced of the feasibility of the procedure, he later

complained that he could get no other case ". . . as medical opinion was solidly against such attempts." It was not until the late 1940s that further attempts along these lines were revived by Dwight Harken of Boston, Charles Bailey of Philadelphia, and Lord Brock of London. The great interest stimulated by their successes led other surgeons to make technical improvements in the operation, and within a few years, the procedures were widely adopted for certain forms of mitral and pulmonary stenosis.

Although as early as 1907, John Munro of Boston had proposed tying off a patent ductus arteriosis, the treatment for congenital abnormalities of the heart remained ineffective. In 1937, Ashton Graybiel, John Strieder, and N. H. Boyer of Boston made an unsuccessful attempt to ligate a patent ductus arteriosus. The next year, however, Robert Gross of Boston performed the procedure successfully, and thus initiated great interest in the surgical attack on certain congenital anomalies. This was further enhanced by the successful surgical treatment of coarctation of the aorta by Clarence Crafoord of Stockholm in 1944, and by Robert Gross of Boston shortly thereafter. Additional impetus was provided by the successful "blue baby" operation by Alfred Blalock and Helen Taussig of Baltimore in 1945, consisting in anastomosing the subclavian artery to the pulmonary artery, in order to increase the blood flow through the lung and thereby obtain a higher blood oxygen content.

Congenital defects, such as patent ductus arteriosus and coarctation of the aorta, were amenable to surgical correction because the surgeon was operating on blood vessels outside of the heart. Beyond these abnormalities were all those congenital and acquired cardiac diseases and injuries that could be corrected only by opening the heart. Until a safe way to open the heart could be discovered, the vast range of cardiac diseases remained beyond the surgeon's skill.

The primary obstacle to further progress was how to maintain circulation of the blood to the rest of the body, particularly the brain, with its need for a constant supply of oxygenated blood, while interrupting the work of the heart for a few hours. The brain will survive for approximately four minutes without permanent damage if its supply of oxygenated blood is blocked.

To gain sufficient operating time, surgeons experimented with *hypothermia,* a procedure in which the patient is packed in ice or wrapped in refrigerated blankets to cool the body well below the normal temperature. Experiments on animals had shown that hypothermia reduces cardiac output, pulse rate, blood pressure, and oxygen consumption. Cells, including those of the brain, survive longer when chilled. But cooling and then warming the body

often resulted in serious adverse effects. In some patients, ventricular fibrillation developed—instead of the muscle fibers of the heart uniting in coordinated contraction and relaxation, a rapid flutter of separate strands of muscle occurred. The dispersion of effort by heart muscle that is too weak to pump blood causes immediate death.

The possibility of extracorporeal circulation, that is, circulating the patient's blood outside the body to keep it supplied with oxygen while stopping the pumping heart, became the objective of an intense search. Such a mechanical device would need to perform two complicated functions: the steady pumping of blood that did not damage delicate cells and adequate oxygenation of blood. Efforts to construct such a machine date back to 1885. For a brief time, scientists toyed with the idea of using a lung removed from an animal and aerated by artificial respiration to oxygenate blood, but that approach was considered unsuitable for humans. Others experimented and a few actually used a human donor temporarily connected to the patient for cross circulation, but none of these methods proved a satisfactory solution to the problem.

In the United States, the development of the heart-lung machine owes much to the pioneering work of John Gibbon of Philadelphia. In 1931, while a Resident in a Boston hospital, he treated a 53-year-old woman dying from a series of blood clots that blocked her pulmonary artery. In a letter to a friend, Gibbon recalled,

> During the 17 hours by this patient's side, the thought constantly recurred that the patient's hazardous condition could be improved if some of the blue blood in the patient's distended veins could be continuously withdrawn into an apparatus where the blood could pick up oxygen and discharge carbon dioxide and then be pumped back into the patient's arteries. Such a procedure would also lend support to the patient's circulation while the embolectomy (removal of the clots) was performed.

During an emergency operation on the woman, the surgeon removed the emboli in only six and one-half minutes, but the patient died on the operating table, for lack of a life-supporting system as Gibbon described.

Three years later, Gibbon began to design a heart-lung machine at the Massachusetts General Hospital. He reminisced, "I bought an air pump in a second hand shop down in East Boston for a few dollars, and used it to activate the . . . blood pumps." To test his apparatus, he experimented with cats.

Gibbon eventually proved that animals could survive 30 to 40 minutes of complete bypass of their own hearts and lungs while supported by his machine. Most of his animals died, however, a few hours after their own circulation was restored.

Apparently, the pumping mechanism seriously damaged blood cells, and thus produced fatal clots.

During this period, Michael DeBakey designed a roller pump to study the pulse wave and later to facilitate direct transfusions of blood from donor to patient. This pump's rollers moved blood without injury to its cellular components. DeBakey suggested to Gibbon that he try this pump, which he then installed in his machine and found to be highly effective. Since then, it has become the standard pump for heart-lung machines. Still, the oxygenation process seemed to be insufficient for the needs of an animal, to say nothing of a human. World War II delayed further research, but in 1945 Gibbon resumed work on this project. He convinced International Business Machines to assign some of its technicians and engineers to help him construct a heart-lung machine.

In 1950, about 19 years after Gibbon's initial effort to develop a life-supporting mechanical system outside of the human body, he decided his machine was ready for use. His first patient, a 15-month-old baby, died shortly after the operation. Instead of the atrial defect originally diagnosed, the infant had a large patent ductus arteriosus. Gibbon's second attempt on May 6, 1953, was on an 18-year-old girl with an atrioseptal defect. The heart-lung machine functioned beautifully, and the operation was a total success. It seemed that the feasibility of the total heart-lung bypass had been proved, and this encouraged others to perfect the oxygenating component of the machine.

The principle of the heart-lung machine, or, as it is termed medically, cardiopulmonary bypass, is relatively simple (Figure 15.9). It consists essentially in diverting all the venous blood returning to

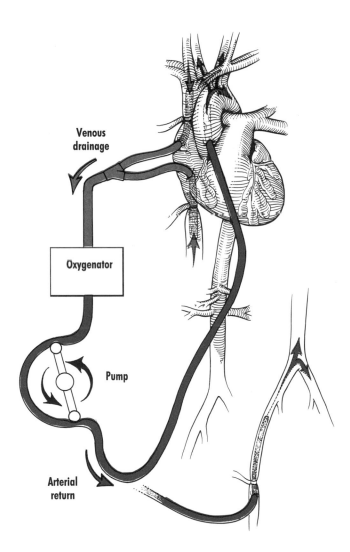

Venous drainage

Oxygenator

Pump

Arterial return

Figure 15.9. The heart-lung machine, or cardiopulmonary bypass, oxygenates the venous blood from the patient and then pumps it throughout the arterial system via the ascending aorta or the common femoral artery.

the heart to the artificial lung of the heart-lung machine, where oxygen is added and carbon dioxide is removed. The refreshed oxygenated blood is then pumped into the arterial system of the patient. In this way, the functions of the heart and lungs are temporarily assumed by the machine. Thus, life-supporting circulation is provided to the rest of the body while certain types of corrective surgical procedures are performed within the heart or on one of its vessels.

The procedure is usually performed by inserting two plastic cannulas through the wall of the right atrium into the upper and lower venae cavae, the two major veins returning blood to the heart. By encircling and tightening two cotton tapes placed around the venae cavae and around the inserted plastic tubes, all blood from the venae cavae is shunted into the heart-lung machine. After passing through the artificial lung, the blood is returned to the patient by means of the pump through a plastic tube inserted into one of the major arteries in the groin or into the ascending aorta. Some variations in this procedure may be necessary, depending on the patient's condition and specific problems.

CHAPTER SIXTEEN

Congenital Abnormalities of the Heart

The first major cardiovascular disorders to yield to corrective treatment were congenital defects, and their repair required surgical correction. To comprehend what was involved requires knowledge of the evolution of the heart, from conception to birth.

Toward the end of the first month of fetal life, the heart begins to develop (Figure 16.1). During four more weeks a fully-formed, tiny replica of an adult heart has formed. The process starts with a group of cells organizing themselves into a hollow tube; one end is called the venous and the other, the arterial. The tube grows faster than the space around it. Under the pressure of confinement, the tube bends, first into a "U" and then an "S" shape. The venous end bulges into a pocket that eventually will form both the right and left atria. Meanwhile, the middle section of the original hollow tube expands into a bag shape, which will form the right and left ventricles; clumps of cells arrange themselves into the vital mitral and tricuspid valves.

At the arterial end of the original hollow tube, another division occurs. A partition separates the once-single trunk into two channels: the aorta and the pulmonary artery. Obeying the genetic instructions for human embryonic development, the other cells dutifully build the tissue of the aortic and pulmonary valves.

A bare two months after conception, the fetal heart looks like an adult heart, but a major portion of its functions remains dependent on the mother. This dependence continues even after the fetal heart begins to beat during the later stages of pregnancy. The oxygenation of blood to feed the growing tissue of the fetus and the elimination of waste occur in the mother's placenta (Figure 16.2). Oxygenated blood passes through the umbilical cord into the *ductus venosus* of the fetus, a vessel that bypasses the unborn's liver and leads directly to the inferior vena cava, and hence to the right atrium. Unlike a normal adult, whose blood in the right atrium lacks oxygen, the fetus collects oxygenated blood into this chamber from the inferior

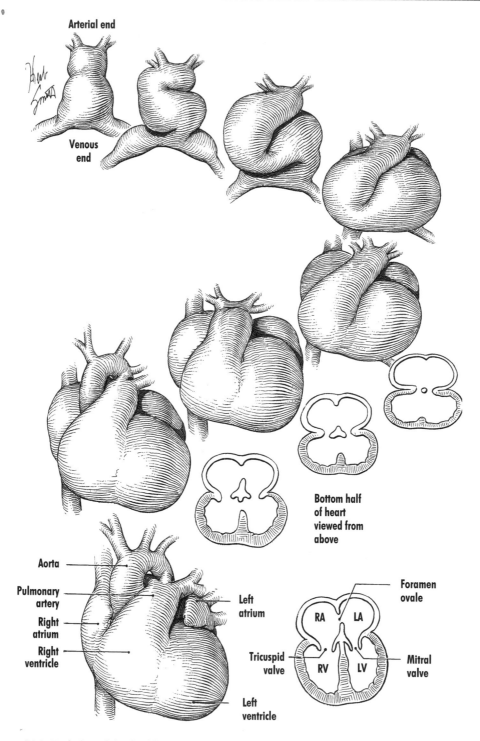

Figure 16.1. Evolution of the fetal heart.

vena cava. Because of the *foramen ovale* (the opening between the atria), some of the oxygenated blood in the right atrium conventionally enters the right ventricle and is pumped out into the pulmonary arteries during systole. But instead of flowing the length of the pulmonary artery, most blood is diverted before it reaches the lungs into the *ductus arteriosus,* a fetal blood vessel that connects the

pulmonary artery with the aorta. The fetal lungs, which do not breathe while inside the womb, require only enough blood to nourish the growing tissue. Meanwhile, the oxygenated blood, flowing through the foramen ovale into the left atrium, reaches the left ventricle and is pumped into the aorta.

At birth, a new circulatory system develops in the infant (Figure 16.3). As the

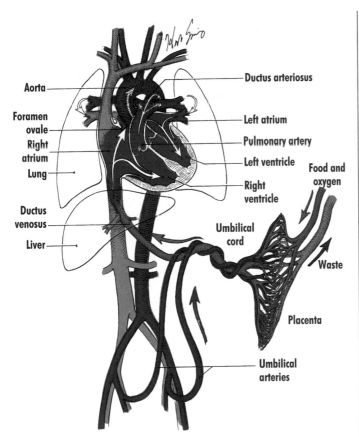

Figure 16.2. During pregnancy, the mother's placenta provides oxygen and food to the fetal circulation and eliminates waste from the fetus.

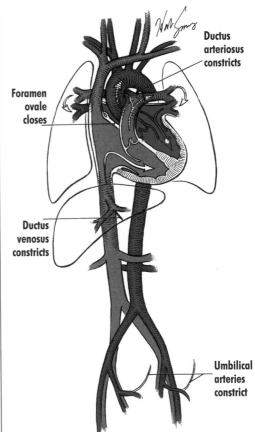

Figure 16.3. At birth the infant's circulatory system becomes self-sufficient.

baby begins to breathe, the ductus arteriosus constricts, and this closes the communication between the pulmonary artery and the aorta. Unused, the ductus arteriosus normally degenerates into a solid cord of tissue called the ligamentum arteriosum. Now blood pumped from the right ventricle can flow into the lungs. It returns to the left side of the heart through the pulmonary veins. During contraction of the heart, the left atrium exerts hydraulic pressure, which prevents the flow of any blood from the right atrium to the left. The foramen ovale is so constructed that this continued high pressure in the left atrium over the period of a year turns the foramen ovale into a flap that seals the prenatal opening. The ductus venosus, the original pipeline from the mother's placenta, also loses its function and turns into a ligament across the lower half of the child's liver.

This complicated mechanism of cellular growth and organization characterizes the development of every human heart. Whereas any manufacturer would be delighted with the remarkably high rate of flawless units that mark human reproduction, the small percentage of imperfections (less than 1 per 1,000) poses grave threats to the lives of those with such congenital defects.

Patent Ductus Arteriosus

The first human congenital cardiac defect to be corrected surgically was patent ductus arteriosus, the fetal vessel between the pulmonary artery and the aorta that fails to close (Figure 16.4). Some researchers believe that German measles in the mother during the early months of pregnancy may cause this condition, which heightens pressure in the pulmonary artery. It is estimated to occur in about one in 2,500 to 5,000 births, and it affects females more often then males.

Symptoms produced by this defect vary depending on the size of the ductus and the amount of blood shunted from the aorta into the pulmonary artery. Most infants with this condition tire more quickly than those without it. Often, the disorder retards growth, and heart failure

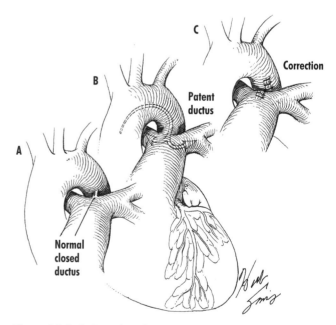

Figure 16.4. A. Drawing showing normal closure of patent ductus arteriosus;
B. Failure of normal closure;
C. Surgical procedure, consisting in division and suture closure.

may also occur. Another threat of patent ductus seems to be that bacterial infection often develops around the defect. Usually, diagnosis can be easily made soon after birth by detection of a characteristic murmur and can be readily confirmed by two-dimensional echocardiography.

As early as 1907, John Munro of Boston proposed a procedure to tie off, or ligate, a patent ductus. He had worked extensively on cadavers, but surgeons were reluctant to attempt the operation on their patients because the diagnosis could not be made with certainty by the available methods of the time. After adequate research had been done to clearly identify the syndrome of patent ductus, a new assault on the defect began. In 1938, a young surgical assistant resident at Boston Children's Hospital, Robert Gross, ligated a 7-year-old girl's patent ductus with a single-braid silk suture. This feat convinced surgeons that the condition could be corrected surgically.

If left uncorrected, a patent ductus can lead to serious complications and early death in most patients. Even if the infant survives the early period in life, pulmonary vascular resistance may occur and cause the condition to become inoperable. For this reason, and because the risk of operation is virtually zero if performed within the first few years of life, surgical correction is the only effective therapy. The procedure consists essentially in division and suture closure (Figure 16.4).

Coarctation of the Thoracic Aorta

Coarctation of the aorta is a relatively common abnormality representing 5 to 10 percent of congenital heart disease and is twice as common in males than females. Associated anomalies may also be present, including particularly bicuspid aortic valve, ventricular septal defect, patent ductus arteriosus, and mitral valve disorders.

The lesion consists in severe narrowing or constriction of the aorta that produces an obstruction to blood flow. Although it may occur at various sites in the aorta, it is most commonly found as a localized constriction at the insertion of the ductus or ligamentum arteriosum (Figure 16.5). More diffuse narrowing, which may also occur, is referred to as *tubular hypoplasia*. It increases blood pressure in the arms and reduces blood flow in the legs. It causes high blood pressure because the heart must pump harder to provide adequate circulation beyond the narrowed segment. Victims of coarctation usually do not live longer than 50 years unless the condition is corrected.

Symptoms of coarctation depend on the location and severity of the narrowing and the presence of other heart defects. When it occurs alone it may cause few symptoms. These children may complain of headache, cold arms and legs, or leg pain on exercise, and over time, the upper body may become more developed than the lower body.

The human body makes a valiant effort to compensate for a disorder such as coarctation of the aorta. Blood vessels branching off the subclavian arteries in the upper half of the body enlarge and communicate with other arteries to provide some circulation to regions below the point of coarctation. Because of this collateral circulation, symptoms of coarctation may not appear early in life, and for some patients the condition goes unnoticed through young adulthood.

The diagnosis can usually be made by clinical examination with such findings as high blood pressure in the arms and much lower blood pressure in the legs, reduced or even absent femoral pulses, and a loud systolic murmur over the upper left side of the chest. Rib notching on the x-ray of the chest is a common finding. The diagnosis can be confirmed by angiocardiography, which provides precise visualization of the location and extent of the narrowing.

Early surgical correction of coarctation is recommended, preferably between the ages of 3 and 7 years, unless early heart failure requires immediate correction. Repair in late childhood or adulthood may be associated with persistent hypertension. Technically, the simplest and most commonly employed procedure consists in clamping the aorta above and below the

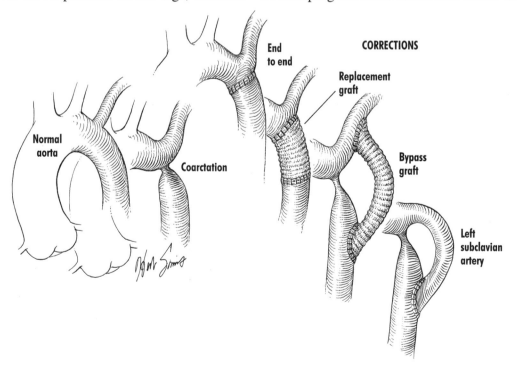

Figure 16.5. Several methods of operative treatment may be used, depending on a number of factors, including particularly extent of the coarctated segment.

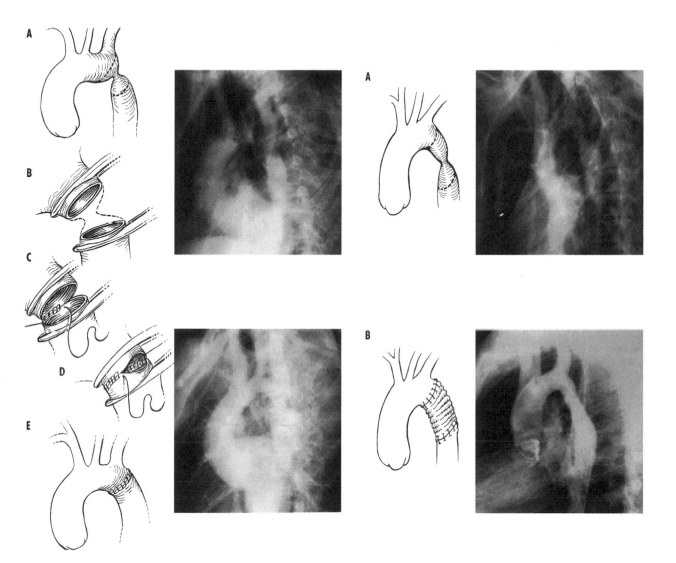

Figure 16.6. A. Drawing showing method of surgical treatment of coarctation of thoracic aorta, consisting in B. excision of coarctated segment between occluding clamps and C., D., and E. suture anastomosis of the two open ends of the aortic wall.
Above: Preoperative aortogram of a 14-year-old boy with typical manifestations of coarctation of the aorta showing severe narrowing in aorta just distal to the origin of left subclavian artery.
Below: Postoperative aortogram shows restoration of normal aortic lumen.

Figure 16.7. A. Drawing and preoperative aortogram of a 14-year-old boy, showing coarctation in the usual site in the descending thoracic aorta just below origin of left subclavian artery.
B. Drawing showing method of surgical treatment, consisting in resection of coarctated segment and replacement with Dacron® graft, and aortogram made 22 years after operation, showing restoration of normal circulation in aorta. Patient remains well now, 33 years after operation.

constriction, excising the coarctated segment, and reattaching the two ends by end-to-end suture anastomosis (Figure 16.6). This was first performed successfully on a 12-year-old boy with coarctation by Clarence Crafoord of Sweden, in 1944. In some patients, the coarctated segment may be of such length that after its excision it is not possible to bring the two ends together for end-to-end anastomosis. Robert Gross and Charles Hufnagel demonstrated first experimentally and then clinically that such a defect could be bridged by means of a homograft, that is, a segment of aorta removed at autopsy. Since then, a Dacron® graft was developed and is used for this purpose (Figures 16.5 and 16.7). Other surgical procedures include the use of patch-graft aortoplasty or turning down the subclavian artery for this purpose (Figure 16.5). Still another method consists in using a bypass Dacron® graft from the left subclavian artery to the aorta below the coarctation (Figures 16.5 and 16.8).

Early surgical correction of coarctation is recommended and, ideally, should be done between the ages of 3 and 7 or 8 years, unless early heart failure requires immediate correction. Today, surgical correction consists essentially in excising the coarctated segment and reconnecting the two ends or in some cases, in which this cannot be done because the resulting defect is too long, by replacing the segment with a Dacron® graft. In some

A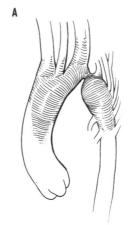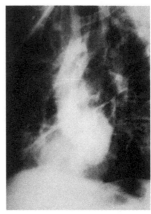

B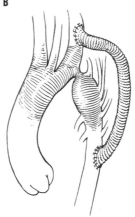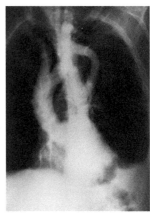

Figure 16.8. A. Drawing and preoperative aortogram showing coarctation of the thoracic aorta in the most common site just below origin of left subclavian artery.
B. Drawing showing method of surgical treatment, consisting in Dacron® graft bypass from left subclavian artery to descending thoracic aorta. Postoperative aortogram shows Dacron® graft restoring normal circulation to aorta below coarctation. Patient remained well for 15 years.

older patients, it may be preferable to use a bypass graft.

In uncomplicated forms of coarctation, the risk of operation is low, about 1 or 2 percent, and the results are excellent. In our own experience with surgical treatment of a large series of patients with follow-up studies extending up to 30 years, the operative mortality rate was 1.6 percent (Figure 16.7). The blood pressure was restored to normal and maintained after operation in 87 percent of patients operated on at age 13 years or younger, whereas in patients older than 21 years, only 47 percent were restored to normal; these statistics emphasize the significance of early operation.

Survival expectancy was also found to be significantly related to age. Thus, among patients operated on at age 13 years or younger, survival expectancy at 30 years was 98 percent, at 13 to 21 years it was 94 percent, but in those older than 30 years, it ranged between 74 and 56 percent. The patient's blood pressure should be monitored regularly since it may be elevated later in life and require medical treatment.

Coarctation of the Abdominal Aorta

Although coarctation of the aorta usually affects the thoracic aorta as described earlier, occasionally it may involve other segments of the aorta, particularly the abdominal aorta, thereby affecting the origins of the major arteries supplying blood to the abdominal organs (Figure 16.9). It has been estimated that this type of coarctation occurs in about 2 percent of the cases. It seems to occur more commonly in females in a ratio of about three or four to one and becomes apparent at an early age, with most cases being diagnosed during the first two decades of life. The coarctated segment varies in extent from a small localized segment, often just above the renal arteries, to longer involvement of the entire abdominal aorta, including the origins of the celiac, superior mesenteric, and renal arteries.

Among the most important signs and symptoms of the condition are severe hypertension (high blood pressure), headache, fatigue after minimal exercise, and decreased blood pressure in the legs. If untreated, the prognosis is poor, with eventual death from heart failure or cerebral hemorrhage.

Treatment is surgical and consists in placing a bypass graft from the descending thoracic aorta to the abdominal aorta. Since the renal arteries are also involved in most patients, it is usually necessary to place additional bypass grafts to these arteries (Figure 16.9). Occasionally, bypasses to the celiac and superior mesenteric arteries are also necessary.

Results of operation are excellent. We have had no deaths, and all of our patients responded favorably, with restoration of normal blood pressure and resumption of normal activities. Many of our patients

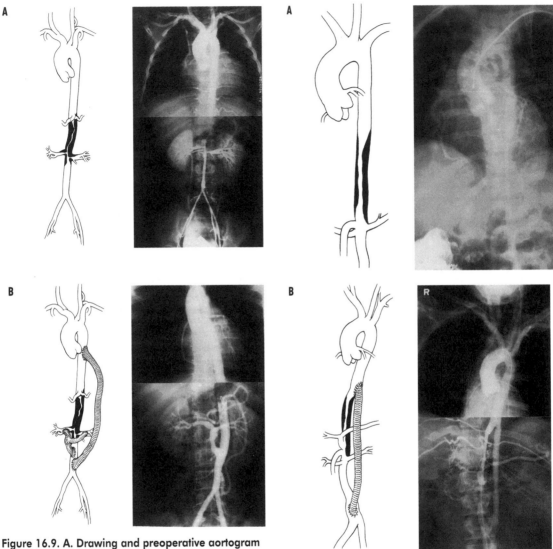

Figure 16.9. A. Drawing and preoperative aortogram of a 7-year-old girl with severe hypertension and absent pulses in legs, showing coarctation of abdominal aorta with severe narrowing of abdominal aorta below celiac artery and extending to involve origin of the renal arteries.

B. Drawing showing method of surgical treatment, consisting in a Dacron® bypass graft from descending thoracic aorta above coarctated segment to abdominal aorta below occlusion, and bypass graft to both renal arteries. Aortogram made nine years after operation shows restoration of normal circulation to terminal abdominal aorta and both renal arteries. Patient remains asymptomatic 17 years since operation and has recently graduated from university.

Figure 16.10. A. Drawing and preoperative aortogram of a 5-year-old boy with severe hypertension and cramps in legs on exertion, showing severe abdominal coarctation.

B. Drawing showing method of surgical treatment, consisting in bypass Dacron® graft from descending thoracic aorta to lower abdominal aorta, and aortogram made 28 years after operation, showing restoration of normal circulation through bypass graft. Patient remains well.

followed as long as 30 years after operation have continued to lead normal lives (Figure 16.10).

Anomalies of the Aortic Arch Causing Vascular Rings

In the embryologic development of the aortic arch, certain abnormalities may occur that result in *vascular rings,* which surround the esophagus and trachea and may produce symptoms of obstruction (Figure 16.11). Among the most common of the several varieties of this abnormality are the double aortic arch and the right aortic arch associated with a segment passing behind the esophagus and a left-sided

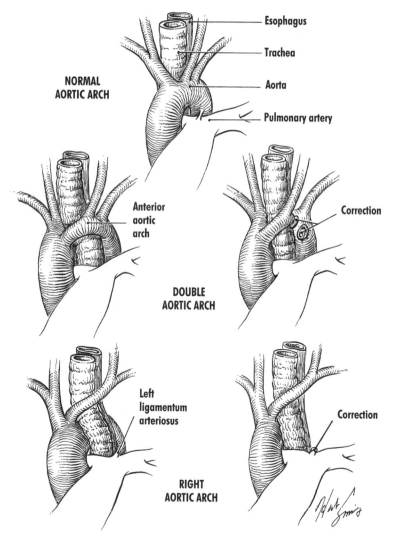

Figure 16.11. Various forms of vascular rings and their surgical treatment.

ligamentum arteriosum. Many patients with this type of abnormality remain asymptomatic and appear to lead normal lives. Under these circumstances, no treatment is necessary. If symptoms develop, they usually occur in infancy or early life and are manifested by noisy respiration, difficulty in swallowing, and repeated pulmonary infections. Under these circumstances, surgical treatment is recommended, consisting in dividing and ligating or closing the ends of the smaller of the two aortic arches or the left-sided ligamentum arteriosum. Results of operation are excellent, with little or no risk.

Tetralogy of Fallot

In 1888, a French physician, Etienne-Louis Arthur Fallot, described a four-fold congenital malady of the heart, tetralogy of Fallot, which bears his name. Although four separate problems are recognized in this condition, the primary defects are a narrowed pulmonary valve and an opening in the septal wall between the ventricles (Figure 16.12). In addition, there is biventricular origin of the aorta and right ventricular hypertrophy. The defective valve prevents an adequate amount of blood from being pumped through the pulmonary artery to

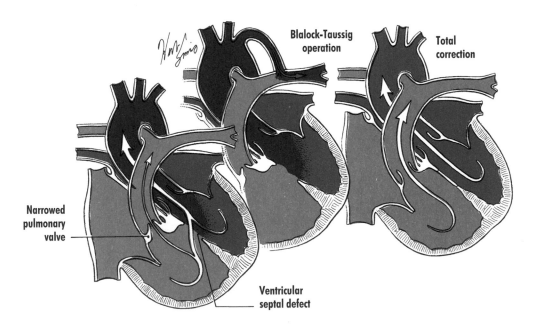

Figure 16.12. Anatomic abnormalities of the heart in tetralogy of Fallot, consisting in stenosis of pulmonary valve, ventricular septal defect, biventricular origin of the aorta, and hypertrophy of the right ventricle, and methods of surgical treatment.

the lungs, and the hole in the septum permits unoxygenated blood to mix with the normally oxygenated supply in the left ventricle. As a result, the child receives a grossly inadequate supply of oxygenated blood, which is often manifested by a bluish tinge called cyanosis—a sign that has popularized the abnormality as the "blue baby" disease. Apart from the bluish tinge, symptoms of the malformation include clubbing of fingernails, particularly as the child grows older; labored breathing; frequent fatigue; and stunted growth.

Helen Taussig proposed a method of surgical treatment to improve this condition. In charge of a cardiac clinic at Johns Hopkins Hospital in Baltimore at the time, she noticed that children with tetralogy of Fallot actually faired better if they also had a patent ductus arteriosus. From this observation, she deduced that the patent ductus supplemented the supply of oxygenated blood by rerouting some of it back to the lungs before it could make its way into the general circulatory system via the aorta. She reasoned that an artificially created shunt from one of the nearby arteries to the pulmonary artery might provide an even more efficient means of bypassing the narrowed pulmonary valve (Figure 16.12). She discussed her idea with Alfred Blalock, and together they devised the surgical procedure named the *Blalock-Taussig* operation after its creators, con-

sisting essentially in joining the subclavian artery to the pulmonary artery.

Few patients with uncorrected tetralogy of Fallot will survive beyond the first or second decades of life. Moreover, their growth is greatly impaired, and they are subject to serious, even fatal, complications such as pulmonary hemmorhages, cerebral infection, and episodes of severe anoxia. For these reasons, surgical treatment is recommended. The procedure of total correction of tetralogy of Fallot using the heart-lung machine and hypothermia (Figure 16.12) is now considered the preferable procedure. This procedure consists in closure of the ventricular septal defect; relief of right ventricular outflow tract obstruction by dividing the parietal band; and using, if necessary, a pericardial patch; and relief of pulmonary stenosis.

Most experienced surgeons in this field recommend primary one-stage repair in early infancy. Best results in such cases are obtained in institutions equipped for specialized neonatal cardiac surgery and with an experienced team of pediatric cardiologists and cardiac surgeons. Palliative procedures such as the Blalock-Taussig shunting procedure between the subclavian artery and the pulmonary artery, the Potts procedure of anastomosis between the descending thoracic aorta and the left pulmonary artery, or the Waterson procedure of anastomosis between the ascending aorta and the right pulmonary artery may be

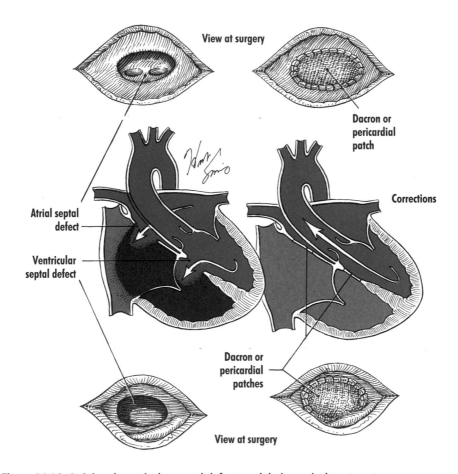

employed. Other systemic-to-pulmonary artery connections may be used in some patients in whom there is increased risk of early repair or in other circumstances in which total correction is not feasible.

The results of the operation are excellent. The surgical risk in most experienced centers is less than 6 percent, even in patients requiring operation at an early age. Studies on patients 10 to 20 years after complete repair have provided grati-

fying results, with more than 90 percent alive, well, and leading productive lives.

Defects of the Septum

Defects of the *septum*, or wall between the right and left chambers of the heart, often referred to as a "hole in the heart," are among the most common congenital abnormalities. They may occur in the septum between the two upper chambers

View at surgery

Dacron or pericardial patch

Corrections

Atrial septal defect

Ventricular septal defect

Dacron or pericardial patches

View at surgery

Figure 16.13. Atrial and ventricular septal defects and their surgical treatment.

of the heart (*atrial septal defects*) or between the two lower chambers (*ventricular septal defects*) (Figure 16.13).

There are several different kinds of atrial septal defects, the most common being the type in which, despite the size of the opening, there is a remnant of the septum around the defect. In some patients, this remnant may be partially absent, usually on the back side of the heart. Another variation, termed *sinus venosus,* occurs in the upper part of the right superior pulmonary vein, which allows blood to flow directly into the right atrium instead of the left atrium. Still another, termed *ostium primum,* is a partial form of a defect called *common atrioventricular canal*, in which the mitral valve is cleft.

The defect between the two upper chambers of the heart allows blood to flow in either direction. In most patients, however, blood flows from the left atrium into the right, to create what is termed a left-to-right shunt because of the increased pressure on the left side. Depending on the size of the opening, the shunt may cause a several-fold increase in the blood flow to the lungs and thus increase the burden on the heart. Occasionally, because of elevation of pressure in the right atrium due to other complications of the condition or to an increased resistance in the lungs, blood flows from the right to the left. Indeed, this may take place because of pulmonary

vascular changes that cause an initially left-to-right shunt to become reversed. This sometimes is the consequence of allowing a large left-to-right shunt to remain uncorrected. Surgical treatment may then become contraindicated.

Most patients with atrial septal defects tolerate the abnormality so well that disabling symptoms do not develop until adulthood. Growth and development are usually normal, although occasional heart failure and retardation of growth occur in infancy. There may be some symptoms of mild fatigability and shortness of breath during periods of exertion, and the heart might be slightly or moderately enlarged.

Surgical correction of the defect is advisable. Although it may be necessary to operate at an early age, ideally operation should be done on patients between 2 and 6 years of age. This provides sufficient time to determine whether the closure will take place normally. However, good results of surgical corrections can be achieved even in patients over 60 years of age.

The operation is performed with use of the heart-lung machine, and the defect may be corrected by one of several ways, depending on the type of defect. Some can be closed simply by suturing the edges of the defect together. Most others require a patch of Dacron® or pericardium sutured and placed in proper position to close the defect and to divert the pulmonary venous flow into the proper chamber, the left atrium (Figure 16.13). In other patients, the mitral valve may also require repair.

Results of operation are excellent, with virtually no deaths in uncomplicated cases involving children and young adults. Even in older patients, the risk of operation is only about 5 percent. Survival expectancy in patients operated on early is similar to that of the normal population.

Ventricular septal defects consist in an opening or hole between the two lower chambers of the heart, the right and left ventricles (Figure 16.13). They are among the most common types of congenital heart disease. The defect varies in position and size, but in most cases it produces a left-to-right shunt because of the higher pressure in the left ventricle. This causes a greatly increased blood flow to the lungs and puts a burden on the heart. Other anomalies not infrequently associated with ventricular septal defects are coarctation, occurring in about 12 percent of patients, and a patent ductus arteriosus, occurring in about 6 percent. They have been found more frequently in infants coming to surgery at 3 months of age or younger.

The effect of this condition on the patient varies, depending on its type and size, as well as blood flow through the defect. Spontaneous closure may occur in some patients with small defects, and for this reason, such patients, who are without symptoms, should be observed over a period of several years. On the other hand,

some infants with greatly increased blood flow through large defects may die in the early months of life. Others who survive infancy may develop progressive *pulmonary vascular disease* that sometimes becomes so severe that the condition becomes inoperable.

Surgical correction of a large ventricular septal defect is indicated during the first two years of life when growth is severely retarded and heart failure or progressive pulmonary hypertension develops. With more moderate-sized defects, the operation may be delayed until the child is 4 to 6 years of age. Children with smaller defects may be observed longer to see if the defect closes without surgical correction. If the defect persists beyond the age of 10 years, an operation may be advisable.

The defect is corrected surgically with use of the heart-lung machine. It is closed with a Dacron® patch, depending on the type and size of the defect (Figure 16.13). Results of the operation are excellent, with a risk of only about 1 or 2 percent. Survival expectancy is excellent, particularly in patients on whom operation is performed before the child is 2 years old.

Aorticopulmonary Window or Septal Defect

This type of rare congenital abnormality consists in an opening between the ascending aorta and the pulmonary artery (Figure

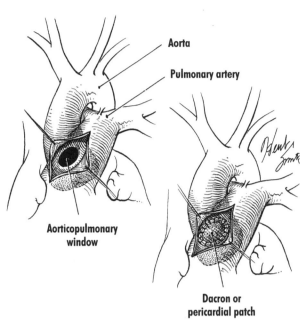

Figure 16.14. Aorticopulmonary window and surgical correction.

Transposition of the Great Arteries

This is one of the most severe congenital malformations of the heart, and most of these infants do not even survive one year. Although it is a rather complex condition with a number of variations, the basic abnormality is the transposition of the aorta and the pulmonary artery (Figure 16.15). Thus, instead of the normal relation of the aorta to the left ventricle and the pulmonary artery to the right ventricle, the aorta arises from the right ventricle and the pulmonary artery from the left ventricle. Some of these infants survive for a few months or even for some years because of the shunting or mixing of venous and arterial blood through associated anomalies such as septal defects or patent ductus arteriosus. Most of the infants suffer from cyanosis (as in the "blue baby"), a blue tinge of the skin resulting from lack of oxygen in the blood, retarded growth, and shortness of breath.

16.14). Because pressure is greater in the aorta, blood is shunted from the ascending aorta into the pulmonary artery (a left-to-right shunt); this creates an additional burden on the heart and ultimately causes severe pulmonary vascular disease and heart failure. For these reasons, operation should be done as soon as possible, preferably before the age of 2 years. The operation is performed with use of the heart-lung machine and closure of the window by means of suture or, in most cases, a patch of Dacron.® The risk involved in the operation is relatively small, and results are good.

Surgical treatment usually is recommended within the first five months of life. Under some circumstances, it may be preferable to perform a palliative operation first and postpone the definitive repair for some months or a few years. Several types of definitive procedures for surgical repair have been devised for this purpose and are designed to restore proper circulation of arterial and venous blood. Results of the operation are generally good, with an operative mortality ranging from 5 to about 10 percent, depending on the various types of abnormalities that may be present. Survival expectancy is good, being about 90 percent at 15 years after operation.

There are several different forms and variations of transposition. These include corrected transposition, a condition in which transposition of the ventricles accompanies the transposition of the aorta and pulmonary artery (Figure 16.16). The normal location of the left ventricle is occupied by a ventricle that has the morphologic (structural) characteristics of the right ventricle, and vice versa. In this situation, the morphologic right ventricle receives blood from the left atrium and pumps it into the aorta. The morphologic left ventricle receives blood from the right atrium and pumps it into the pulmonary artery. Thus, blood follows a normal pathway through the heart, hence the term corrected transposition. The presence of associated lesions, such as ventricular septal defects and pulmonic stenosis, determines the prognosis and the need for surgical correction.

Total Anomalous Pulmonary Venous Connection

Normally, the pulmonic veins return oxygenated blood from the lungs to the

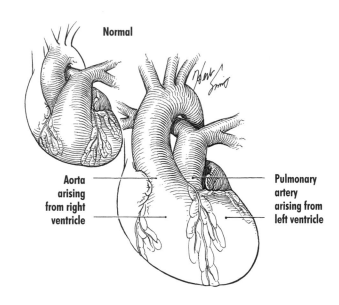

Figure 16.15. Anatomic abnormalities in transposition of the great arteries.

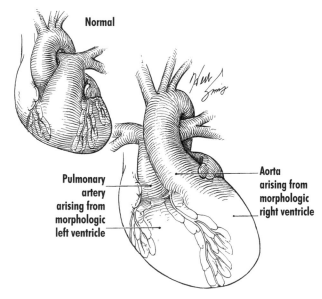

Figure 16.16. Corrected transposition of the great arteries.

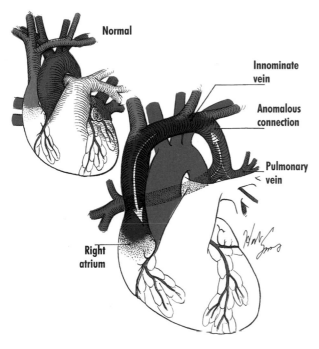

Figure 16.17. Total anomalous pulmonary venous connection.

left atrium of the heart. In the abnormality termed *total anomalous pulmonary venous connection,* the pulmonary veins fail to communicate with the left atrium; instead, they discharge their blood into the right atrium by way of the major systemic veins (Figure 16.17). The condition is accompanied by an atrial septal defect or a large foramen ovale; this allows the mixed venous and oxygenated blood to be shunted into the left atrium and permits temporary survival of these infants. Patent ductus arteriosus is also present in 25 to 50 percent of the patients.

Symptoms develop shortly after birth in most infants with this condition. They include rapid respiration, shortness of breath, feeding difficulties, and frequent respiratory infections. If left uncorrected, heart failure and death usually occur within the first year of life. The corrective surgical procedure should be performed as soon as the diagnosis is made, even within the first few days of life.

Depending on the nature of the anomaly, certain variations in the surgical procedure may be required but are designed to restore the normal return of oxygenated blood from the lungs to the left atrium. The more common procedures consist in making an anastomosis between the left atrium and pulmonary vein or through an opening in the right atrium, and suturing a pericardial patch over the openings of the pulmonary veins to an enlarged atrial septal defect in order to direct the pulmonary venous blood into the left atrium. The risk of operation ranges between 5 and 15 percent, and long-term results are excellent.

Aneurysm of the Sinus of Valsalva

This condition is caused by a congenital weakness in the wall of the aorta just above the aortic valves near the origin of the coronary arteries. It may also be acquired usually secondary to bacterial endocarditis or less frequently to cystic medial necrosis.

This weakness in the wall gradually balloons out to form a wind-sock appearance (Figure 16.18). Symptoms develop if the aneurysm impinges on surrounding structures, especially if it ruptures. Depending on the size of the ruptured opening, symptoms vary from mild manifestations to sudden shortness of breath and even rapid heart failure and death.

Surgical treatment is suggested as soon as the diagnosis is made, even in patients who are relatively asymptomatic. The condition is corrected surgically with use of the heart-lung machine, and consists in excising the aneurysm and repairing the defect by suture closure or in most cases, a Dacron® patch. For more extensive aneurysms, an albumin-coated Dacron® tube graft is used after the diseased segment is excised and is anastomosed proximally to the aortic root and distally to the normal ascending aorta. If necessary, the coronary arteries are implanted in the sides of the graft. In some patients the aortic valve may require replacement. Results of operation are excellent, with an operative risk of less than 5 percent and excellent long-term survival.

Truncus Arteriosus

This form of congenital anomaly is characterized by the absence of direct

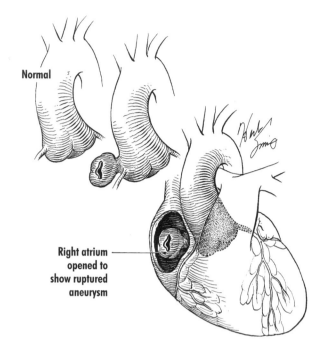

Figure 16.18. Aneurysm of the sinus of Valsalva.

anatomic continuity between the heart and the pulmonary arterial system. There are several types and variations. In the most common form, the pulmonary artery arises from the ascending aorta, where the pulmonary blood flow originates (Figure 16.19). A large ventricular septal defect is always present. There are several types of this anomaly, and in one unusual type there are no identifiable pulmonary arteries, and pulmonary blood flow is by way of the bronchial arteries, which arise from the descending aorta to supply blood to the tissues of the lung.

Most infants with this form of congenital heart disease die within the first year of

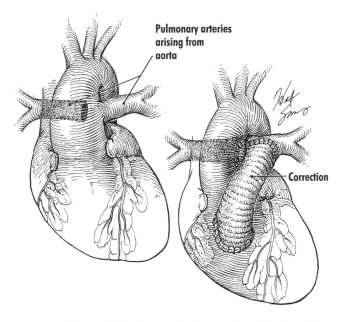

Figure 16.19. Anatomic abnormality of the heart in truncus arteriosus and surgical correction.

life. A few survive beyond this time but usually develop severe pulmonary vascular disease that renders this condition inoperable.

Until relatively recently, no satisfactory surgical procedure was known for this problem. The surgical procedures that have been developed seem to provide good results. The operation consists in disconnecting the pulmonary artery from the ascending aorta, repairing the defect, closing the ventricular septal defect, and connecting the right ventricle to the pulmonary artery by means of an aortic *homograft* or *synthetic graft*. The mortality rate is relatively low, about 12 to 15 percent.

Congenital Aortic Stenosis

In this type of congenital heart disease, the flow of blood from the left ventricle into the ascending aorta is obstructed (Figure 16.20). The blockage may be produced by partial narrowing of the aortic valve itself or by a circumferential ridge of tissue in the ascending aorta just above the valve, termed *supravalvular aortic stenosis*, or in the outflow tract just below the aortic valve, termed *subvalvular aortic stenosis*. Still another form of obstruction may be produced by massively hypertrophied muscle in the outflow tract of the left ventricle, termed *idiopathic hypertrophic subaortic stenosis* (IHSS).

Depending on the type and severity of the obstruction, infants with this condition may develop acute left ventricular failure and die, or may have few symptoms until early childhood, when chronic left ventricular failure may occur. Later, others may develop angina or chest pain and attacks of weakness or fainting. Sudden death may occur, presumably from ventricular fibrillation. Many patients survive into adult life and then develop increasing obstruction with calcification and progressive symptoms. Coarctation of the aorta is not an uncommon associated anomaly.

For neonates and very sick, small infants with critical stenosis, as evidenced by a pressure gradient of greater than 50 mm Hg, balloon dilation may be used first as the procedure of choice to tide the patient over this critical period until more definitive surgical correction can be performed. Surgical treatment is indicated in patients with congenital aortic stenosis who have symptoms and evidence of left ventricular failure. The procedure is performed with use of the heart-lung machine. In infants and children particularly, it is usually possible to divide the fused commissures of the stenotic aortic valve. In adults it is often necessary to replace the diseased valve with an artifi-cial valve (for more detail, see the section on valvular disease in Chapter 22).

The risk of operation depends on the severity of the lesion and associated anomalies. The operative mortality rate in infants less than one year of age may range from 10 to 30 percent, whereas in children older than one year of age, the risk is very low. Most children later require repeat operations, and not infre-quently, aortic valve replacement.

In supravalvular stenosis, the procedure consists in excision of the ridge of tissue

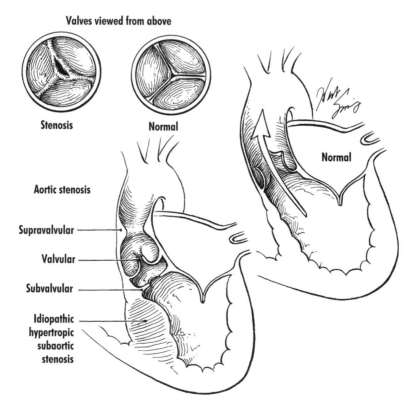

Figure 16.20. Types of congenital aortic stenosis.

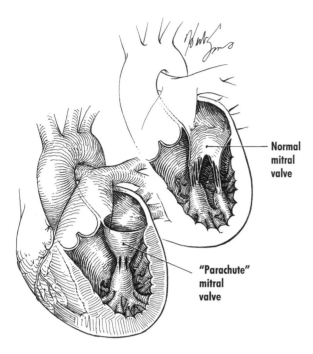

Figure 16.21. Congenital mitral valve disease.

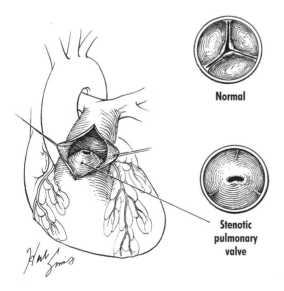

Figure 16.22. Pulmonary valve stenosis.

and repair of the opening in the ascending aorta with a patch of Dacron® to widen the lumen to normal size. In subvalvular stenosis, the ridge of tissue causing the obstruction is excised. In idiopathic hypertrophic subaortic stenosis, medical treatment is tried first, and if symptoms are not controlled adequately, it may be necessary to excise a part of the hypertrophic muscle. Results of the operation are generally excellent, with very low risk.

Congenital Mitral Valve Disease

Congenital malformation of the mitral valve may produce narrowing (stenosis) or incompetence of the valve, or a combination of these effects (Figure 16.21). This condition is often associated with other congenital malformations of the heart such as *endocardial fibroelastosis,* coarctation of the aorta, patent ductus arteriosus, and aortic stenosis. Patients with severe types of malformations are usually gravely ill in infancy and do not survive early childhood. Patients with milder forms of the disease may reach adulthood. Surgical treatment is directed toward repair of the valve, when it is possible. Occasionally, replacement is necessary, but this usually requires reoperation later because the child outgrows the valve. Results of repair are reasonably good, with freedom from reoperation of 75 percent at 10 years.

Pulmonary Valve Stenosis

This congenital malformation of the pulmonary valve, lying between the right ventricle and the pulmonary artery, consists in a narrowing of the valve, which produces an added burden on the right ventricle (Figure 16.22). If there is an associated opening in the atrial septum (a patent foramen ovale or an atrial septal defect), cyanosis may develop. Depending on the severity of the lesion, patients may die in early infancy, or soon thereafter, from heart failure. In mild forms of the condition without a septal defect, the patient may have few or no symptoms and tolerate the abnormality quite well.

Treatment is indicated in patients with symptoms, including particularly cyanosis, dyspnea on exertion, and moderate to severe stenosis. Percutaneous balloon valvuloplasty is now the preferred procedure for initial treatment. This consists in inserting a catheter with a balloon at the tip, usually through the femoral vein in the groin, directing it to the pulmonary valve, and then expanding the balloon to widen the valve. Results of this method of therapy have been found highly successful. In some patients, however, surgical valvulotomy may be necessary. The operation is performed with use of the heart-lung machine and consists in opening the valve with an incision. Sometimes hypertrophied muscle in the outflow of the right ventricle must be excised. If an atrial septal defect exists, it is closed. Results of the operation are excellent, with virtually no operative risk.

Congenital Tricuspid Atresia

This is a serious congenital abnormality in which the tricuspid valve is absent; the right ventricle is very small; and there is an atrial septal defect (Figure 16.23). There may be some variations in the abnormality. These infants are usually gravely ill and become moderately to

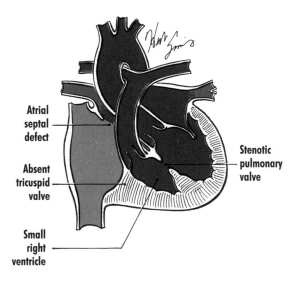

Figure 16.23. Congenital tricuspid atresia.

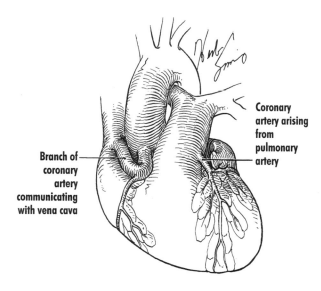

Coronary artery arising from pulmonary artery

Branch of coronary artery communicating with vena cava

Figure 16.24. Congenital coronary artery disease.

severely cyanotic. Most will die within the first few months of life unless operation is performed, but this is usually only palliative treatment rather than definitive correction, and is directed toward increasing pulmonary blood flow. Infusion of prostaglandin E is often first used in treating these severely cyanotic infants to restore patency of the ductus arteriosus. This form of medical treatment has improved the surgical results in cyanotic newborns requiring a shunt operation. Several techniques may be used, including making connections (*anastomoses*) with use of a graft between the left subclavian artery and the pulmonary artery, the superior vena cava and the right pulmonary artery, or between the aorta and the left pulmonary artery. Results after these operations are good, with relatively low risk. A more corrective type of operation, referred to as the Fonton procedure or some modification of it, may also be used in patients in early childhood with increasing cyanosis.

Congenital Coronary Artery Disease

There are two forms of this congenital anomaly of the coronary arteries (Figure 16.24). In the first type, a large branch of a coronary artery communicates directly with the vena cava, the right atrium, the right ventricle, or the pulmonary artery. Blood thus flows from the arterial system directly into the venous system. If this flow is great enough, symptoms will appear and ultimately lead to heart failure. An operation is therefore necessary and consists essentially in closing the anomalous artery by ligation.

The second type is characterized by the left coronary artery arising from the pulmonary artery. Unless corrected, most of these infants will not survive the first year of life. The operation in this case consists in closing off the artery by ligation and transplanting its origin to the ascending aorta directly or with the use of a vein graft or anastomosis to the internal mammary artery. Results are good in all of these operations.

What the Future Holds

The outlook for children born with heart defects has improved dramatically during the past 20 years. Improved diagnostic techniques and microsurgical procedures now allow abnormalities to be detected and oftentimes corrected in the smallest infants.

For others, palliative procedures buy time for a young child, relieving life-threatening symptoms and enabling corrective procedures to be delayed until an age when they are more likely to be successful.

All children born with a heart defect require regular monitoring throughout life. Even successfully corrected abnormalities may increase the risk of developing other heart problems in adulthood.

What about family planning? The dramatic strides being made in human genetics will continue to increase our understanding of how and why normal heart development sometimes goes awry. Genetic explanations for many of the heart defects that puzzle us now will likely be found in the years to come. For example, a

great deal of progress has been made in identifying several genetic defects that can result in IHSS.

Genetic counseling is advisable both for the parents of an affected child, if they would like to have another baby, and for the adults who were born with a heart defect and are now contemplating parenthood. Genetic counseling, although not able to provide all the answers, can rule out many genetic flaws and provide a good measure of peace of mind for many people.

Finally, the medical profession and the public have come a long way in their understanding of how alcohol, cigarettes, viruses, x-rays, medications, and environmental toxins can damage an unborn child.

Not too many years ago, doctors mistakenly believed that the placenta was a perfect barrier that screened out harmful substances and protected the fetus. Today, however, we realize how vulnerable the developing baby really is.

The best hope for preventing congenital heart defects is knowledge. Prevention will depend on our constantly expanding understanding of genetics and human development—and on our ability to educate parents-to-be about the need to avoid harmful substances (even before conception) and the importance of good prenatal care.

CHAPTER SEVENTEEN

Coronary Artery Disease

Coronary arteries are the blood vessels that supply the heart with the blood it needs to function. What that blood provides to the heart are life-giving oxygen and nutrients. Partial or complete blockage of one or more coronary arteries may decrease blood flow to the heart muscle. When the blockage is mild, the blood flow may be adequate to support the heart's functions at rest but unable to support them under conditions of stress or exercise.

This blocking, or coronary occlusion, can be caused by an atherosclerotic plaque (see Figure 13.1), a blood clot, a temporary spasm or contraction (coronary vasospasm) of the artery, or any combination of these factors. Plaque is the most common form of blockage; thrombosis (clot formation) nearly always occurs on preexisting plaque. What results is *ischemia,* a deficiency of blood or oxygen to the heart caused by poor circulatory supply. Ischemia may be "silent" and unidentified

by symptoms or may be clearly associated with chest pain (angina).

When any one of the coronary arteries is blocked completely, blood flow to that portion of the heart supplied by the artery stops. If it stays cut off, a heart attack—a *myocardial infarction*—results. This term means literally "death of heart muscle" (see below).

The heart, to some extent, has its own emergency medical system for clogged or blocked coronary arteries. The collateral circulation is a system of small vessels connecting two segments of the same artery (Figure 17.1) or two different arteries. These small vessels offer blood an alternate route, a detour, in case of blockage. By traveling these passageways, the blood can continue to arrive at its destination. But not everyone's collateral circulation is operable. Myocardial ischemia can prompt its development, and the vessels can grow and compensate to some degree

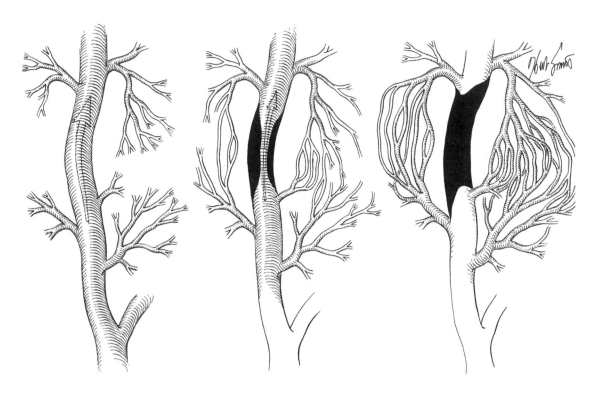

Figure 17.1. Nature can compensate for vessels occluded by atherosclerotic disease with collateral circulation, a network of small arteries and capillaries that detour around the obstruction, connecting two parts of one vessel or connecting different vessels.

for what is lost to coronary artery disease. The compensation may not be enough to sustain normal function. Exercise may also stimulate growth of collateral vessels. (For a fuller discussion of collaterals, see pp. 461–462.)

Anatomy

Understanding how these arteries encircle the heart helps make clear how they nourish it. Of the two main coronary arteries, the right one and the left, both have branches important to heart health (Figure 17.2). An early anatomist called them "coronary" arteries because they "crown" the heart, extending from the aorta and encircling the heart's uppermost part (the Latin word *corona* means "wreath" or "crown"). With their spreading branches, they bring to mind a garland, an encircling wreath, or an upside-down crown. On the left are the left main coronary artery and its extensions—the left circumflex coronary artery and the left anterior descending coronary artery. On the right is the right

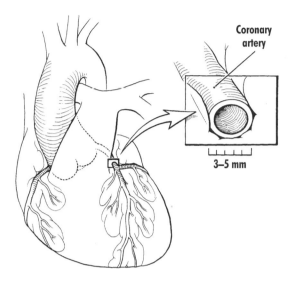

Coronary artery

3–5 mm

Figure 17.2. The left and right coronary arteries extend from the aorta's base near the aortic valve. From the left main coronary artery, the left circumflex coronary artery and the left anterior descending coronary artery both extend. The right coronary artery runs along the front of the heart near the right atrium. Not visible from this view of the front of the heart is a branch of the right coronary artery. These arteries, with a diameter of 3 to 5 millimeters (see inset, enlarged to show detail), supply the blood bearing the oxygen and nutrients that keep the heart going—about 3.5 gallons every hour.

coronary artery, whose main muscular branch runs alongside the atrium and whose marginal branch spreads outside the right ventricle. On the opposite side of the heart is the right coronary artery's posterior interventricular branch.

The major coronary arteries in adults are on average $2/16$ to $3/16$ of an inch in diameter, measured on the inside of a vessel. The diameter may be about 10 percent smaller in women than in men. The arterial wall, which surrounds the channel through which the blood flows, has three layers (see Figure 3.2). The outer layer, made up of connective tissue and nerve fibers, is called the *adventitia* and is itself nourished by a network of blood vessels called the vasa vasorum. The thickness of the outer layer dictates how flexible the vessel can be. Pulmonary arteries are more compliant than the aorta, but both have thick outer layers. The middle layer of a coronary artery, or *media,* is made of smooth muscle that can tense in response to stimulation by nerves, hormones or other chemical substances, or drugs. This middle layer is sheathed on both inner and outer surfaces with an elastic membrane. The inner layer, or *endothelium,* is also very responsive to stimulation and can itself release vasodilators that enlarge the vessel, or vasoconstrictors that cause the lumen, or passageway, to narrow.

Coronary Corridors

The coronary arteries are the corridors or passageways through which the blood passes on its mission to ensure oxygenation and nutrient supplies for the heart. The main obstacles to free passage are atherosclerosis (see Chapter 13) and thrombosis (clot formation), which is often related to atherosclerosis. Arterial constriction can aggravate the effects of atherosclerosis or thrombosis, as in coronary artery spasm, which can result in a myocardial infarction.

The effect of coronary artery disease is to reduce the amount of blood that the heart receives. Sometimes that reduction is not even noticed by an individual, who manages to participate in normal activities without any breathlessness or pain. When the obstruction or constriction or both become more pronounced, the patient experiences chest pain (angina pectoris) when attempting activities that require moderate exertion. The location of the blockage, its severity, the number of vessels, and the areas of blockage are determinants of ischemia. When a clot joins with arterial constriction or atherosclerosis to block, or occlude, an artery, a portion of the heart is deprived completely of the oxygen and nutrients it needs and the affected heart muscle cells die. A heart attack is what physicians call a myocardial (heart muscle) infarction (cell death from lack of local blood supply). It is like leaves that wither when the branch they are on is cut from a tree.

This is why prompt action when a heart attack hits is so very important. Any delay may increase chances of heart damage and hurt chances of survival. Unfortunately, for some people who have heart attacks, sudden cardiac death is the first indication of underlying heart disease. But ischemia means the existence of coronary heart disease and places a patient at very high risk for experiencing a heart attack. Aggressive changes in lifestyle, diet, and health care need to be made to prevent "the big one."

When Your Heart Is Deprived of Oxygen: Ischemia

Silent Ischemia

Although there is ample evidence that people who know that they have coronary artery disease can learn how to cope with it, how do you adjust diet and other lifestyle habits when you don't know what you've got?

Silent ischemia is a type of coronary artery disease that is called *silent* because the person who has it experiences no symptoms. Disease may have narrowed an artery, making it unable to supply an area of the heart muscle with the oxygen and nutrients it needs. Without them, as noted, that part of the heart muscle eventually dies. The person's light activity profile may prevent him or her from being challenged enough by exertion to experience symptoms—usually angina—or the ischemia may "speak" visually by angiograms or only by angina during some episodes of ischemia but not in others. The American Heart Association estimates that as many as three to four million Americans may have had ischemic episodes and not known it. Some people experience a "silent" infarct, a heart attack that occurs without symptoms that is eventually detected by diagnostic testing performed for reasons unrelated to the attack.

Angina

Myocardial ischemia's natural voice is the chest pain known as *angina pectoris*. Maybe you have a friend who has experienced angina when you were in a restaurant or on an athletic field together, or maybe you yourself have experienced the pain that characterizes it: pressing chest pain, numbness, center-of-the-breastbone squeezing sensation, and/or pain radiating to the left neck, jaw, and shoulder and into the left arm. Patients often use a clenched fist at their breastbone to indicate the feeling. After eating, angina is sometimes mistaken for indigestion or gas pain.

Usually angina, which lasts for about five minutes or less, is brought on by taxing the heart beyond its limits by exertion, emotional stress, eating, exposure to cold, or some combination of these factors. In other words, the heart's demand for oxygen outpaces its supply. Relief for angina is available with nitroglycerin or rest within two to five minutes.

The American Heart Association estimates that almost seven million people in the United States experience angina and that 350,000 new cases occur annually. The older you are, the more likely you are to have it. Twenty-seven percent of all men 80 to 84 years old, and 25 percent of all women age 85 and older have it. Statistics reported by the American Heart Association indicate that the crude prevalence of angina is higher in women than in men, and higher in blacks and Hispanics than in whites (Table 17.1).

Table 17.1. Percentage of American Population Experiencing Angina

Group	Black	White	Hispanic
Women	5.2%	4.1%	4.6%
Men	2.6%	3.4%	3.4%

SOURCE: National Health and Nutrition Examination Survey III data reported by the American Heart Association.
NOTE: Figures are measures of crude prevalence (i.e., raw data without age or other adjustments for comparison).

Stable Angina

Angina that over several weeks or months is predictable—that is, it occurs predictably and responds to nitroglycerin or rest predictably—is called stable angina. Atherosclerotic plaques are most typically to blame for stable angina. Vasoconstriction caused by exposure to cold also can decrease oxygen delivery.

Any type of angina requires careful medication evaluation and follow-up. Of course, this type of pain should not be ignored or simply made manageable by accommodation. A physician should be monitoring symptoms. Vigorous efforts should be made to reduce elevated low-density lipoprotein levels and to correct any other coronary artery disease risk factors.

Unstable Angina

Angina that is more frequent, is more intense, brings discomfort at rest or with light exertion, and increases in severity is known as unstable angina. There are now more hospital admissions for unstable angina than for myocardial infarction (heart attack). Unstable angina carries a greater risk for heart attack than stable angina and is sometimes called *preinfarction angina*. In fact, unstable angina associated with electrocardiographic changes is considered to be a significant clinical event. In this situation, aspirin is highly effective in reducing the likelihood of myocardial infarction and death from coronary disease. Other causes include coronary artery spasm or constriction.

You do not have to have had stable angina in order to have unstable angina. It can be the first indication of any coronary artery disease. It is a medical emergency that requires prompt medical care. If you know you have coronary artery disease and you are familiar with the characteristics of your angina attacks, you may need guidance about when it is necessary to seek medical attention. The U.S. Public Health Service suggests that your chest pain is an emergency when one of the following occurs:

- Pain or discomfort is very bad, gets worse, and lasts longer than 20 minutes.
- Weakness, nausea, or fainting accompanies the pain and discomfort.
- Three prescribed nitroglycerin tablets fail to take away the pain or discomfort.
- Pain or discomfort exceeds limits of former bouts with heart discomfort.

Call an ambulance and then call your doctor.

Variant Angina

Both the cause and symptoms of variant angina set it apart from stable and unstable angina. Spasm of a coronary artery is most often its cause, and its symptoms generally occur at rest. A partner associated with the pain is an exaggerated slowing down, delay, or cessation of the electrical signal the atria transfer to the ventricles (atrioventricular block) or perhaps a speeding up of ventricular beats (ventricular tachycardia). Electrocardiography records variant angina as a dramatic elevation of the ST phase (see pp. 29–31 for an explanation of electrocardiography phases). Nitroglycerin brings relief from the symptoms.

Heart Attack

It is no wonder heart attack is referred to as "the big one." It is responsible for more deaths every year than any other single disease or cause, taking about half a million Americans' lives. That would be more people than the entire population of Kansas City, Missouri. The American Heart Association estimates that about every minute of every day, heart attack claims a life. That means that the 20-minute ride into work could be counted as 20 lives lost. That during your lunch hour, 60 people died. That round the clock any day, about 1,400 hearts that are beating at its beginning will be quiet at its end.

Included in these statistics are some who survived a heart attack initially. Almost 13.5 million people living today have experienced angina, a heart attack, or both and are alive to tell about it. But alive though they are, their risk of illness or death can be as much as nine times more than someone who has never experienced heart attack. In the aftermath of a heart attack, only about one-third of those who survive have a complete recovery. Those who survive may experience the complications that come with a weakened or injured heart, such as congestive heart failure or heartbeat rhythm abnormalities. Angina may become a common companion, and stroke and sudden death rise as threats to be reckoned with.

Causes of Heart Attacks

Most heart attacks are caused by a clot that joins with atherosclerotic plaque to block or occlude an artery and deny oxygen-giving blood to part of the heart. The clot may arise from the plaque because the plaque has cracked or fissured, allowing clotting factors from the blood into the artery's wall. *Platelets,* which are important in blood coagulation, cluster in response; this clustering combines with an inability of the atherosclerotic artery to relax and a tendency to constrict, resulting in the obstruction of blood flow. The "culprit" plaque, or lesion, may block only 30 to 50 percent of the artery's lumen (channel), but it has special features (see pp. 186–188).

Warning Signals

More than 60 percent of heart attack victims experience classic indicators of heart difficulty days to weeks before the heart attack occurs (Figure 17.3). They may have unstable angina that is accompanied by shortness of breath and a pervasive feeling of being extremely tired. Ways to identify a heart attack are the frequency of occurrence of the chest pain, its duration, its intensity, and its resistance to relief. Chest pain that lasts 20 minutes or longer suggests a heart attack or unstable angina and demands immediate transport to a hospital. In angina attacks, by contrast, pain goes away with rest. One-fifth of heart attacks are painlessly silent and may go unidentified by patients.

As many as 20 percent of men and women with diabetes mellitus may experience silent heart attacks. Others who have these initially unrecognized attacks include patients who develop coronary

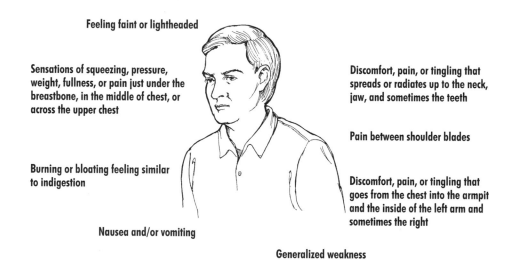

Feeling faint or lightheaded

Sensations of squeezing, pressure, weight, fullness, or pain just under the breastbone, in the middle of chest, or across the upper chest

Discomfort, pain, or tingling that spreads or radiates up to the neck, jaw, and sometimes the teeth

Pain between shoulder blades

Burning or bloating feeling similar to indigestion

Discomfort, pain, or tingling that goes from the chest into the armpit and the inside of the left arm and sometimes the right

Nausea and/or vomiting

Generalized weakness

Figure 17.3. Classic warning signals of a heart attack experienced by men and women include pain, sweating, nausea, sensations of indigestion or burning, and feeling faint. Women, research has revealed, are slower to attribute these signals to a heart attack and are more likely to postpone seeking help during this critical period. Their symptoms may also be less severe.

artery disease after heart transplantation, those with neuromyopathic abnormalities, and even those who appear otherwise normal.

Discomfort and pain associated with heart attack but not necessarily present in every case include:

- Sensations of squeezing, pressure, weight, fullness, or pain just under the breastbone, in the middle of the chest, or across the upper chest.
- Discomfort, pain, or tingling that spreads or radiates up to the neck, jaw, and sometimes the teeth.
- Discomfort, pain, or tingling that goes from the chest into the armpit and the inside of the left arm and/or sometimes the right.
- Burning or bloating feeling similar to indigestion.
- Feeling faint or lightheaded.
- Unexplained pervasive weakness.
- Nausea and/or vomiting.
- Sweating.

Women may be more likely than men to describe a feeling of tightness in the chest that comes and goes, with no particular precursor. Weakness, lethargy, breathlessness, or nausea may be their key symptom. There may be a sense of inhaling cold air. Men may be more likely to report that the pain gets better with rest. Remember that no one should feel foolish for having gone to an emergency room unnecessarily. It is the medical staff's responsibility to take care of you.

Responding to a Heart Attack

If someone you know experiences sensations that may indicate a heart attack, transport that person to the hospital or call an emergency service. Some emergency services, usually those in large cities, can begin to help the patient immediately because of equipment on board emergency vehicles or the capability of performing certain tests whose results will expedite treatment once the ambulance arrives at the hospital. In other situations, the emergency service provides only fast transport. If you or someone you love or work with is at risk for a heart attack, make sure you know which hospitals have 24-hour emergency cardiac care units and which are closest to home and work. Keep their phone numbers handy. If you need to call an emergency service to take you to the hospital, call the service first and your doctor second. Don't delay obtaining help because you are unable to reach your doctor for advice. Every minute counts.

It has been said that women who have heart attacks sometimes die of surprise—they are unaware that they are at risk for coronary artery disease and fail to seek help. One study showed women to be many hours slower in seeking help and in recognizing their symptoms for what they were. Grandmothers, mothers, daughters, sisters, aunts, and nieces all need to remind one another that the risk for coronary artery disease and heart attack is real and to seek promptly proper monitoring of their hearts in trouble-free times and proper treatment when there is disease or an emergency.

Sudden Cardiac Death

Sudden cardiac death occurs in a wide range of cardiac disorders. Although about 90 percent of adults in whom sudden cardiac death occurs have coronary artery disease, sudden cardiac death is also a feature of a variety of cardiac electrical disorders, the cardiomyopathies, and hypertensive disease. Most deaths in adolescents and young adults during exercise represent cardiac deaths due to congenital defects such as hypertrophic cardiomyopathy. About half of deaths due to coronary artery disease in the United States occur within an hour of the onset of symptoms and before the patient can reach the hospital. That's about 250,000 deaths each year.

Twenty-five to thirty-three percent of those suffering sudden cardiac death fall dead instantaneously or are found dead

by others. The remainder may experience symptoms for minutes, a few hours, or longer. But emergency intervention with cardiopulmonary resuscitation (CPR) and defibrillation (delivering a strong electrical shock to restart the heart's beating regularly), along with advanced care options, can make the difference between life or death if it can be started within a few minutes of the beginning of the symptoms.

Life after a Heart Attack

Having a heart attack damages the heart—some of the cells die and can no longer function—but when a person survives, the rest of the heart keeps working. The aftermath of a heart attack can be difficult if you are like most and do not recover completely. The first six months after a heart attack are important while your heart readjusts to its work load and you cope with fatigue.

The heartbeat pattern is disturbed in more than 90 percent of initial heart attack survivors, and these arrhythmias are in evidence within the first 24 hours afterward. These types of problems are responsible for about half of deaths after a heart attack. With them comes the threat of cardiac arrest—the cessation of heart contractions. Sometimes associated with a heart attack linked with damage to the front (anterior) wall of the heart is a ventricular aneurysm, a balloonlike protrusion that occurs in the heart wall thinned and damaged by lack of oxygen. An aneurysm of this sort generally will not rupture but may be associated with low cardiac output and congestive heart failure.

Part of the heart's impaired function may include poorer pumping ability. About 30 percent of people who experience a heart attack find they must manage heart failure afterward (see Chapter 8). Its cause most often is failure of the left ventricle.

This impaired pumping ability of the left ventricle sometimes permits the mitral valve to regurgitate blood from the ventricle back to the atrium. When the functioning of the left ventricle myocardium declines to the point that blood pressure falls to dangerously low levels, compensatory reactions such as tachycardia and fluid retention result, and cardiogenic shock (shock resulting from decreased cardiac output) may ensue. More than 65 percent of patients who have cardiogenic shock die. Other life-threatening difficulties encountered following a heart attack include perfora-tion or rupture of the septum dividing the ventricles, and clots formed in the left ventricle that can be released into the bloodstream and cause a stroke.

Patients ask not only, "Is there life after a heart attack?" but also, "Is it worth living?" The answer to both questions is yes. Eventually, most patients who survive a heart attack return to a normal lifestyle. Confidence in knowing recovery is possible undergirds progress. Honestly communicating to physicians, family, and friends about fears helps those who have experienced a heart attack dispel worries about the future and their place in it. Worries about returning to a normal lifestyle, including work and home life, can cast a long shadow.

The heart attack victim finds life forever changed, because of the lifestyle changes brought about by the event and because of the change in perspective wrought by it. Early anxiety may be replaced by depression. Openness allows sharing of the burden, and oftentimes discussion brings forth facts that can eliminate problems. Psychological counseling may help.

CHAPTER EIGHTEEN

Surgical Treatment of Coronary Artery Disease

The surgical treatment for coronary artery disease began more than 70 years ago when Professor Thomas Jonnesco performed a sympathectomy (interrupting some of the nerve supply to the heart) to treat angina pectoris. This proved to be so strikingly successful that it caused great enthusiasm for surgery of the sympathetic nervous system. Since that time, surgeons have been interested on and off in surgical treatment of coronary arterial disease. From time to time during the next several decades, numerous other indirect procedures designed to increase collateral circulation were developed. Among these, the only procedure which offered some encouragement was the operation promoted by A. Vineberg, which consisted in implanting the internal mammary artery into the myocardium. Although the implanted artery sometimes remained patent (suggesting some blood flowed to the myocardium), the magnitude of blood was so inadequate that this operation was also finally abandoned. Accordingly,

surgeons soon lost enthusiasm and interest, largely because of inconclusive and disappointing results.

In the early 1960s, interest was revived in surgical treatment geared toward a direct approach to the problem. Two major factors were responsible for this breakthrough. The first was the development of coronary arteriography (Figure 18.1), which is the keystone for surgical treatment because it provides visualization of the arterial lumen, and thus revealing the precise location of the nature and extent of the obstruction (Figure 18.2). Indeed, this was the key that opened the door to surgical treatment for other forms of arterial disease in the early 1950s. But its safe application to the study of coronary arterial disease was delayed for about a decade.

The second major factor was concerned with the development of surgical procedures designed to restore normal circulation in an artery beyond an obstruction. Experience with the procedures developed for treating occlusive disease of the aorta

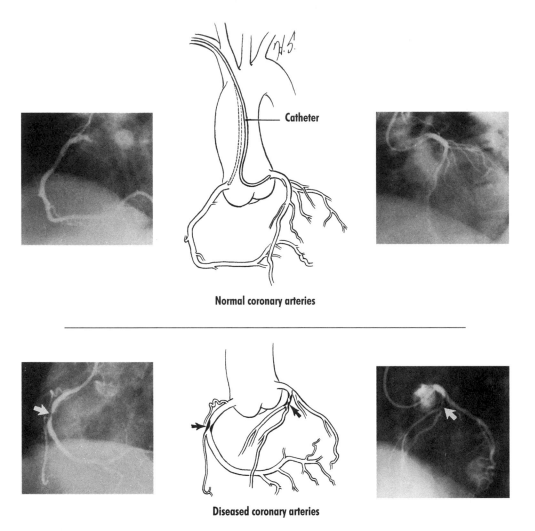

Normal coronary arteries

Diseased coronary arteries

Figure 18.1. (above) Drawing and photograph of normal coronary arteries. Coronary arteriography is performed by making a cine-roentgenogram while a radiopaque dye is injected into the coronary arteries via a catheter inserted into a peripheral artery in the legs or arms. (below) Drawing and photographs show severe, well-localized obstruction in the right and left anterior descending coronary arteries.

and major arteries (see Chapter 19) encouraged surgeons to consider applying these techniques to similar diseases of the coronary arteries, once arteriography was developed as a safe diagnostic procedure.

Accordingly, surgeons in this country and in Europe conducted intensive research on animals to evaluate various surgical technical vascular procedures, such as segmental excision and vein replacement,

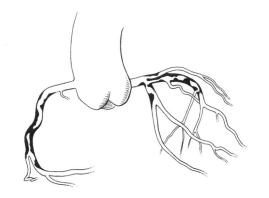

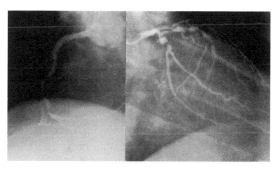

Figure 18.2. Drawing and coronary arteriogram of a 58-year-old man with angina, showing precise location and extent of severe, well-localized, stenotic disease in both the right and left coronary arteries. Particularly significant is the presence of relatively normal vessels distal to the occlusion, thus permitting bypass operation.

patch-graft angioplasty, and the bypass concept, with use of both veins and anastomosis to the coronary arteries of the arterial branches arising from the aortic arch, such as the carotid, subclavian, and internal mammary artery. In 1961, we summarized our experience with the coronary bypass procedure in experimental animals with the conclusion that it was successful in about 50 percent of the cases, which was similar to results obtained in other laboratories. Our concluding statement at that time was ". . . that more intensive investigations of this approach toward relief of coronary occlusive disease are fully justified."[1]

In the first attempts to apply one of these direct surgical approaches, endarterectomy and patch-graft angioplasty were used (Figure 18.3). Although such procedures could be highly successful (indeed, we have some patients who have survived as long as 20 years after operation), as many as one-half of our cases were failures, and the risk of operation was relatively high. This somewhat discouraging picture was changed by two important developments: the bypass technique and improvements in the heart-lung machine in preserving heart muscle function. On April 4, 1962, David Sabiston[2] at Duke University performed the first application of a saphenous vein autograft as a bypass graft from the ascending aorta to the right coronary artery on a 41-year-old man with severe angina on whom coronary endarterectomy had been performed. Symptoms recurred one year later, and occlusion of the previous endarterectomized segment was demonstrated by

[1] *Circulation* 23:111–120 (January, 1961).
[2] *Johns Hopkins Medical Journal* 134:314 (1974).

A.

B.

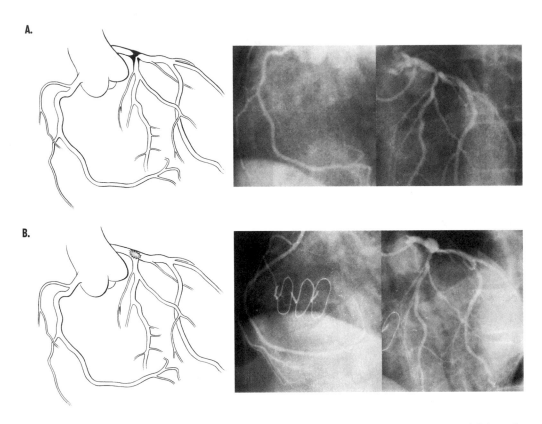

Figure 18.3. A. Drawing and preoperative coronary arteriogram of a 45-year-old man complaining of severe angina, showing an occlusive lesion in the left main coronary artery near the origin of the left anterior descending coronary artery.
B. Drawing and postoperative coronary arteriogram showing correction of occlusive lesion almost 20 years after operation, during which time the patient remained asymptomatic.

coronary arteriography. The procedure consisted in end-to-end anastomosis to the right coronary artery distal to the occluded segment and end-to-side anastomosis of the proximal end of the vein graft to the ascending aorta. Unfortunately, a cerebrovascular accident (stroke) developed in the postoperative period, and the patient died three days later.

The first successful coronary artery bypass operation was performed by us at The Methodist Hospital in Houston, Texas, on November 23, 1964.[3] This was also done on a 42-year-old man with severe incapacitating angina whose coronary arteriogram showed severe localized stenosis in the left main and proximal segment of the left anterior descending coronary arteries, with

[3] *Journal of the American Medical Association* 223:792–794 (February 12, 1973).

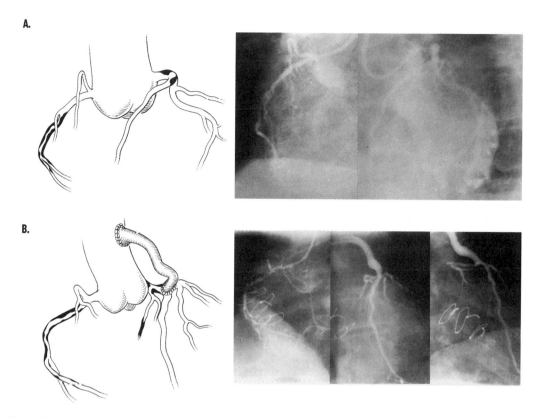

Figure 18.4. A. Drawing and coronary arteriogram made preoperatively of a 42-year-old man complaining of angina, showing almost complete occlusion of the left main coronary artery and severe stenosis of the right coronary artery.
B. Drawing and coronary arteriogram in same patient made seven years after operation, showing patency of the saphenous vein bypass graft from the ascending aorta to the left anterior descending coronary artery.

diffuse disease throughout the right coronary artery. The procedure consisted in a bypass saphenous autograft from the ascending aorta by end-to-side anastomosis to the left anterior descending coronary artery distal to the occlusive lesion by end-to-side anastomosis. The patient recovered, was completely relieved of symptoms of angina, and resumed normal activities. He was readmitted to the hospital on September 17, 1968, complaining of intermittent claudication of the legs, and on aortography was found to have complete obstruction of the terminal abdominal aorta just below the bifurcation. Operation consisting in endarterectomy and patch-graft angioplasty was performed, with restoration of normal circulation in the legs.

He remained asymptomatic and returned periodically for evaluation. On September 9, 1971, approximately 7 years after operation, coronary arteriography was performed, which showed complete occlusion of his left main coronary artery and patency of the vein bypass graft (Figure 18.4).

According to A. S. Olearchyk,[4] whose first report was published in 1988, Professor V. I. Kolessov, who was Chairman of the Department of Surgery at the first Leningrad Medical Institute between 1953 and 1976, performed end-to-end anastomosis between the internal mammary artery and the coronary artery in 1967, and the next year, he performed end-to-side anastomosis on another patient. According to Olearchyk, Professor Kolessov performed this procedure on 132 patients during his tenure from 1953-1976, most of which were done on a beating heart. In 1968, R. G. Favoloro at the Cleveland Clinic reported highly successful results with 55 patients who had interposition autogenous vein replacement by end-to-end anastomosis proximally and distally for segmental occlusive disease of the right coronary artery, in order to overcome the unfavorable results after pericardial patch reconstruction. Two years later, Favoloro and Donald Effler and associates reported using the autogenous saphenous vein as a bypass from the occluding ascending aorta to the coronary arteries by end-to-side anastomosis. Further impetus to the more widespread use of the coronary bypass procedure was given by W. Johnson and his associates in Milwaukee, Wisconsin, after their report in 1969 of the application of this procedure to the left coronary artery in 301 patients, with an operative mortality rate of 12 percent. Since then, numerous investigators in this country and in Europe have improved and perfected the procedure, with the indications for its application being continuously reassessed for more precise definition.

The selection of patients for surgical treatment depends on the careful assessment of the cardiac function and precise arteriographic evaluation of the atherosclerotic occlusive process. Assessment of cardiac function is based on taking a detailed history from the patient, physical examination, and special laboratory tests, including treadmill exercise testing. Other special tests include echocardiography with exercise and radionuclide angiocardiography. If these procedures indicate coronary artery disease and the patient has angina pectoris, coronary arteriography may be indicated. Other potential indications for coronary arteriography are atypical chest pain of undetermined origin, congestive heart failure of undetermined cause, angina after a myocardial

---

[4] *Journal of the Ukrainian Medical Association,* 35:3 (1988).

infarction, and valvular heart disease with chest pain.

Depending upon the results of these tests, surgical treatment may be recommended. Important factors are the site and extent of the obstructing lesions (Figures 18.1 and 18.2), the function of the left ventricle, and the general clinical condition of the patient. Particularly important is the nature of the obstructive process, which may produce varying degrees of narrowing or even total obstruction of the arterial lumen. Narrowing of more than 60 or 70 percent of the lumen is considered of significance in causing decrease in blood flow. The extent and pattern of the obstructing lesion is particularly important. Fortunately, in many patients the pattern tends to be localized, with a relatively normal artery distal to the lesion. Regardless of how severe or extensive the obstructing lesion is, if there is a sufficiently normal distal arterial segment and if left ventricular function is not too severely impaired, it is possible to perform surgical treatment. In general, the following are considered indications for operation:

1. Left main artery stenosis of 50 percent or greater;
2. Proximal left anterior descending stenosis of 70 percent or greater associated with other significant coronary stenosis;

3. Stenosis of 60 percent or greater in the proximal segments of the right, left anterior descending, and obtuse marginal coronary arteries;
4. Multiple stenosis of 50 percent or greater associated with moderate to severe left ventricular impairment as evidenced by an ejection fraction of 0.35 to 0.45 (see Chapter 5);
5. Angina of such severity as to interfere with daily activities or associated with severe ischemia by exercise testing. Patients with unstable angina are included in this group;
6. Patients with acute evolving myocardial infarction who are not successfully treated by thrombolytic therapy and balloon angioplasty;
7. Patients with significant obstructive lesions of the coronary arteries who also require surgical correction of valvular heart disease or an aneurysm of the ascending aorta or of the left ventricle;
8. As an emergency procedure for patients undergoing balloon angioplasty in which serious complications occur, such as acute occlusion or rupture of the artery.

Not all patients with coronary heart disease need or should have surgical treatment. Indeed, there are certain forms of the disease in which surgical treatment is of no value or are not amenable to surgical treatment. For example, patterns that are characterized by diffuse involvement, sometimes with calcification or with extensive and diffuse narrowing of the distal arterial segments, do not lend themselves to surgical treatment. In instances when the muscle of the left ventricle is severely damaged or extensively scarred from previous myocardial infarction so that poor left ventricular function results, as evidenced by an ejection fraction of 0.25 or less, an operation usually is not indicated. In such patients the risk is very high, and it is extremely doubtful that the patient will be much improved. In addition, patients with associated diseases such as cancer and severe pulmonary or renal diseases, with severe debility and restricted activity, are not candidates for operation.

Age, in itself, however, is not a contraindication to surgical treatment. Our own experience and that of others have shown that properly selected patients in their 70s and 80s, who otherwise are in reasonably good general condition, may be successfully operated on without a very high risk. Other indications may involve special circumstances that require the professional judgment of the cardiologist and cardiac surgeon. Such a decision is made jointly by the physicians and the patient after his being fully informed of the various factors associated with the problem, and is based primarily on the severity of the manifestations, the extent of the coronary lesions, and left ventricular performance. After the patient is informed, his wishes must be respected. Some patients may express the desire to proceed immediately for surgical treatment, since they may not wish to accept prolonged pharmacologic therapy and are desirous of avoiding the potential sudden future development of an acute myocardial infarction.

Of the two basic surgical procedures used for the treatment of coronary occlusive disease, endarterectomy and bypass, at present, endarterectomy is used mostly to supplement the bypass procedure and to open distal segments that can then be attached to a bypass graft. Endarterectomy consists in removing the atheromatous plaque by separating it from the remainder of the arterial wall (Figure 18.5). It usually is applied for extremely well-localized lesions, although in some circumstances it can be used in longer lesions. The operation is performed by making a longitudinal incision in the artery from well above to well below the occlusive lesion. A cleavage plane is then found between the atheromatous lesion and the remainder of the arterial wall, and the lesion is separated carefully from the wall in a similar way one would peel the covering of an orange from the inner fruit. The lesion is completely removed, after which a vein graft may be attached to the opening in the artery by end-to-side anastomosis, or the

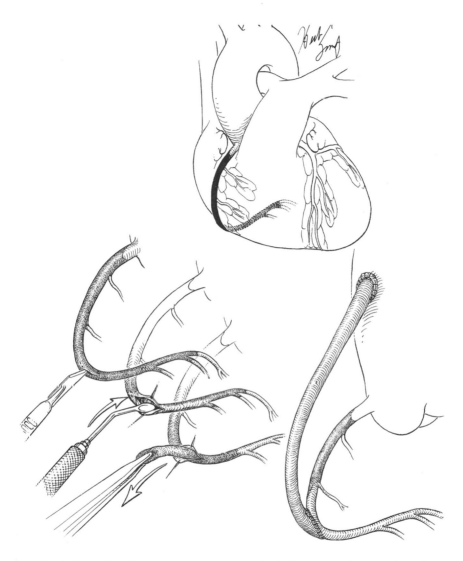

Figure 18.5. Technique of endarterectomy, showing method of removal of obstructive atheromatous plaque from a distal segment of right coronary artery, following which an autogenous saphenous vein bypass graft is performed.

incision may be closed by using a small piece of vein as a patch graft (Figure 18.6).

The bypass operation has proved to be the procedure of choice in most patients for whom surgery is indicated. This opera-tion is performed under general anesthesia using the heart-lung machine to support the patient during actual performance of the bypass. A segment of the saphenous vein, a fairly large superficial vein in the

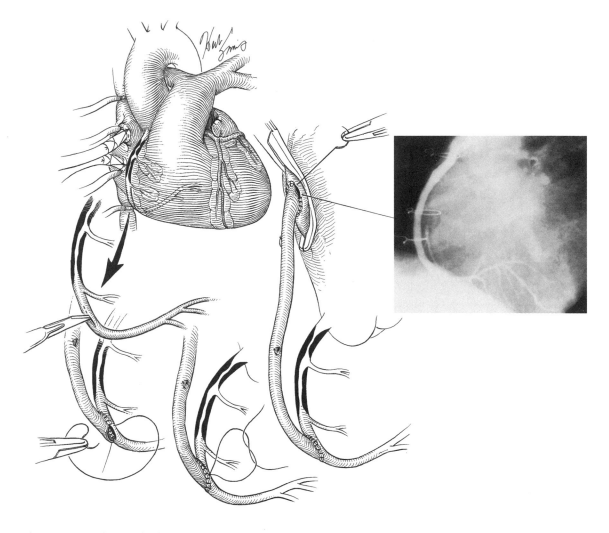

Figure 18.6. Technique for bypass using an autogenous saphenous vein removed from the patient's leg and attached to an opening in the right coronary artery distal to the obstructing lesion by end-to-side anastomosis, and then attached to an opening in the ascending aorta by a similar anastomosis. To the right is a photograph of the arteriogram performed five years after operation, showing the graft functioning normally.

leg, is removed. Removal of the vein causes no circulatory disturbances in the leg since there are sufficient other veins to replace its function. The vein graft is prepared by ligating, or closing off by suture, its small branches. Because of its valves (see Figure 3.8 in Chapter 3), it will be attached so that blood will flow through it in the same direction as when it functioned in the leg. The heart is exposed by a median sternotomy, a longitudinal incision that is made through the breastbone with an electrical saw. Since the coronary arteries are on the surface of the heart, it is relatively easy to identify and isolate the proper segment for attachment of the graft as determined by the arteriogram. The patient is connected to the heart-lung machine, and in most instances, the heart function is stopped by occluding the ascending aorta and stopping blood flow to the heart through the coronary arteries with the use of a cardioplegic drug. This provides a quiet heart that facilitates the delicate suture connection of the graft to a coronary artery. The left internal mammary artery, which arises from the left subclavian artery and lies along the lateral part of the breastbone, is mobilized from its attachment to the chest wall. It is then divided inferiorly at about the level of the sixth intercostal space, and the distal end is occluded by ligature. The proximal opening is then tailored to be anastomosed by end-to-side anastomosis to the opening in the coronary artery, usually the left anterior descending or some branch of the circumflex coronary artery, depending upon the location of the occlusive process.

A longitudinal incision, about a quarter of an inch in length, is made in a reasonably normal segment of the coronary artery beyond the obstructive lesion (Figure 18.7). The distal end of the mobilized internal mammary artery is bevelled and trimmed to fit the opening in the artery, and then it is attached to the edges of the incision by fine plastic sutures. If other coronary arteries require bypass grafts, an autogenous saphenous vein, which has previously been removed from the leg, is used for this purpose. A similar end-to-side anastomosis of the end of this vein is attached to an opening in the coronary artery as previously described, and the proximal end of the vein is attached to an opening in the ascending aorta by end-to-side anastomosis.

When all such attachments are completed, the aortic clamp is removed to allow blood flow through the coronary arteries to resume. In a few seconds the heart starts to beat again. Sometimes the heart goes into ventricular fibrillation and requires an electrical shock to convert it to a normal rhythm.

The risk of operation ranges between 1 and 4 percent, depending on a number of factors, including severity of disease, ventricular function, and other associated conditions. The operation results in excellent relief of chest pain. During the past three decades, we have performed more than 25,000 coronary artery bypass operations with highly gratifying results. The risk of operation is now only about 2 or 3 percent, and more than 90 percent of the

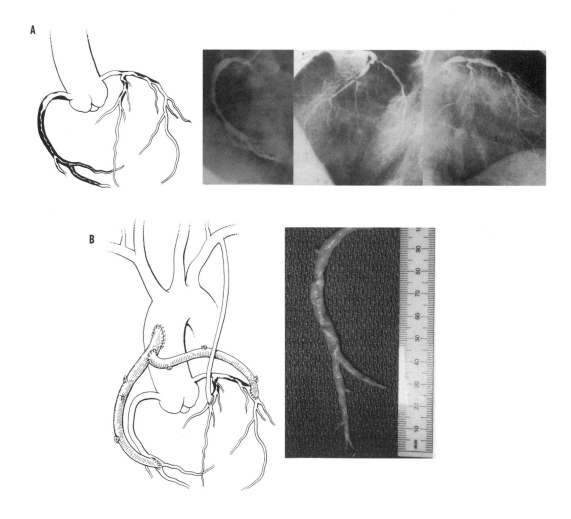

Figure 18.7. A. Drawing and coronary arteriogram showing occlusive lesions in the right, left anterior descending, and circumflex coronary arteries.
B. Drawing showing method of surgical treatment, consisting in a bypass to the left anterior descending coronary artery using the left internal mammary artery, and bypass to the circumflex coronary artery and right coronary artery after endarterectomy, for removal of an extensive obstructing plaque, shown in photograph on right, using autogenous vein.

patients are significantly improved. Indeed, most of them are completely relieved of chest pain and resume normal activities. Some actually resume work that involves considerable physical activity.

Long-term results are also excellent, with recurrence of symptoms in only about 3 or 4 percent a year. A number of studies including our own have shown that survival expectancy after operation is about 90 percent at 5 years, about 80 percent at 10 years, 55 percent at 15 years, and 40 percent at 20 years. Patients may remain free of angina for long periods, but after about 10 years angina recurs in about 40 percent of patients, usually not as severe as it was preoperatively, and in most cases it can be satisfactorily controlled medically (Figure 18.8).

Restenosis and occlusion of the vein grafts begin to appear within 5 to 10 years after operation. This takes place at a rate of about 3 or 4 percent a year so that about 40 percent of grafts will be severely stenosed, or obstructed, in 10 years. The internal mammary graft remains patent for a much longer period of time. Re-operation is highly successful in some patients whose symptoms recur after graft occlusion. The question of whether or not the operation prolongs life has been undetermined until recently when some evidence

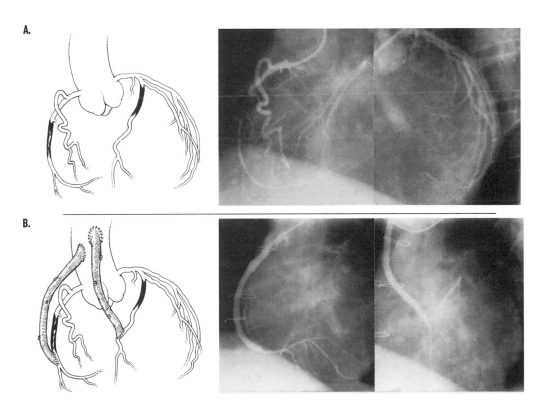

Figure 18.8. A. Drawing and photograph of coronary arteriogram of a 54-year-old man complaining of severe angina, showing well-localized obstructive lesions in proximal segments of both the right and left anterior descending coronary arteries.
B. Drawing showing method of surgical treatment, consisting in autogenous saphenous vein bypass from ascending aorta to right and left anterior descending coronary arteries. Photograph of coronary arteriogram at right shows both grafts functioning normally 10 years after operation.

has become available to suggest it does. Although reduction of the mortality rate is important, the primary reason for the operation is to relieve disabling symptoms and to restore the patient to reasonably normal functional activity.

Most patients with acute myocardial infarction can be successfully treated medically with thrombolytic therapy and angioplasty. Surgical treatment, however, may be recommended for some patients with severe infarction complicated by shock that resists medical treatment and is associated with severe arrhythmia. Under these circumstances, the patient is usually placed on some kind of a mechanical heart support device, in most instances the intra-aortic balloon (see Figure 24.4 in Chapter 24) or the heart-lung machine, and an emergency coronary arteriogram is performed. If the pattern of the occlusive disease is amenable to surgical treatment, the patient is immediately taken to the operating room, where the appropriate bypass operation is performed. Approximately 80 percent of such cases are successful.

Surgical treatment may also be suggested for patients with left ventricular aneurysm after a myocardial infarction.

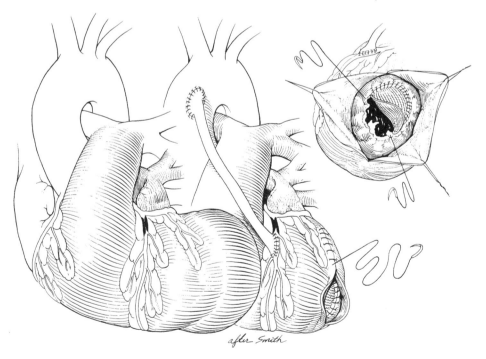

Figure 18.9. Drawing on left showing left ventricular aneurysm following myocardial infarction and on right, method of surgical treatment, consisting in incisional opening of aneurysm with Dacron® patch to correct defect and covering with suture closure of wall of aneurysmal sac.

This complication is produced by scar formation that replaces the damaged muscle of the left ventricle during the healing process. The scarred area is unable to resist the pounding pressure of repeated ventricular contraction. The weakened ventricular wall balloons out, sometimes growing larger than the ventricle itself. In opposition to the contracting ventricle, the aneurysm interferes with left ventricular function and leads to heart failure. Under these circumstances, operation is recom-

mended. With the patient supported by the heart-lung machine, the scarred area is incised and may be partially excised, and the opening in the left ventricle is repaired by suturing the edges together or by using a Dacron® graft to repair the defect (Figure 18.9). In patients with occlusion of the coronary arteries, vein bypass also may be performed. Results of this operation are excellent, with a better-than-90-percent recovery rate.

Mitral insufficiency, or incompetence of the mitral valve, occurs as a complication of myocardial infarction when the heart is damaged at the site of attachment of the chordae tendineae from the papillary muscles (Figure 18.10). These string-like attachments to the edges of the valve cusps resemble the ropes attached to the edges of a parachute. Rupture of these attachments after infarction allows the cusp of the mitral valve to flop back and forth uselessly, and often results in heart failure. Surgical treatment usually consists in replacing the damaged valve with an artificial one and sometimes placing a vein bypass to the coronary arteries. Results of the operation are good, with a relatively low risk.

Ventricular septal defect may also be a complication of myocardial infarction (Figure 18.11). This occurs from infarction damage to the ventricular septum and death of the tissues so that they are no longer able to tolerate the pressure in the

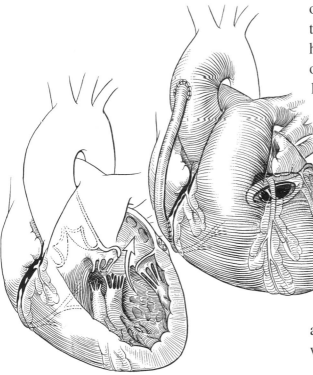

Figure 18.10. Drawing on left showing incompetence of a mitral valve occurring as a complication of myocardial infarction. Drawing on right showing method of surgical treatment, consisting in valve replacement and in appropriate cases, coronary bypass.

left ventricle. If the resulting opening is large enough, acute severe heart failure develops and is usually fatal. Surgical correction of the defect, usually with a Dacron® patch, is performed in much the same manner as for congenital ventricular septal defects, and results of the operation are reasonably good.

In recent years, efforts have been made to utilize minimally invasive surgery in performing the coronary bypass operation. This consists essentially in exposing the heart through a flap incision over the left anterior chest wall about the level of the junction of the third and fourth costal cartilages, which are then excised. This permits visualization of the left internal mammary artery, which can be mobilized from its attachment to the sternum and then used for attachment by end-to-side anastomosis to the left anterior descending coronary artery. This suture anastomosis is made on a beating heart using traction suture to facilitate the suture anastomosis. It is obviously limited in its application to a small number of cases requiring only one or two anastomoses. The great majority of patients require three or more bypasses that cannot be performed by this minimally invasive procedure.

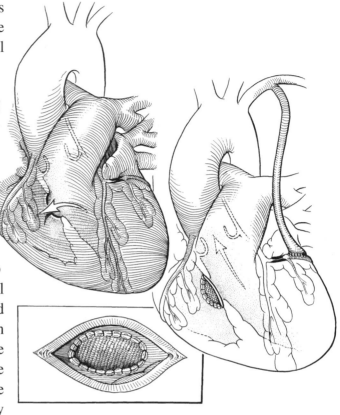

Figure 18.11. Drawing, upper left, showing left ventricular septal defect occurring as a complication of myocardial infarction. Drawing on right showing method of surgical treatment, consisting in Dacron® patch graft used to close ventricular septal defect (shown in insert) and coronary bypass when appropriate.

CHAPTER NINETEEN

Arterial Occlusive Disease

Occlusive Disease of the Legs

Arteriosclerosis or atherosclerosis is the underlying lesion in most patients with occlusive disease of the legs. The disease tends to assume distinctive patterns of location and extent. It may be confined completely to the terminal abdominal aorta and its major branches, the common iliac arteries, with relatively normal arteries below (Figure 19.1). This pattern of the disease is often termed the Leriche syndrome after the late French surgeon René Leriche, who originally described it (Figure 19.2). As the atheromatous process progresses, it narrows the lumen of the lower abdominal aorta or its major branches, the common iliac arteries, and this decreases blood flow to ultimately cause complete obstruction. A second pattern of the disease involves the main arteries in the thighs, the superficial femoral arteries. Here again, the disease is localized, usually in the mid-portion of the thigh with relatively normal arteries above

and below. The disease begins with gradual narrowing of the lumen of the artery and progresses to complete obstruction, sometimes because of superimposed clotting. Some patients have a combination of these two patterns, with localized involvement in the abdominal aorta, iliac arteries, and superficial femoral arteries in the thighs (Figures 19.3 and 19.4). Still another pattern of the disease involves the arteries below the knee. This is the most serious pattern because it usually does not lend itself to effective treatment.

Occlusive disease of the legs occurs most often in men (in a ratio of about 10 to 1), usually between the ages of 40 and 70 years. It may, however, occur in patients in their 20s or in some older than 80 years of age. In women, it occurs more often after the age of 60 years.

Symptoms depend on the site and extent of the disease and its speed of development. Gradual development of the disease allows time for collateral circulation to occur; in such cases, symptoms are minimal at first and progress slowly. If the

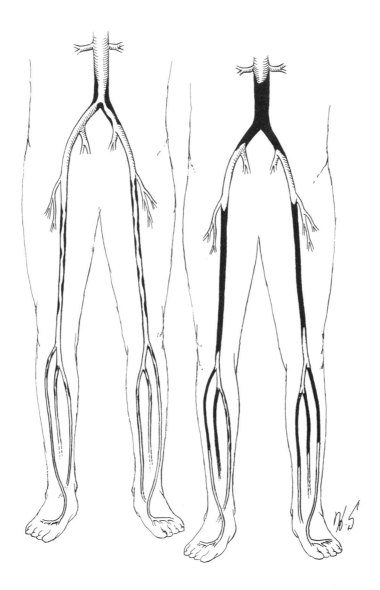

Figure 19.1. Typical patterns of occlusive disease of the abdominal aorta and vessels to the legs. The athero-sclerotic lesion tends to occur in the terminal abdominal aorta and common iliac arteries, in the superficial femoral arteries, and in the distal branches of the popliteal arteries. Usually there is a gradual progression from mild to moderate stenosis to complete obstruction (right).

disease strikes without time for develop-ment of collateral circulation, distal circu-lation may suddenly become impaired. In

most patients, however, symptoms develop gradually. In patients with the aorto-iliac pattern of the disease, the most common

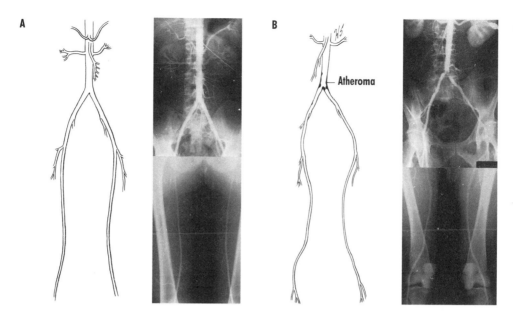

Figure 19.2. A. Drawing and aortogram, showing normal abdominal aorta and its branches in the legs. B. Drawing and aortogram of a 50-year-old man complaining of intermittent leg and buttock pain on exercise and impotency (Leriche syndrome), showing severe well-localized obstruction in the terminal abdominal aorta and origin of common iliac arteries.

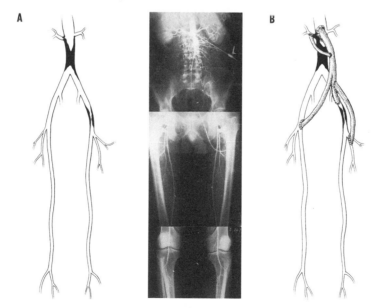

Figure 19.3. A. Drawing and preoperative aortogram of a 44-year-old man with intermittent claudication and hypertension showing complete obstruction of terminal abdominal aorta and well-localized stenosis in left external iliac artery.
B. Drawing showing method of surgical treatment, consisting in Dacron® bifurcation bypass graft to the right common femoral, left external iliac, and left common femoral arteries and to the right renal arteries.

A   B

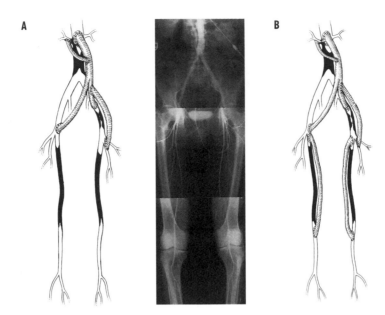

Figure 19.4. A. Drawing and preoperative aortogram of same patient as shown in Figure 19.3, three years later now complaining of intermittent pain on exercise in both calves because of progressive development of atherosclerotic obstructing disease in both superficial femoral arteries, as demonstrated by aortogram, which also shows patency of grafts to the right renal and femoral arteries.
B. Drawing showing method of surgical treatment, consisting in bilateral Dacron® femoral-popliteal bypass grafts. Patient has remained asymptomatic for 23 years.

complaint is pain in the buttocks, thighs, and legs during exercise. The pain is relieved with rest and renewed on walking or exercising. This is termed *intermittent claudication.* With gradual progression of the disease, the patient finds that he can walk only a few blocks or less before the pain becomes so severe that he must stop and rest before walking again. The aorto-iliac pattern of the disease often causes male patients to become impotent. Patients whose superficial femoral arteries in the thighs are affected complain of tightening-like pain in the calves of the legs during walking or exercise. As both patterns of

the disease worsen, claudication becomes more severe; the ability to walk becomes more limited; and eventually pain is felt even at rest. Simultaneously, the patient develops atrophy of the muscles in the legs, wasting of the subcutaneous tissues, coldness of the feet, loss of hair, and excessive growth of the toenails. Ultimately, gangrenous changes may occur in the skin of the feet and toes, often precipitated by a slight injury.

The diagnosis usually is readily made from the typical symptoms just described, along with diminution or absence of pulses in the legs. Normally, the systolic blood pressure recorded at the ankle is greater than that in the arm. Accordingly, the ankle/arm index is 1.0 or greater. Progressive narrowing of the arteries and atherosclerotic occlusive disease produce a fall in the ankle/arm index. This is used as a relatively simple diagnostic procedure. Mild to moderate disease will produce values between 0.5 and 1.0, whereas more severe occlusion will result in values below 0.5. In some centers, a diagnostic procedure called plethysmography (see Chapter 5) is used. Doppler flow studies (ultrasonic) of the extremities can readily confirm the diagnosis. Arteriography, however, is required to provide more precise information, particularly to determine the pattern of the disease so that the most appropriate method of treatment can be selected. Arteriography is performed by injection of a radiopaque substance into the aorta or artery above the occlusive process followed by roentgenography (x-ray studies). This is a relatively simple procedure that is performed usually with local anesthesia by inserting a catheter through the femoral artery in the groin or through the artery in the arm into the abdominal aorta. This procedure permits visualization of the normal lumen of the aorta and its major branches and the exact site and extent of the occlusion (Figures 19.2 and 19.3). The risk associated with this procedure is extremely low, as evidenced by our experience in which

significant complications occurred in only one patient out of three or four thousand.

Treatment is directed toward restoration of normal circulation by one of several procedures, depending on the pattern of the disease. One of these procedures is percutaneous transluminal angioplasty (Figure 19.5). It is performed after induction of local anesthesia by inserting a balloon catheter into the artery through a small opening and directing the catheter to the stenotic area by a guide wire under fluoroscopic control. When the balloon of the catheter is properly placed in the stenotic area, it is inflated to a predicted diameter. This dilation enlarges the lumen by compressing and fracturing the atheromatous plaque and causing some dehiscence of the intima from the media. In some cases a stint is used following the dilatation to assure maintenance of the dilated lumen. The procedure is preferably indicated in relatively short focal lesions no longer than 3 or 4 centimeters in the abdominal aorta, and iliac, femoral, and popliteal arteries. The early results of this procedure are quite satisfactory, with restoration of circulation in over 90 percent of patients (Figure 19.6). After one or two years, however, about 30 percent of these patients have a recurrence. Certain complications, occurring in 5 to 7 percent of patients, include thrombus or clot formation and embolism, arterial rupture and perforation, and loss of life. About 2 to 3 percent of patients may

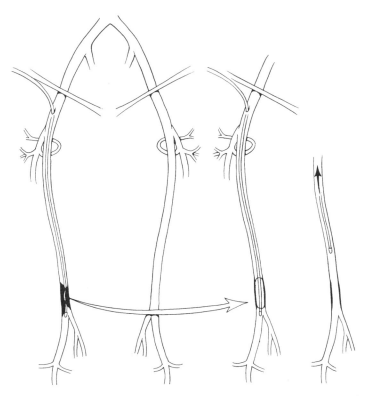

Figure 19.5. Technique of transluminal angioplasty, consisting in insertion of a balloon-tipped catheter to the site of the stenotic lesion (left). The balloon is then inflated to dilate the area (right), following which the catheter is removed.

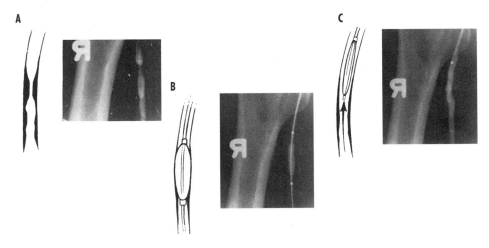

Figure 19.6. A. Right femoral arteriogram of a 68-year-old man complaining of intermittent pain in right calf on exercise, showing well-localized occlusive lesion in upper segment of right superficial femoral artery. B. Right femoral x-ray showing dilatation of balloon. C. Right femoral arteriogram made after angioplasty, showing relatively normal lumen.

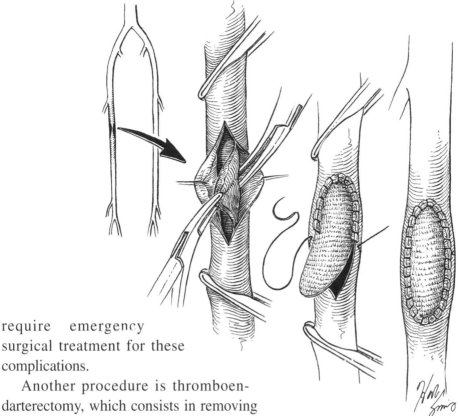

Figure 19.7. Surgical technique of endarterectomy and patch-graft angioplasty for localized occlusive lesion of the superficial femoral artery.

require emergency surgical treatment for these complications.

Another procedure is thromboendarterectomy, which consists in removing the atheromatous lesion by dissecting, or separating, it from the arterial wall (Figure 19.7). The incision in the artery is often repaired with a patch to avoid constriction of the lumen after closing the incision. This technique is used in extremely well-localized lesions, perhaps no more than one or two inches long.

A third method is application of a bypass graft. In most of our patients with disease of the terminal abdominal aorta and common iliac arteries, the bypass graft has proved to be the most satisfactory. The trunk of a Y-shaped Dacron® graft is attached by end-to-side anastomosis to an opening made in the aorta above the obstructive lesion, usually just below the origin of the renal arteries (Figure 19.8). The two limbs of the graft are attached by end-to-side anastomosis to the main arteries below the obstruction. By this means, circulation is shunted through the graft around the obstructed segment in the legs. In some patients in whom the

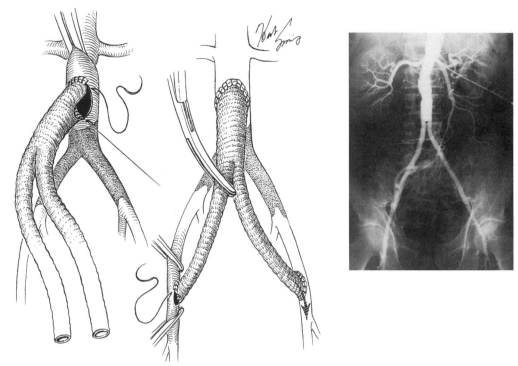

Figure 19.8. Surgical technique for bypass graft from the abdominal aorta to the external iliac or common femoral arteries. Aortogram shows graft functioning with restoration of normal circulation 20 years after operation.

occlusive process produces complete obstruction of the abdominal aorta from the origin of the renal arteries to the bifurcation, it is necessary to perform thromboendarterectomy to provide an opening in the lumen of the aorta to which the Dacron® graft can be attached.

Results of this operation are excellent, with successful restoration of circulation in about 98 percent of the patients. Long-term results are good; many patients maintain relatively normal and even vigorous physical activity for 10 to 25 years (Figure 19.4). The risk of operation is minimal,

with an operative mortality rate of only 1 or 2 percent.

For the second pattern of disease, in which the superficial femoral artery in the thigh is involved, the bypass procedure has also proved to be the most satisfactory, particularly for those long occluded segments (Figure 19.9). In this procedure, a small incision is made in the groin to expose the common femoral artery, and a longitudinal incision is made in the artery between temporary occluding clamps. One end of a Dacron® graft is attached to this opening by end-to-side anastomosis. The

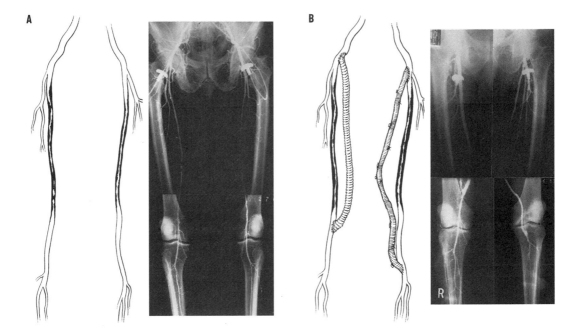

Figure 19.9. A. Drawing and preoperative arteriogram of a 72-year-old man complaining of intermittent pain in both calves upon exercise, showing well-localized complete occlusion in both superficial femoral arteries with relatively normal popliteal arteries below the occlusion.
B. Drawing showing method of surgical treatment, consisting in Dacron® bypass graft from right common femoral artery to popliteal artery above the knee and autogenous saphenous vein bypass graft from left common femoral artery to popliteal artery below the knee, and postoperative arteriogram showing restoration of normal circulation to legs through both grafts. Patient has remained asymptomatic for 20 years.

vessel below the obstruction, the popliteal artery, then is exposed by an incision on the inner side of the leg just above the knee. The other end of the graft is brought down to this incision through a tunnel under the skin and is attached to an opening made in the popliteal artery by a similar end-to-side anastomosis. Circulation is thus shunted through the graft into the main artery of the lower leg. In some patients, particularly when the obstructive lesion extends for a short distance below the knee, it may be prefer-able to use a segment of the saphenous vein removed from the leg, instead of a Dacron® graft, as a substitute.

Results of operation are excellent, with restoration of circulation and normal activities in more than 90 percent of the patients (Figure 19.9). The risk of operation is small, with an operative mortality rate of less than one percent.

In some patients with a combination of aort-oiliac and superficial femoral occlusive disease, it may be desirable to use both types of grafts (Figure 19.10). In

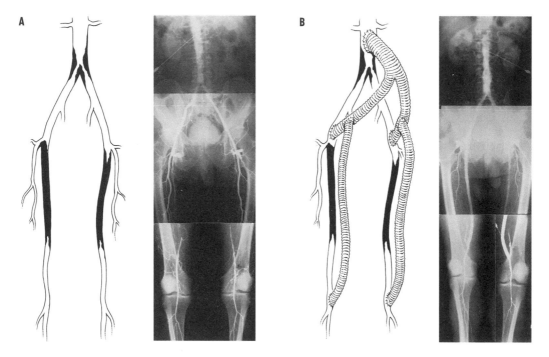

Figure 19.10. A. Drawing and preoperative aortogram of a 65-year-old man with severe intermittent claudication in both legs, showing severe atherosclerotic occlusive disease in terminal abdominal aorta and both superficial femoral arteries.
B. Drawing showing method of surgical treatment, consisting in bypass Dacron® bifurcation graft from abdominal aorta to both common femoral arteries and from these limbs of the bifurcation graft to both popliteal arteries with use of 8 mm tubular Dacron® grafts, and aortogram made 12 years after operation showing restoration of normal circulation. Patient was completely relieved of claudication symptoms.

others, sympathectomy may be indicated. This procedure consists in excising a small segment of the lumbar sympathetic nerve ganglia in order to interrupt the nerve impulses that cause constriction of the muscle in the wall of the arteries of the legs. Its purpose is to permit widening of the lumen of the arteries, particularly the smaller arteries, and thus enable more blood to flow through these small arteries and a greater degree of collateral circulation to develop in the lower leg. The method of treatment selected should be based on the type, nature, and extent of the obstructive disease. Men should be aware of the possibility of being unable to ejaculate after the bilateral lumbar sympathectomy.

With the third pattern of occlusive disease, the type in which the obstructive process involves the major arteries below the knee with relatively little or no occlusion in the arteries above this level, it is often not possible to perform effective treatment by endarterectomy or bypass graft. Sometimes, the procedure of lumbar

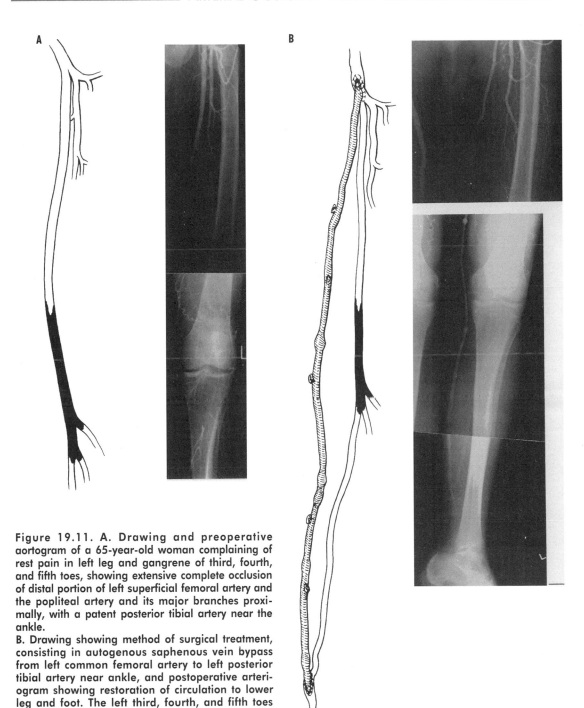

Figure 19.11. A. Drawing and preoperative aortogram of a 65-year-old woman complaining of rest pain in left leg and gangrene of third, fourth, and fifth toes, showing extensive complete occlusion of distal portion of left superficial femoral artery and the popliteal artery and its major branches proximally, with a patent posterior tibial artery near the ankle.

B. Drawing showing method of surgical treatment, consisting in autogenous saphenous vein bypass from left common femoral artery to left posterior tibial artery near ankle, and postoperative arteriogram showing restoration of circulation to lower leg and foot. The left third, fourth, and fifth toes were then successfully amputated. About six weeks after operation, the patient fell and fractured her hip, requiring surgical correction.

sympathectomy may provide some improvement; however, in some patients with this pattern of disease and with patent segments of the arteries around the ankle and foot, it may be possible to use a vein bypass graft from the femoral artery above to one of these patent segments in the ankle area. In a small proportion of our patients, this procedure has been reasonably successful in relieving discomfort and even in preventing early amputation (Figure 19.11).

Transluminally placed endovascular grafts, as described in Chapter 23, have also been used recently in the treatment of occlusive lesions of the arteries in the legs.

Occlusive Disease of the Arteries to the Abdominal Organs

The arterial blood supply to the abdominal organs, such as the liver, spleen, stomach, intestines, and kidneys, comes from arteries that arise from the abdominal aorta. Thus, the kidneys receive their blood supply from the two arteries, termed the right and left renal arteries. The remaining abdominal organs receive their blood supply from the celiac, superior mesenteric, and inferior mesenteric arteries. Aside from congenital abnormalities, such as coarctation (discussed in Chapter 16), certain acquired diseases may develop in these arteries

and cause disturbances in circulation and function.

There are two major causes of occlusive disease in the renal arteries (Figure 19.12). The first, and by far the most common, is atherosclerosis, which is well localized in the proximal portion of the artery, with a relatively normal distal segment. The second, which is much rarer, is fibromuscular hyperplasia; it is characterized by multiple areas of thickening of the middle layer of the arterial wall and consequently, narrowing of the lumen (Figure 19.13). This condition occurs most often in relatively young women in their 20s and 30s. A most important consideration in both of these occlusive diseases is that they are

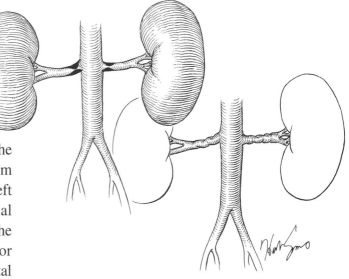

Figure 19.12. Patterns of occlusive disease of renal arteries, with atherosclerotic occlusive disease (left) and fibromuscular hyperplasia (right).

A

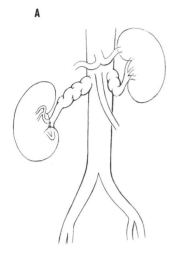

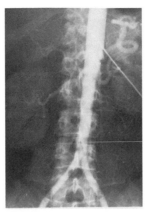

B

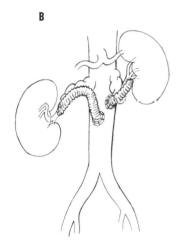

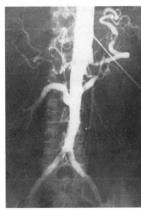

Figure 19.13. A. Drawing and preoperative aortogram of a 45-year-old woman with severe hypertension not controlled by medical treatment, showing occlusive disease of both renal arteries from fibromuscular hyperplasia.
B. Drawing showing method of surgical treatment, consisting in bypass Dacron® grafts to both renal arteries, and aortogram made 23 years after operation, showing restoration of normal circulation to both renal arteries. Patient remains well now, 32 years after operation.

often associated with hypertension. This is believed to be caused by diminution in blood flow and pulse pressure, triggering the production of a chemical, termed renin, in the kidney, as discussed in Chapter 11 on hypertension. Experience has shown that a causal relation does exist in many patients with hypertension and renal artery occlusive disease. Some patients, however, have this occlusive lesion but do not have hypertension.

Atherosclerotic occlusive disease of the renal arteries occurs predominantly in men, most often between the ages of 50 and 70 years of age. Associated arteriosclerotic disease of other major arteries of the body occurs in about one-third of these patients, and involvement of both renal arteries occurs in about one-third of the patients. A history of sudden onset of hypertension or unresponsiveness to antihypertension drugs highly suggests occlusive disease in the renal arteries. The diagnosis usually can be made by special laboratory tests of kidney function, and confirmed by arteriography, which shows the location and extent of the occlusive lesion. Evaluation of renal hypertension is discussed in Chapter 11.

Initial treatment in most patients is medical, including antihypertensive medication. In patients whose blood pressure is poorly controlled on medication, especially young patients and those with signs of progressive renal impairment, angiography is indicated. Percutaneous balloon angioplasty may be used particularly in well-localized stenotic lesions in the main renal artery. The long-term results and incidence of recurrence after this procedure remain undetermined.

For young patients with severe, uncontrolled hypertension and progressive loss of renal function, and for those with bilateral disease involving the ostia or origin of the renal arteries from the aorta, restoration of normal circulation to the kidney is preferably achieved by one of two surgical procedures, namely, endarterectomy with patch-graft angioplasty or the bypass graft. We have had extensive experience with both procedures, and for most patients we prefer the bypass graft (Figure 19.14). This is performed by attachment of an albumin-coated Dacron® tube graft by end-to-side anastomosis to an opening in the side of the abdominal aorta and then to the renal artery just distal to the occlusive lesions by similar anastomosis.

Results of surgical treatment have been highly satisfactory, with an operative mortality rate of about 1 or 2 percent. In our experience with more than 3,000 patients, blood pressure was restored to normal in more than 80 percent. Long-term results are also good, and survival expectancy is also reasonably good, with best survival in young patients (30 years or younger) being more than 90 percent at 15 years. Even in patients younger than 50

A

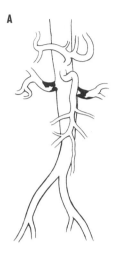 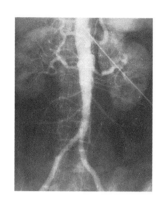

B

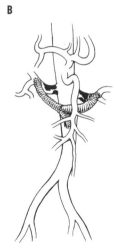 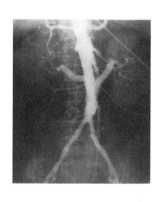

Figure 19.14. A. Drawing and preoperative aortogram of a 45-year-old woman with severe hypertension, despite medical treatment, and headaches, showing bilateral atherosclerotic occlusive lesions in renal arteries.
B. Drawing showing method of surgical treatment, consisting in Dacron® bypass graft from abdominal aorta to both renal arteries, and aortogram made about 15 years after operation, showing restoration of normal circulation to both renal arteries through the Dacron® grafts. Patient has remained well for over 30 years since operation.

years, it was about 80 percent at 10 years (Figure 19.13). In occasional patients with irreversible damage to one kidney, nephrectomy may be indicated.

The clinical syndrome of abdominal angina (also termed chronic mesenteric vascular insufficiency, intestinal angina, or splanchnic ischemia) usually is caused by atherosclerotic occlusive disease, primarily of the celiac and superior mesenteric arteries, but occasionally of the inferior mesenteric arteries, which supply blood to the gastrointestinal tract. In most patients,

the atheromatous lesion is well localized in these arteries just beyond their origin from the aorta. Most patients with abdominal angina have involvement of at least two of the arteries, mostly the celiac and superior mesenteric.

This disease is relatively rare, as evidenced by the fact that our own series of cases is limited to about 150 patients. Occlusion of the celiac and mesenteric arteries occurs most often in persons between the ages of 50 and 70 years. The chief complaint is cramp-like pain in the

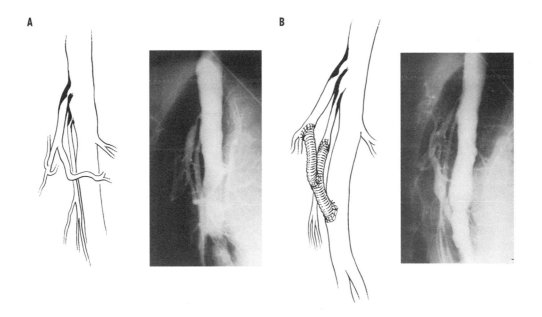

Figure 19.15. A. Drawing and preoperative arteriogram of a 52-year-old woman complaining of abdominal cramp-like pain, especially after eating, and 50-pound weight loss during the past year, showing well-localized atherosclerotic stenotic lesions at origin of celiac and superior mesenteric arteries.
B. Drawing showing method of surgical treatment, consisting in Dacron® bypass graft from abdominal aorta to celiac and superior mesenteric arteries, and postoperative arteriogram showing restoration of normal circulation through Dacron® grafts. Shortly after operation, patient was completely relieved of symptoms and began to gain weight.

upper part of the abdomen shortly after meals. This pain may last for several hours and often radiates to the back. The patient associates the pain with eating, and therefore tends to eat less; the result is significant weight loss. The patient may also complain of bloating, diarrhea, constipation, nausea, and vomiting. Associated arteriosclerotic disease in other arteries of the body is not uncommon. The diagnosis is made by arteriographic demonstration of the occlusive disease (Figure 19.15).

Treatment is surgical and is directed toward restoring normal circulation in the affected arteries. Although endarterectomy may be employed, in our experience, the bypass graft procedure has been found to be more satisfactory (Figure 19.15). Because the occlusive lesion is usually well localized, with a relatively normal artery beyond the lesion, it is possible to attach a Dacron® graft from the abdominal aorta to the distal artery. Blood is thereby shunted through the graft to the celiac and superior mesenteric arteries beyond the occlusive disease. Results of this type of operation, providing restoration of normal circulation to the gastrointestinal tract, have produced excellent relief of the patients' symptoms.

In advanced disease, in which irreversible hypoxic damage to the intestine has occurred, the results are much less favorable, and the mortality rate is high. Irreversible shock, gangrene of the intestine, and peritonitis may occur in terminal cases resulting from ischemia of the intestine.

CHAPTER TWENTY

Stroke

Medical Aspects

by John P. Winikates, M.D.

Stroke is perhaps the most feared of vascular diseases. For many people, it is a devastating illness: it paralyzes and robs them of strength, speech, memory, and, perhaps worst, independence. The very name for it, *stroke*, suggests its suddenness and severity. Hippocrates (460–370 B.C.) called it *apoplexy* — "to be struck down by violence or paralysis." In his original description, he recognized the loss of speech and development of numbness and paralysis; he also observed a poor prognosis in most patients. About 500,000 to 600,000 strokes occur annually in the United States, about 1,400 daily, or about one stroke each minute. Roughly, one-fourth of these are fatal, accounting for about 150,000 deaths each year. This makes stroke the third leading cause of death in the United States, after heart disease and cancer from all causes. Stroke is the most common neurologic illness and the leading cause of neurologic disability in our society, affecting 2 to 3 million stroke survivors. The annual cost of stroke in the United States is estimated between $16.2 billion and $25 billion. As the population ages, the scope of this problem is expected to increase. Medical research and advances in medical and surgical treatment for stroke are improving the outlook for millions of people with this dread disease.

Risk Factors

Observations in patients during the past several decades have clarified the risk factors for stroke. The most significant risk factor is age. The risk of stroke doubles for every decade of life over 55 years; 72 percent of all strokes occur in people over the age of 65 years. More men experience strokes than women, in a ratio of about 1.3 to 1. The incidence of stroke among black Americans is twice that of white Americans, in part because of the higher incidence of hypertension in the black population. Hypertension, or high blood pressure, is the most common treatable risk factor for stroke. About one-fourth to one-third of adult Americans have high blood pressure. This increases stroke risk by four to six times. Studies have shown that improved detection and treatment of high blood pressure are effective in decreasing the incidence and mortality rate of stroke. Diabetes, another treatable risk factor for stroke, increases risk by three times. An elevated cholesterol level is also of great importance and can be treated by proper diet and medication. Smoking accelerates vascular damage and magnifies the effect of other risk factors. In the past, some controversy existed about the true role of smoking as a risk factor for stroke. Recent review of multiple studies over many years (meta-analysis) has finally shown conclusively what was long thought to be true, that smoking is clearly another major risk factor.

Heart disease also increases risk of stroke. The nature of the increased risk depends on the nature of the underlying heart disease. The greatest risk is associated with the abnormal heart rhythm of atrial fibrillation, especially if it is the result of heart valve damage from rheumatic heart disease. Recent myocardial infarction and congestive heart failure also increase the risk of stroke. History of a previous stroke or transient ischemic attack increases the risk of subsequent stroke by ten times. A bruit in the arteries of the neck and sufficient narrowing of

these arteries indicate an increase in stroke risk. Less important risk factors include a family history of stroke (especially in the patient's mother), peripheral vascular disease, polycythemia (high red cell count), and a history of gout. Identification of risk factors and the thorough and thoughtful remediation of those factors that are modifiable can significantly reduce the chance of stroke. Regular monitoring of blood pressure, blood sugar level, and cholesterol count and stopping smoking are fundamental parts of any health maintenance program.

Causes of Stroke

The brain depends on a continuous, secure flow of blood and nutrients. The human brain weighs only about 1.5 kilograms (about three pounds), and accounts for only 2 percent of body weight. Yet 15 percent of the cardiac output goes directly to the brain, which consumes 20 percent of the oxygen used by the entire body. A stroke, or cerebrovascular accident (CVA), results from disruption of the normal blood flow to a portion of the brain, causing damage to that particular region of brain tissue.

About 15–20 percent of strokes are caused by hemorrhage. A break in the wall of a cerebral artery allows blood to push out into normal brain tissue and directly damage the brain. About 80–85 percent of strokes are ischemic. In ischemic stroke, normal blood flow through one of the cerebral arteries is blocked, usually by a blood clot, and this blockage prevents delivery of vital oxygen, glucose, and other nutrients. Such a blood clot may form within a cerebral artery already narrowed by plaque. This type of stroke is called *thrombotic stroke.* The blood clot may also form within the heart or on the wall of the aorta and then break off and travel to a cerebral artery. This is termed an *embolic stroke.* These types of strokes tend to involve the larger arteries within the cerebral circulation. Small branch arteries within the brain, called *penetrating arteries,* are subject to a special form of thickening of the walls, narrowing, and eventually blocking the arteries. Still another form of ischemic stroke is caused by atherosclerotic occlusive disease involving the major arteries supplying blood to the brain, including particularly the common carotid arteries at their bifurcation, as discussed in the section concerned with surgical treatment. This type of stroke is called a *lacune.* Published series indicate that thrombotic stroke is the most common, accounting for about one-half of all strokes, followed by embolic stroke (about 20 to 30 percent) and lacunar stroke (about 15 percent). A variety of other diseases of the cerebral veins and arteries cause another 5 percent.

Symptoms

The symptoms of stroke depend on the area of the brain affected. The brain is highly organized; each specific part of the brain performs a specific task. When blood flow is disrupted in a specific blood vessel during a stroke, the symptoms reflect loss of the specialized function performed by that part of the brain. For example, if the motor control area on the right side of the brain (the right hemisphere) is damaged, weakness or paralysis of the left side of the body develops.[1] Damage to the language areas (usually in the left hemisphere of the brain) leads to difficulty in understanding or producing speech, and dizziness or diplopia (double vision) may occur if the base of the brain (the brain stem) has been damaged.

The single most common symptom of stroke is paralysis, which is usually focal, involving one side of the body or the other. Speech is also commonly affected. The speech disorder may be due to weakness of one side of the mouth or weakness of the tongue, causing slurring of speech.

[1] This phenomenon was recognized by Egyptian physicians about 5,000 years ago as recorded in the Edurin Smith Egyptian papyrus, which is believed by some historians to have been written by Imhotep, the Pharaoh's grand vizier [prime minister], whose status and reputation became so great that he was eventually declared to be a god, Ptah.

This disruption of articulation is called *dysarthria*. The other pattern of speech disturbance is called *aphasia*. In this pattern, the ability to understand language is impaired or the ability to produce words themselves. Less commonly, sensation on one side of the body is affected, and the victim complains of numbness. Just as weakness of the facial muscles can affect articulation, weakness of facial and oral muscles can cause difficulty in swallowing *(dysphagia)*. Vision can be affected in a variety of ways. Vision in one eye can be lost, or part of the field of vision may be blurred or lost. Patients can also experience double vision or impaired focusing.

Loss of coordination or loss of balance may be the result of stroke. Dizziness is less common in stroke and can result from a large number of other causes as well. When, however, dizziness occurs along with other signs, such as weakness, slurred speech, swallowing difficulty, or double vision, the likelihood of stroke is much greater. Sometimes the signs of stroke are more subtle; the patient may have difficulty performing a particular mental task like calculations, have trouble dressing, or appear to have forgotten how to use silverware. The patient may ignore one side of his body. In rare instances, the first signs of stroke may be general confusion or lethargy.

Some strokes occur during sleep; a patient may go to bed well and awaken with symptoms. A stroke may also occur during the day, in the midst of normal activities. The sudden development of any of these symptoms should cause concern about the possibility of stroke and lead the patient to seek immediate medical investigation.

About 10 percent of strokes are preceded by a temporary deficit called a *transient ischemic attack* (TIA). In such an event, the patient experiences symptoms of a stroke, such as paralysis or speech disturbance, but these symptoms resolve spontaneously. The TIA can last up to 24 hours, but most resolve in five minutes or less. The brief nature of the symptoms leads many patients to defer seeking medical attention; less than 50 percent of patients experiencing a TIA seek treatment within 24 hours. Patients with TIAs, however, have a tenfold increased risk of suffering a major stroke; 50 percent will have a stroke within one year. Of these, 20 percent will have a stroke within the month of the initial TIA. Therefore, a TIA is an important opportunity to identify the cause and begin medical treatment or to perform vascular surgery to prevent a completed stroke from occurring. The brief nature of the episode should not be taken as a sign that there is no further risk of stroke, nor should the hope that the attack will resolve on its own lead a patient to delay seeking medical care from appropriate specialists.

In addition to control of risk factors, use of blood thinners and surgical treatment are important means of stroke prevention in patients who have had TIAs or a previous stroke. The most effective treatment depends on the type of stroke or TIA the patient has had (thrombotic, embolic, or lacunar) and the other stroke risk factors that may be present. Aspirin has become the most basic drug for stroke prevention. Recommended doses have ranged from a very low dose (75 to 100 mg daily) to a high dose (1,300 mg daily). The optimum aspirin dose for stroke prevention has not yet been determined; further studies are needed to establish it. Ticlopidine is another drug that decreases the risk of recurrent stroke or TIA. It appears to be more effective than aspirin, especially in women and patients with hypertension and diabetes mellitus (both important risk factors for stroke), patients whose symptoms arise from the brain stem (the vertebrobasilar system), and patients in whom aspirin has failed.

Both these drugs act in different ways to slow blood clotting by inhibiting the activity of blood platelets. Platelets are cell fragments in the blood stream that play a key role in initiating blood clot formation in a vessel whose wall has been damaged. These drugs are therefore often called *antiplatelet agents*. In the case of aspirin, it is necessary to choose a basic dose and adjust it according to side effects, such as abdominal pain. Ticlopidine requires a complete blood count about every two weeks during the first three months of treatment to watch for a fall in the white blood count. The risk of a decreased blood count is about one in one thousand during the first three months of treatment. Afterwards, the increased risk returns to baseline. The most common side effect of ticlopidine is indigestion. In about one to four patients some form of indigestion occurs and often necessitates discontinuation of the drug. Patients with artificial heart valves, atrial fibrillation, or intracardiac clot are given warfarin as a preventive against stroke.

Patients with significant narrowing in the carotid arteries should be considered for surgical removal of the blockage. Recent studies have shown what had been suspected—that patients with 60 percent or more narrowing should undergo carotid endarterectomy to prevent recurrent stroke, especially when the plaque is ulcerated. This approach is combined with aspirin and treatment of any other stroke risk factors to achieve maximum success in prevention. The general benefit from surgical treatment depends on the skill and experience of the surgeon. Surgical candidates should be referred to the most experienced surgeon possible.

Physiology

A relatively large volume of blood is delivered through four major vessels to the brain: the carotid arteries in the front of the neck and the vertebral arteries traveling up the back of the neck; the carotid arteries, which branch near the angle of the jaw into the external carotid artery, which supplies the skin and muscles of the face; and the internal carotid artery, which passes through a special channel in the skull to supply the brain (Figure 20.1). The vertebral arteries enter the skull through the foramen magnum, the hole at the base of the skull through which the spinal cord

passes. As these arteries travel up the front of the brain stem, the lower portion of the brain, they fuse to form the basilar artery. All these major arteries come together deep under the brain to form a ring of blood vessels called the circle of Willis. The arteries then branch out from this central circle to spread over the surface, or cortex, of the brain.

The main blood supply to the cerebral hemispheres comes from the internal carotid arteries, through the circle of

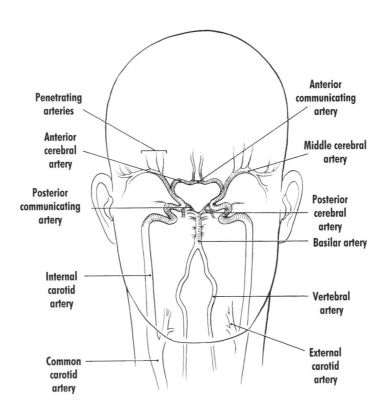

Figure 20.1. Drawing showing blood supply to the brain.

Willis, to the anterior and middle cerebral arteries. This portion of the cerebral circulation is often called the *anterior circulation*. Blood flow to the back of the hemispheres and to the brain stem comes from the vertebrobasilar artery system (called the *posterior circulation*). The majority of blood flow goes to the cortex, or gray matter, the site of the cell bodies of the nerve cells, or neurons, that compose the brain. The long, wirelike processes of the neurons (the *axons*), travel in bundles (called *tracts*), forming the white matter. This portion of the brain is supplied by blood vessels called penetrating arteries, very fine branches off the main arterial trunks of the middle cerebral artery and the basilar artery.

The activity of the brain shifts from one part of the brain to the next as we go from one task to the next—taking a walk, planning a trip to the store, or reading these pages. The brain automatically adjusts blood flow to different areas as the activity of that part of the brain varies. It also automatically maintains an even flow of blood to the brain as a whole, even if the body's blood pressure varies. This is called *autoregulation*. Through autoregulation and with the help of the circle of Willis, the brain maintains a constant overall blood supply, adjusting its distribution throughout itself.

Normal blood flow to the brain is about 750 ml/min, or about 55 ml/100 g of brain tissue/min. This guaranteed supply of oxygen, glucose, and nutrients gives the neurons the energy they need to integrate incoming information from other neurons and to maintain an electrical charge on the neuron cell membrane. This neuron is then ready to fire off a nerve impulse—a minute electrical discharge like a current—down the axon, to signal the next cell. This action ultimately allows you to turn this page.

What happens to a neuron when this guaranteed flow is interrupted depends on the degree of compromise to the flow and how long that decrease lasts. A decrease to about one-third to one-half of normal stops the chemical machinery that maintains the neuron's charge. The neuron fires, or is depolarized, but is unable to reestablish its charge. It becomes unable to signal and is electrically silent; its function is interrupted. When blood flow increases back to normal, the cell can regulate its charge, start signaling once again, and function returns. If blood flow stops completely for as little as four minutes, even more basic chemical machinery of the cell is damaged. The cell membrane begins to leak (membrane pump failure); the cell starts to swell; and the neuron will die. Neurons can survive intermediate degrees of decreased flow if full flow is reestablished promptly (within a few hours). Studies in experimental animals and more recent trials in patients have shown that this period of reversible injury is less than six hours and probably less than three hours. Also, evidence shows that within an ischemic area of the brain, there are varying degrees of decreased flow. In the center closest to the arterial blockage is an area of absent flow in which cell death occurs very rapidly—a core zone of infarction where cell death is virtually certain. Surrounding this area is a shadow region in which flow is decreased but not completely lost, partially maintained by collateral flow from vessels around the margins of the ischemic area. This zone is called the *ischemic penumbra*. The neurons will survive and regain function if the flow is reestablished within hours; if not, these cells too will die, enlarging the area of permanent damage from the stroke. The specific neurologic symptoms in a stroke, then, depend on the specific territory of the artery blocked, the function of the area of the brain supplied, the condition of collateral flow from the surrounding area, and the duration of the blockage.

Evaluation and Treatment

When symptoms of a stroke develop, immediate medical attention and, generally, hospitalization are in order. The goals of treatment at this stage are to stabilize the neurologic damage, prevent complications, and, if possible, identify the stroke type. From this, the physician can plan any further testing that may be needed, begin rehabilitation, and prevent recurrence.

Initial evaluation begins with a history and physical examination. This must be performed quickly and efficiently, with special attention to the neurologic examination and to the heart and blood vessels in the neck. The pattern of deficits on the neurologic examination help the neurologist or other physician identify the part of the brain involved and the mechanism of damage. A computed tomography (CT) scan of the brain is one of the earliest investigations necessary in an acute stroke. The CT scan is very sensitive to signs of hemorrhage; hemorrhagic strokes require a different approach from ischemic strokes. The initial CT scan may also show early signs of swelling in the ischemic region or may show signs of earlier events and provide clues to the type of stroke in progress. The actual blood clot that is causing the acute ischemia is generally too small to be directly seen on the CT scan. Often, the initial CT scan will show no or only minimal changes. The changes caused by stroke may take days to evolve, so that a normal or minimally abnormal CT scan does not rule out stroke as the cause of the patient's symptoms or predict the size of the stroke that may occur later.

Once hemorrhage has been ruled out, treatment may sometimes be started with a blood thinner such as heparin. This drug is administered by injection, usually as a constant slow infusion in a vein. The best use of heparin, and newly developed related drugs called *heparinoids,* is a subject of ongoing research. These drugs do not dissolve the blood clot already present but stabilize the clot by keeping it from enlarging. This helps minimize the size of the ischemic area. They also prevent new clots from forming within the heart or other vessels, so that further emboli that could lead to another stroke do not develop. Aspirin may also be useful during the acute phase of a stroke. No single approach to the treatment of acute stroke applies to all patients. The proper choice of specific treatment must be individualized for the particular patient's needs and the type of stroke that patient has had.

Acute Care/ Thrombolytic Therapy

The most important breakthrough in acute stroke care is thrombolytic therapy. Whereas heparin, warfarin, aspirin, and ticlopidine slow the formation of new clots or the enlargement of existing clots, these drugs, known as *thrombolytic agents,* actually dissolve existing clots. The goals of thrombolytic therapy are to break down the blood clot occluding the cerebral artery and reestablish normal flow, goals that will limit damage resulting from the original

occlusion. Thrombolysis has been effectively and safely used in the treatment of acute myocardial infarction for longer than 10 years. Initial attempts at thrombolysis in stroke were unsuccessful. One reason for this lack of benefit was an increase in cerebral hemorrhage caused by thrombolysis. Animal research revealed that for thrombolysis to be effective in limiting infarct size in experimental strokes, it had to be used within 3 hours of the onset of vascular occlusion. This observation led to patient trials emphasizing much earlier treatment.

In 1995, the National Institutes of Health in the United States announced positive results from a trial of thrombolysis in a study of some 600 patients with acute ischemic stroke. This was the first trial showing positive results with the use of thrombolysis. Patients were evaluated within 3 hours of onset of symptoms and were randomized to placebo or treatment with alteplase (tissue plasminogen activator, or tPA). After performing a CT scan of the brain to ensure that symptoms were not due to a cerebral hemorrhage, physicians administered tPA intravenously. Treated patients showed less disability and greater independent function 3 months after treatment than did the controls.

These were impressive results. The study group showed that stroke patients can be effectively evaluated and treated within the first few critical hours after the onset of ischemic symptoms. They also showed that such early intervention may indeed improve the outcome. Several points must be emphasized as this treatment becomes increasingly available to larger numbers of people. Treatment within three hours is imperative to be successful. Later treatment may be ineffective or even dangerous since it may increase the risk of hemorrhage. For many patients, their first awareness of stroke symptoms is on arising from sleep. In such cases, the precise time of onset is unknown, and thrombolytic treatment may not be possible. Moreover, many patients do not seek medical attention within those first critical hours, waiting for spontaneous improvement. If thrombolysis and other treatments still in development are going to help the greatest number of stroke patients, the public should seek treatment within the first few hours of an attack.

Hemorrhage also remains a serious problem, since patients treated with thrombolysis have more frequent hemorrhages. These hemorrhages are often severe and may contribute to death. Whether one thrombolytic agent is safer than another has not been established but will eventually need to be determined. In a previous tPA trial in Europe, the risk of hemorrhage increased in patients who had subtle signs of cerebral edema on their initial CT scan of the brain. Future brain imaging technology may help to identify patients who are most likely to benefit from thrombol-

ysis and also those most at risk of the complications.

A variety of new drugs are in development through continuing animal experiments and clinical trials in patients. Stroke is obviously a complex cascade of events, triggered by the ischemic occlusion that evolves during minutes, hours, and days. Each of these newly discovered biochemical steps in the evolution of stroke offers a possibility for drug intervention to protect individual neurons from the damage triggered by ischemia. This cytoprotection may also prolong the time that cells can withstand ischemia, and this prolongation increases the effectiveness of thrombolysis.

Once an acute ischemic stroke begins, the patient's condition may fluctuate significantly during the first hours and days. Careful observation of the patient is especially important during this period. Patients are often admitted to an intensive care unit or to a special acute stroke care unit. A regular care unit, sometimes with electrocardiographic (ECG) monitoring, may be appropriate for the patient with less severe stroke or a more stable deficit. Cardiac monitoring is often used, not only because an irregular heart rhythm may have caused the stroke, but also because the stress of the acute illness may cause a new cardiac arrhythmia or coronary symptoms.

Early in an acute stroke, blood pressure may be elevated, even in a patient with no prior history of hypertension. In a hemorrhagic stroke, aggressive control of the blood pressure may help limit the size of the hemorrhage. In an ischemic stroke, however, this early blood pressure elevation may be part of the body's adaptation to the acute change in cerebral blood flow. A gentler approach to blood pressure management for acute ischemic stroke may help to protect some of the area of the brain with less secure perfusion, and thus limit the degree of damage. In either case, careful monitoring of the blood pressure and close observation of the response to any treatment are essential during the first days of an acute stroke.

Many patients with stroke have difficulty swallowing. As a result, food or secretions may enter the lungs and may cause pneumonia. Oral intake may need to be withheld altogether initially or limited to oral medications alone while the degree of swallowing difficulty is assessed. Some patients with persistent trouble may require a feeding tube, either through the nose or through the stomach wall, to ensure proper nutrition during this period. As the patient improves, special diets with soft foods and thickened liquids may be given.

Patients with stroke often have some kind of associated heart disease, such as coronary artery disease, heart valve abnormalities, or cardiac rhythm disturbances. Regular heart and lung examinations such as ECG, chest x-ray, and rhythm moni-

toring, are basic to initial stroke care. An echocardiogram is often part of the evaluation of stroke patients to assess the cardiac output and heart valves, as well as to identify blood clots within the heart. Echocardiography can be done with use of a sound transducer on the chest wall (transthoracic echocardiogram, TTE) or one passed through the esophagus (transesophageal echocardiogram, TEE). These provide a view of the aorta and the back wall of the heart. They may be necessary for full evaluation of a source of embolism and to help determine the long-term need for warfarin (an anticoagulant) to prevent further strokes.

Investigation for coronary disease may be important to assess the patient's overall health status, as well as to determine the safety of different physical therapy approaches. Cardiac stress testing with radionuclide scanning and drug injection, rather than the traditional exercise stress test, may be necessary, since the patient may be unable to perform any sort of exercise test. Consultation from a cardiologist is often beneficial to guide the testing and recommend appropriate medication.

One of the most serious complications during a stroke is brain swelling, or cerebral edema. Since the brain lies inside the rigid skull, swelling can increase intracranial pressure, which can lead to symptoms of drowsiness and lethargy, as well as damage to a previously uninjured part of the brain. In a large stroke, this swelling can be severe, even life threatening. Vigorous treatment with ventilator support, steroids, and other medications may be necessary. This cerebral edema is a temporary phenomenon, which runs its course over several days and gradually resolves in most patients. Maintaining normal blood sugar, blood electrolyte balance, kidney function, lung function, and fluid balance are also part of early stroke management.

Rehabilitation

Once the patient's neurologic and medical condition has stabilized during the first few days, rehabilitation therapy can be started. Different types of therapy are directed at the different needs of the patient. Physical therapy may begin with simple range of motion exercises of the paralyzed limb to maintain flexibility, followed by strengthening exercises for areas of major motor weakness, eventually focusing on walking and mobility. Occupational therapy involves fine motor control as is needed for performing daily tasks, such as dressing and using silverware. These are referred to as activities of daily living (ADLs). Speech therapy focuses on articulation, understanding of language, and word choice. Speech therapists also sometimes assist in the evaluation and treatment of swallowing problems. They may address other mental functions compromised by the stroke, such as memory or calculating.

Therapy can begin as soon as the patient's physical condition allows and is intensified as the patient's recovery progresses. Many patients benefit from consultation with a rehabilitation specialist who can direct the therapists and help focus the goals of treatment. Once the acute phase of the stroke is over, transfer to a rehabilitation unit for continuing the multidisciplinary approach to therapy is appropriate for some patients, whereas others are better served by discharge home and an outpatient therapy program. Addressing the rehabilitation needs of stroke patients is important in order to maximize their eventual recovery and to allow each stroke victim to achieve his highest level of independence after the stroke.

The goal of acute care in stroke is to minimize the damage caused by the ischemic event, prevent the many complications that can occur, and begin rehabilitation to maximize the recovery of every patient. Despite the best currently available treatment, about 25 percent of stroke victims die; 15 to 25 percent worsen after hospital admission; and many stroke survivors are left with significant disabilities, many severe. Current research in stroke, both in animals using experimental models of stroke and in more recent treatment trials in patients, is giving new hope that effective treatment can safely improve the outcome in acute ischemic stroke. New treatment approaches will change the face of acute stroke care during the next decade.

Biochemical Events of Stroke

A wide range of biochemical events occur during ischemia. One of the most fundamental cellular processes is the maintenance of water balance. Because body cells, including neurons, concentrate so many proteins and other molecules within the cell, water tends to be drawn in from the surrounding tissues. Because too much water damages the cell, water needs to be continuously pumped out. This is accomplished by a molecular pump in the cell membrane called the ion pump (or, more technically, the sodium-potassium ATPase). This pump uses energy derived from oxygen and glucose stored in the molecule adenosine triphosphate (ATP) to move sodium and potassium ions across the membrane, moving water with them. When delivery of oxygen and glucose for energy production is stopped, the neuron cannot make ATP; the ion pump cannot operate; excess water cannot be moved out of the cell; and the neuron swells with water and dies. This energy production failure leads to pump failure. This is the fate of cells in the central core of the infarction. Drugs blocking the membrane channels may help maintain the ion and water balance longer, and thus prolong the life of the cell.

Neurons in the ischemic penumbra, where they are receiving some flow, can maintain their ion pumps and water content, but other normal cell functions are impaired. A neuron maintains a certain electrochemical charge, or polarization, across its cell membrane. When a neuron is stimulated, or excited, the membrane depolarizes, and a nerve impulse travels down the axon to the next neuron in line. The axon does not, however, connect directly with the next cell. Instead, there is a specialized structure called the *synapse*. On one side, the axon ends in a bulb-like structure known as the *synaptic bouton*. On the other side, the neuron has special molecules called *receptors*. In between is a narrow gap, called the *synaptic cleft*. When the wave of depolarization reaches the axon terminal, the synaptic bouton releases a packet of neurotransmitters, chemicals that travel across the synaptic cleft and combine with the receptors on the other side. Each receptor is linked to an ion channel, a tubelike structure that passes through the cell membrane. This channel contains a gate. When the receptor is stimulated by the neurotransmitter, the gate opens and allows one of several ions (sodium, potassium, calcium, or chloride) to pass into or out of the cell. Depending on which ion is moving, the cell polarization increases, or hyperpolarizes, an action that inhibits firing of a nerve impulse. Once the cell depolarizes, it must be repolarized (recharging it so it can fire again).

Such channels controlled by a neurotransmitter and its receptor are called *ligand- gated ion channels.* Other channels in the neuron membrane open and close according to the charge, or voltage, across the membrane. These are called *voltage-gated ion channels.* Maintaining these channels, resetting them, and recharging the membrane, all require energy. In addition, the neuron must keep the rest of its chemical machinery going, synthesizing the neurotransmitters, packaging them, transporting them to the axon terminal, manufacturing membrane components, and maintaining the enzyme systems needed to convert oxygen and glucose into ATP energy to run everything.

Calcium has a key role in all this activity. The intracellular concentration of calcium is carefully controlled by the neuron as one of the means by which different phases of this cellular machinery is regulated. Calcium may enter the cell through ion channels or be released within the cell from special stores, and then it is collected within these stores to keep its concentration correct for the current activity needs of the neuron.

The relatively decreased blood flow in the ischemic penumbra can affect a neuron in a variety of ways. Neurons tend to depolarize when made ischemic. Once depolarized, they waste energy on recharging the membrane. Some of these neurons are inhibitory, some excitatory. During ischemia, excitatory influences tend to predominate, stimulating other neurons to fire, further consuming scarce energy and oxygen. The neurons excessively stimulated in this way will then start to falter. This process is called *excitotoxicity.*

The key neurotransmitter causing excitotoxicity is called *glutamate.* Glutamate opens a ligand-gated ion channel for calcium, leading to excessive calcium buildup within the excited cell. Since intracellular calcium must be kept in strict control to keep the cell functioning normally, all this unwanted calcium influx is deleterious. The chemical machinery of the cell is misdirected, leading to a kind of self-inflicted damage to vital systems within the cell and to the cell membrane itself. During ischemia, abnormal levels of calcium build up within the cell, resulting in damage to the normal chemical systems within the cell and cell death. Drugs blocking glutamate action can prevent damage otherwise caused by excitotoxicity, and calcium channel–blocking drugs may keep excessive calcium out of the cell to maintain more normal intracellular calcium balance.

Ischemia also triggers the neuron to make a group of highly reactive chemicals called *free radicals*. These free radicals damage the cell membrane and components of the intracellular machinery. Ischemic neurons make a substance called *nitric oxide*. Although beneficial to the neuron it normally conditions during ischemia, this substance aggravates the damage caused by other processes such as excitotoxicity. Formation of free radicals and nitric oxide can be blocked, and thus prevent a portion of this damage.

Ischemia prompts cells to begin manufacturing substances called ischemic cell adhesion molecules (ICAMs). These ICAMs attract white blood cells, or leukocytes, into the area of ischemia. The resulting inflammation increases the amount of brain tissue damaged. These ICAMs can be blocked by antibodies, and this inflammatory component of the stroke can be limited. Ischemia triggers some cells to make proteins that actually take apart the cell's own DNA. This permanently disrupts the cell's function, and the neuron dies. This process is called programmed cell death, or *apoptosis*. Nerve growth factors can alter this protein synthesis and stop programmed cell death.

As can be seen from this discussion, the damage caused by cerebral ischemia evolves in many directions over the minutes, hours, and days following the original ischemic event. Research in experimental animals is increasing our understanding of these events and can lead to the development of new drugs that can block some of these damaging processes in the hope of limiting the damage from a stroke and speeding patient recovery. Some of these new drugs are beginning to be tried in patients with stroke. Future stroke treatment will emphasize early intervention within hours of the onset of symptoms, and will probably combine multiple treatments in varying combinations to achieve better stroke survival, more complete recovery, and patient independence.

The Surgical Treatment of Stroke
by Michael E. DeBakey, M. D.

Experience at Baylor College of Medicine with the surgical treatment of stroke began on August 7, 1953, when Michael E. DeBakey performed the first successful carotid endarterectomy (Figure 20.2) on a 53-year-old man complaining of transient episodes of weakness of the right arm and leg, hesitancy and difficulty in speaking, and difficulty in writing clearly.[2] For 19 years after the operation, he remained free

---

[2] M. E. DeBakey, "Successful Carotid Endarterectomy for Cerebrovascular Insufficiency. Nineteen Year Follow-up," *Journal of the American Medical Association* 233:1083 (1975).

of these symptoms and resumed a normal life until his death from a heart attack (coronary occlusion). Before this operation, a number of investigators, based on observations at autopsy showing obstructive lesions in the carotid arteries in patients who had died from stroke, had indicated the causal relation between the lesions and the strokes. After this successful operation, accumulated experience from many medical centers, including our own, established the conceptual relation of the obstructing lesions to the development of stroke. From this experience the indications and contraindications for the operation have been established.

The surgical treatment of stroke is directed toward the prevention of ischemic damage to the brain, since once that has actually occurred, surgical treatment will not restore brain function. Obstruction to blood flow to the brain, which results in most cases from arteriosclerosis or atherosclerosis, if not corrected surgically, leads to a major stroke.

Particularly important considerations in determining treatment are the nature and location of the obstructing lesions in the arteries supplying blood to the brain. In most patients, these occlusive lesions are well localized to certain segments of the arteries, often not more than one-half to a little more than one inch in length, and the remainder of the artery above and below the lesion is normal. The most common

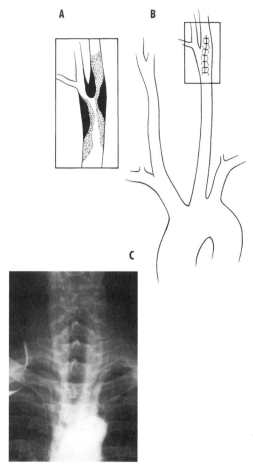

Figure 20.2. A. Drawing showing severe constricting lesion at bifurcation of left common and origin of internal and external carotid arteries in a 53-year-old man with transient ischemic attacks.
B. Drawing showing method of surgical treatment consisting in endarterectomy.
C. Postoperative carotid arteriogram showing restoration of normal circulation in left carotid artery.

location of these obstructive lesions is in the common carotid arteries, where they divide into the external and internal carotid arteries just below the angle of the jaw (Figure 20.3). The next most common site is in the vertebral arteries just as they arise

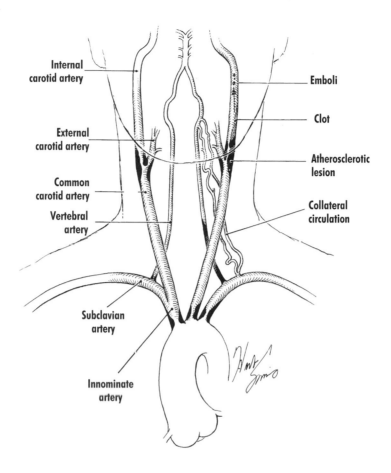

Internal carotid artery

External carotid artery

Common carotid artery

Vertebral artery

Subclavian artery

Innominate artery

Emboli

Clot

Atherosclerotic lesion

Collateral circulation

Figure 20.3. Patterns of occlusive disease in the major arteries supplying blood to the brain. A clot may form at one of these lesions, and pieces may break off to form emboli, which can pass through the blood stream to block important vessels in the brain and cause a stroke. During slow onset of occlusive disease, collateral circulation may develop to provide for the flow of blood around the occluded artery.

from the subclavian arteries. The third most common location is in the innominate, left common carotid, and left subclavian arteries near their origin from the aortic arch.

Arteriosclerosis or atherosclerosis is most often the cause of these patterns. There are, however, some less common forms of obstructive lesions. One of these is called *fibromuscular hyperplasia,* characterized by a thickening and thinning of the arterial wall, producing a screwlike appearance. Another is termed *arteritis,* which is a peculiar inflammatory condition of undetermined etiology. Both of these types of occlusive disease occur more often in relatively young females. In about one-half the patients, only one of the four major arteries is affected; in the remaining patients, two or more of these arteries are affected.

Arteriosclerotic or atherosclerotic occlusive disease of the carotid and vertebral arteries occurs most commonly in men between the ages of 50 and 70 years. Symptoms vary considerably, depending on the extent of obstruction and the arteries involved. In general, a decrease in blood flow from the obstruction of the internal carotid artery produces symptoms resulting from functional impairment of the front part of the brain—the area concerned with memory, speech, control of muscular movements, and the appreciation of sensations such as touch, temperature, and pain. A variety of symptoms may then occur including weakness, paralysis, numbness, and tingling on the side of the body opposite the occluded vessel, since each side of the brain controls the opposite side of the body. In most people, however, speech is controlled by the left side of the brain and is therefore usually affected only by obstruction of the left internal carotid artery.

Atherosclerotic lesions of the carotid artery also may produce strokelike symptoms by a process other than actual obstruction of blood flow. In such cases, the lesion may be ulcerated on its inner surface with deposits of a thrombus or clot. Small particles of this clotted material or even of the cholesterol and fatty deposi-

tion in the atheromatous lesion may break off and then be swept up in the blood stream to block circulation to a segment of the brain. This is called *embolization.* Symptoms of this type of occlusion usually occur suddenly. Again, depending on the adequacy of collateral circulation, symptoms may be transient with complete recovery.

Symptoms produced by vertebral artery obstruction may be extremely variable depending on the section of the brain affected by the inadequate circulation. The vertebral arteries supply blood to the upper part of the spinal cord, the base and back part of the brain, and the cerebellum. Since, for example, the back part of the brain controls vision, the patient may have difficulty in seeing. Such visual disturbances usually occur in both eyes, in contrast to patients with obstruction of the internal carotid artery, who will have difficulty with only one eye.

Inadequate circulation to the cerebellum produces vertigo (dizziness) and inability to perform fine, delicately coordinated movements. Impaired blood flow to the brain stem or base of the brain produces disturbances in sensation and weakness or paralysis on both sides of the body, rather than on one side, as occurs in obstruction of the internal carotid artery.

The pattern, variety, and severity of symptoms depend on a number of factors, including particularly the site and severity of obstruction, the number of arteries affected, and the amount of blood supplied by collateral circulation. If, for example, the artery is not completely blocked, there may be enough circulation through it and through collateral circulation to maintain normal function most of the time. Symptoms may, however, be precipitated by several contributing factors such as reduction in blood pressure, which further reduces the flow of blood through the partially blocked artery. Reduced blood pressure may occur from drugs, a shift in position from lying to sitting to standing, or changes in heart function. The patient may then have brief attacks or small strokes (TIA) during which he experiences slight weakness, or even paralysis, difficulty in speech, or partial blindness. He may recover completely in a few seconds, minutes, or hours. The term transient ischemic attacks (TIA) is often used for these attacks. In spite of this recovery, such seizures often precede further attacks, which may ultimately result in permanent brain damage or even death.

Obstruction of the main arteries arising from the aortic arch (the innominate, common carotid, and subclavian arteries) produces a wide variety of symptoms, since the entire brain and both arms receive their blood supply from these major arteries. Because two of these arteries, the left subclavian and innominate arteries, which give rise to the right subclavian artery, supply blood to the arms as well as the brain, obstructive lesions in these arteries may produce inadequate circulation to the arms, resulting in cramps in the arms or hands during exercise and coldness and pain in the hands and fingers. In rare cases, even gangrene of the fingers may occur. If symptoms are accompanied by the absence of a pulse at the wrist, or diminished blood pressure in one or both arms, the obstructions are in the subclavian arteries.

The diagnosis of obstructive or ulcerative lesions can usually be suspected from the symptoms of the patient and further refined by a careful physical and neurologic examination. Although not always present, a particularly significant sign of occlusive lesions in the carotid artery is the presence of a *bruit,* or murmur, heard through a stethoscope placed on the neck just below the angle of the jaw. This is a swishing noise, synchronized with the heartbeat, and is produced by the blood as it rushes through the narrowed part of the artery. Sometimes the patient himself may hear the sound in his own ears.

After the patient's condition has been thoroughly evaluated by clinical and neurologic examinations that indicate the probable diagnosis of occlusive disease, which can be made by ultrasound imaging (color Doppler flow), a precise diagnosis can then be made by arteriography (Figure 20.4). The procedure can be performed

A

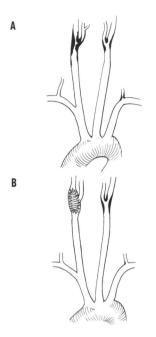

B

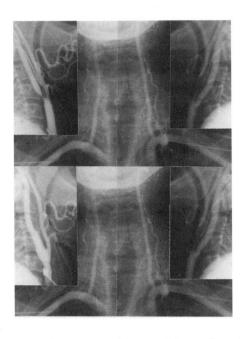

Figure 20.4. A. Drawing and carotid arteriogram of a 45-year-old man with manifestations of transient ischemic attack (TIA), showing severe, well-localized, stenotic disease at origin of right internal carotid artery. B. Drawing showing surgical procedure, consisting in endarterectomy with Dacron® patch-graft angioplasty of left common carotid artery, and arteriogram made 15 years after operation, showing restoration of normal lumen and circulation in common internal and external arteries.

with use of a local or light general anesthetic. Carotid and subclavian arteriography accurately shows the location of the obstruction and also provides information necessary for determining the need and the type of surgical treatment. In our experience at the Cardiovascular Center of The Methodist Hospital with thousands of cases, the risk of serious complications is extremely small (about 1 per 5,000).

Treatment may be medical or surgical, depending upon a number of factors. Surgical treatment is usually recommended for well-localized obstructive or ulcerative disease involving the carotid artery, the origin of the vertebral arteries, and the major arteries arising from the aortic arch. Surgical treatment may also be suggested for some relatively asymptomatic patients with severe obstruction of the internal carotid artery in the neck. These are usually patients who are found to have such a lesion on routine examination, or who may require an operation for another related condition. In our early experience, we encountered some patients who had a stroke after other operations and were subsequently found to have obstructive disease of the internal carotid artery that could have been surgically corrected before the operation, possibly precluding the development of the stroke. On the basis of this experience, we now perform arteriography on patients who have significant murmurs, or bruits, over the carotid artery, and if the arteriogram demonstrates severe occlusive disease, surgical treatment is recommended.

Surgical treatment is not routine for all patients with occlusive disease of the arteries supplying blood to the brain. Operations are not recommended for patients with occlusive disease of the arteries within the skull, nor for those with complete occlusion of the major arteries in the neck who have a permanent condition, such as paralysis, or develop a speech defect after a period of weeks or months. Under these circumstances, the brain damage is not reversible even if circulation can be restored, although operation may be performed in some such patients as an emergency procedure within a few hours after the stroke occurs. This decision to operate requires careful assessment by the neurologist and the surgeon. Certain associated diseases, such as severe emphysema or heart failure and some debilitating conditions, may also discourage surgical treatment because of the high risk of operation.

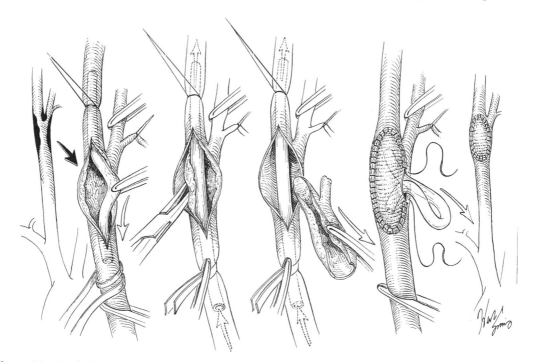

Figure 20.5. Technique of endarterectomy and Dacron® patch-graft angioplasty. After the artery is incised above and below the lesion, a temporary shunt is inserted to provide blood to the brain during the procedure. The lesion is peeled away from the arterial wall, and a Dacron® patch is sewed in the opening. The shunt is withdrawn before the suture is tied.

Circulation is restored by one of two types of operation, namely thromboendarterectomy or the bypass graft procedure. In occlusive and ulcerative disease involving the common carotid artery and the origin of the internal carotid artery, endarterectomy is usually performed (Figure 20.5). These lesions are well localized within a short segment of the artery, and it is possible to separate the lesion cleanly from the remainder of the arterial wall. The artery is exposed through a small incision in the neck, and temporary occluding clamps are applied above and below the lesion. An incision is made through the wall of the artery just below the blockage and continued up through the obstructed segment for a short distance into the normal healthy artery. A temporary shunt consisting in a small plastic tube is then inserted into the opening above and below the obstruction to allow blood to flow to the brain while the operation is being performed. The diseased lesion, termed an *atheroma*, is then removed by separating it cleanly from its

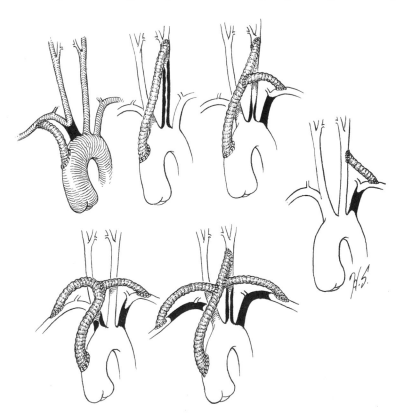

Figure 20.6. Examples of some of the varieties of bypass grafts that can be used in the treatment of occlusive disease in the proximal segment of the arteries arising from the aortic arch.

attachment to the arterial wall. The incision in the artery is then closed by sewing the edges together with a fine suture, or because in most patients this may produce some reduction in the bore of the artery, a

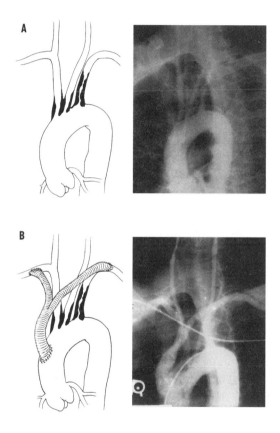

Figure 20.7. A. Drawing and preoperative arteriogram of a 54-year-old man with dizziness and intermittent claudication of the arms, showing well-localized stenotic disease involving the proximal portion of the innominate and left subclavian arteries.
B. Drawing showing surgical procedure, consisting in Dacron® bypass graft from ascending aorta to both subclavian arteries, and arteriogram made 10 years after operation, showing restoration of normal circulation through the Dacron® graft. Patient has remained asymptomatic for 30 years.

small patch of Dacron® fabric is sutured to the edges as a patch graft. Just before the closure is completed, the internal plastic tube shunt is removed, and the final closure is completed. In time, a new intimal lining covers the entire area, including the inner surface of the graft.

In obstructional lesions of the major arteries arising from the aortic arch, the bypass procedure is preferred. In virtually all such patients, the obstructive lesions are well localized, with relatively normal arteries beyond the obstruction in the neck. This, of course, is the reason the bypass graft can be applied so successfully in these patients (Figure 20.6). The operation is performed by exposing the ascending aorta through a small incision at the front of the chest on the right side, usually between the second and third ribs. With a special partial occluding clamp, a small portion of the ascending aorta is pinched off, and an incision is made through the wall of the vessel in this pinched-off segment. A tubular albumin-coated Dacron® graft is attached to this opening by sewing the edges of the graft to the edges of the opening in the aorta. The graft is then passed up into the base of the neck, through a tunnel made in the tissue at the front of the neck where it joins the chest. The appropriate artery beyond the obstruction is exposed by an incision in the neck. The other end of the Dacron® tube is attached, by a similar suture procedure, to an opening made in the

A

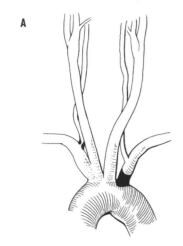

B

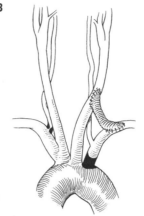

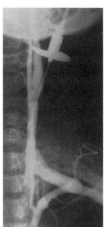

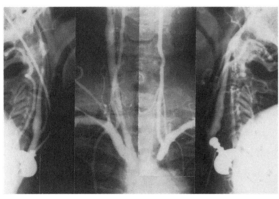

Figure 20.8. A. Drawing and preoperative arteri-ogram of a 58-year-old man complaining of inter-mittent episodes of dizziness, weakness in the left leg and arm, and visual disturbances, showing well-localized complete obstruction in the proximal segment of the left subclavian artery.
B. Drawing showing surgical procedure, consisting in bypass Dacron® graft from left common carotid artery to left subclavian artery, and arteriogram made three years after operation, showing restora-tion of normal circulation to left subclavian artery through the bypass graft. Patient remained asymp-tomatic for 10 years.

artery where it is relatively normal. In this way, blood is shunted from the ascending aorta to the artery beyond its obstruction, and normal circulation is thus restored to the brain (Figure 20.7).

In those patients in whom more than one of these major arteries is obstructed, additional grafts may be attached to the main graft from the ascending aorta. In instances where the occlusive lesion is limited to the left common carotid or subclavian artery, an even simpler opera-tion may be done by employing a bypass graft from the normal artery to the one with the occlusion beyond the obstruction through an incision exposing both arteries in the neck (Figure 20.8).

Results of these operations have been extremely gratifying. The risk of operation is only about 1 or 2 percent, and complica-tions are also minimal—about 2 percent. Long-term results have also been good. Postoperative follow-up studies extending from 10 to 35 years have demonstrated that most patients are completely relieved of symptoms and have few recurrences.

CHAPTER TWENTY-ONE

Diseases of the Pericardium and Myocardium

There are times when the myocardium (the muscular part of the heart wall) is affected by disease. These disorders are not necessarily related to problems of the coronary arteries, the valves, or high blood pressure. In fact, their cause often remains unknown. These *cardiomyopathies,* as they are called, are characterized by an enlargement or stiffening of the muscular part of the heart wall that prevents the heart from functioning as it should. The heart structure may become inflamed; it may be infiltrated with a substance such as iron or with a disease such as cancer; or it may suffer changes to its internal architecture, such as in processes in which the heart muscle is replaced by fibrous connective tissue. Sometimes a blood-related illness (leukemia or sickle cell anemia, for example) may play a part; an allergic reaction may be to blame; or there may be some other cause, such as a viral illness. In South America, a parasite is the major cause. Excessive alcohol intake can be a significant contri-

buting factor. Cardiomyopathy means "an illness of the heart muscle."

The wall of the heart is made of three parts, with outer and inner shells sheltering the muscle layer, which is many times thicker than either of the others (Figure 21.1). The outside layer (epicardium) and the inside layer (endocardium) protect the muscular myocardium that performs the pumping work of the heart.

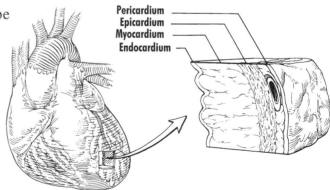

Figure 21.1. This cross-section of the heart wall and pericardium shows how the thick muscular layer of the heart (myocardium) is protected by an interior lining (the endocardium) and an exterior one (the epicardium). The pericardial sac (pericardium) encloses the heart, and its fibrous outer layer anchors the heart within the chest.

Surrounding the heart epicardium is a membrane called the *pericardium*. Made up of a thin inner layer and a tough outer layer, with fluid in between, the flask-shaped pericardium protects the heart. Its inner layer (the visceral pericardium) encloses the heart and any fat around it. The fibrous yet elastic outer layer (parietal pericardium) protects it and secures it within the chest. The fibrous pericardium is loosely anchored by ligamentous structures to the sternal manubrium and xiphoid process. It is firmly attached to the central tendon of the diaphragm. On each side, the pericardium is adherent to the mediastinal pleura. About one-eighth to one-fourth of a cup of clear pericardial fluid creates a buffer between the two layers.

Like the heart's wall, the pericardium can become inflamed because of a viral or bacterial infection, in a reaction to cancer (or radiotherapy for it), or because of some other disorder. You do not have to have the pericardium to live: some people are born without it and others have to have it removed because of disease.

Though their functions are dramatically different, the heart wall and the pericardium will be considered sequentially here both because of their structural proximity and because of the effect pericardial disease can have on heart function (see the section on restrictive cardiomyopathy below).

Cardiomyopathy

Many patients with dilated cardiomyopathy die within five years of diagnosis, and many of these deaths are sudden. In the United States, cardiomyopathies claimed 24,573 lives in 1992, according to the American Heart Association, and were responsible for about 33,000 hospitalizations in 1993. According to hospital discharge survey records, cardiomyopathy is more common among blacks than whites and more common among men than women. In one study of a county population, cardiomyopathy was three times more common in men than in women. But the outlook, which depends more on the severity of the disease and the underlying cause than anything else, has improved significantly over the past several years.

Dilated Cardiomyopathy

Almost 90 percent of all cases of cardiomyopathy are of the dilated type. As many as 75 heart diseases can produce the clinical findings linked with the diagnosis of dilated cardiomyopathy. There may be damage produced by a myriad of toxic assaults, metabolic deficiencies or imbalances, and inflammatory processes.

The toxic assault may be from alcohol abuse, other drug abuse, cancer chemotherapy (especially with doxorubicin), or another source. Chronic alcohol abuse can cause widespread abnormalities in the heart's muscle layer, impairing the heart's ability to relax and properly fill with blood. Arrhythmias may result, and the patient may also experience chest pain (angina pectoris).

Metabolic disorders that play a role in dilated cardiomyopathy include nutritional deficiencies caused by inadequate dietary intake of, for example, thiamine (vitamin B1), protein, or selenium. Endocrine imbalances that result in acromegaly (a pituitary gland–related ailment causing hands, feet, and face to enlarge) and thyrotoxicosis (a thyroid gland–related ailment) are also implicated as factors.

Inflammatory processes cited as causes include infectious agents (see discussion of myocarditis below) and noninfectious causes, such as collagen disease and Kawasaki's disease (a malady that most often affects infants and young children). When coronary artery disease produces a myocardial ischemia with symptoms indistinguishable from those of dilated cardiomyopathy, the condition is sometimes referred to as *ischemic cardiomyopathy.* Symptoms are more closely allied to those of heart failure than those such as angina. The loss of blood supply results in a left ventricular myocardium incapable of contracting properly, but the supply, though depressed, is able to sustain tissue

viability. Such a condition is referred to as a "hibernating" myocardium. These and other causes of dilated cardiomyopathy are not simple, and often no single factor can bear all the blame.

Dilated cardiomyopathy of unknown cause occurs more frequently among blacks than whites, and blacks more frequently die of it than do whites. Investigators have speculated about factors influencing these findings—genetic or environmental differences, smoking, or preexisting conditions such as hypertension or asthma, among others. A study in Baltimore found black race and asthma statistically related to the disease.

Dilated cardiomyopathy may be caused by an infection (Inflammation of the cardiac muscle, whether due to an infection or another cause, is called *myocarditis.*) Causative processes include viral, bacterial, rickettsial, fungal, and parasitic infections that initiate an inflammatory response in the myocardium. Often myocarditis will develop after an infection affects the endocardium or the pericardium. Diseases associated with myocarditis include rheumatic fever, diphtheria, trichomoniasis, and influenza. Mild cases entail few symptoms; in more serious cases, identification of myocarditis is obscured by the symptoms of the underlying disease—typically, fever, fatigue, nausea and vomiting, a fast heartbeat, and chest pain. Patients are treated with drugs and rest. Myocarditis can lead to shock and death in those at the vulnerable extremes of the age spectrum, the young and the very old. In some cases of dilated cardiomyopathy, myocarditis is not recognized until after the infection has resolved.

These assaults, most typically an infection, other inflammation, or long-term damage, result in expansion, or dilatation, of the ventricles. When pumping function declines and the amount of blood forced out of the ventricle decreases, the heart tries to make up the deficiency by beating faster.

The symptoms of dilated cardiomyopathy may develop slowly, or they may occur unexpectedly and suddenly. Early in the course of the disease, patients may be completely asymptomatic; when the disease is advanced, patients may, with light physical challenge, experience shortness of breath and easily tire. Veins in their neck will be somewhat distended, their blood pressure somewhat low, and their heartbeat fast. Some patients report a feeling of tightness in their neck. As many as half of these patients complain of chest pain. Others remain without symptoms for months or years.

In the late stages of dilated cardiomyopathy, a patient may have abdominal pain because of swelling of the liver. Swelling of the feet, ankles, and legs, nausea, and loss of appetite are characteristic of advanced disease and indicate that the right side of the heart has been affected.

To make the diagnosis of dilated cardiomyopathy, a physician will perform a physical examination, order a chest x-ray, and ask for studies of blood to detect metabolic deficiencies. Other tests may include clinical electrocardiography, Holter monitoring (electrocardiography using a device worn about during regular activities outside the hospital or clinic), echocardiography, radionuclide ventriculography, cardiac catheterization and angiography, left ventriculography, coronary arteriography, and endomyocardial biopsy. Of all these, echocardiography is the most widely used noninvasive technique for diagnosing dilated cardiomyopathy.

Because its cause often remains a mystery, treatment for dilated cardiomyopathy is directed at reducing fluid retention, deactivating sympathetic nervous system responses, and preventing adverse effects from arrhythmias or blood clots. A physician may prescribe an angiotensin-converting enzyme (ACE) inhibitor (or other dilating agent) plus digoxin and a diuretic (the classic triad in this disorder), antiarrhythmic drugs, or sometimes anticoagulants. In some severe cases, cardiac transplantation may be an option.

Hypertrophic Cardiomyopathy

In hypertrophic cardiomyopathy, the walls of the heart thicken abnormally. This irregular thickening can so skew the geometry of the heart that it fails to perform properly. Wall thickening, which occurs in some areas and not in others, can range from an increase of one-third to two and one-half times. In a subset of these cases, ventricular septal enlargement occurs, which is so dramatic that early investigators thought the abnormal growth had to have been caused by a benign tumor.

Similar thickening may occur within the inner and middle layers of coronary arteries serving the inner walls of the heart in some patients with hypertrophic cardiomyopathy. These intramural vessels fail to deliver the oxygen and blood the heart needs, causing ischemia and further impairing function. Though coronary blood flow is increased, it is more than matched by the increase in myocardial oxygen demand. Mitral valve structure is also affected in about two-thirds of these patients; anomalies include not only enlargement but also other malformations.

Hypertrophic cardiomyopathy may be classified as *obstructive* or *nonobstructive* (Figure 21.2). In obstructive disease, the outflow of blood during the contraction (systolic) phase is partially blocked; the decreased flow is secondary

to an effect that pulls the mitral valve into the left ventricular outflow tract. In nonobstructive disease, ventricular outflow is not

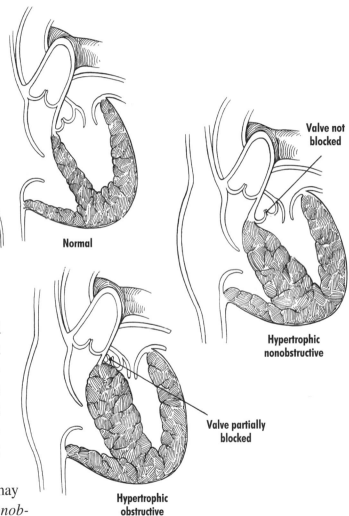

Figure 21.2. In hypertrophic cardiomyopathy, the ventricular septum is abnormally thickened, even more so than the left ventricular free wall. It may be classified as nonobstructive (right) or obstructive (bottom). These conditions contrast with the normal heart (top).

impaired, although a nonobstructive case may progress to an obstructive one.

Hypertrophic cardiomyopathy affects between 0.02 and 0.2 percent of the population. When young athletes die suddenly on the playing field, unrelated to injury, hypertrophic cardiomyopathy may be the cause.

Though hypertrophic cardiomyopathy is rare, it engenders particular interest among physicians because of its diverse and complex nature. It can be symptomatic or asymptomatic; it can be transmitted genetically or acquired; its characteristic hypertrophy can be concentric or asymmetric. One textbook lists 58 names that it says are only part of the more than 75 by which this disorder is known. It can affect both the systolic and diastolic functions of the heart. Eighty percent of patients have problems during the diastolic (filling) phase. The hypertrophic ventricle's stiffness impairs its ability to relax and fill properly. Sometimes problems exist in the left ventricle's ability to eject blood during the systolic phase. This is usually because of obstruction within the ventricle related to the hypertrophied septum and the mitral valve's contact with it. Myocardial ischemia observed in patients with hypertrophic cardiomyopathy may relate to oxygen demand's outpacing the coronary system's supply ability, the impairment of intramural vessels that deliver blood to the heart wall, or factors related to myocardial wall tension.

Although hypertrophic cardiomyopathy is usually identified in adults in their 30s and 40s, it has been initially diagnosed in infants as well as in the elderly. Most instances of sudden death, which may be the first symptom, occur in patients who are ages 15 to 35. Links between wall thickness, mass, and clinical signs and outcome remain too weak to predict how any given case might turn out. While blood pressure and pulse are normal, patients experience angina and shortness of breath with physical challenge. Arrhythmias, infective endocarditis, and sudden death are the most dreaded complications of the disorder.

Earlier calculations of 2 to 4 percent for those with hypertrophic cardiomyopathy who experience sudden death are now thought to be overestimations. Sometimes patients with hypertrophic cardiomyopathy are asymptomatic through the midlife years.

To detect hypertrophic cardiomyopathy, physicians usually use Doppler echocardiography and a chest x-ray. Holter monitoring may be useful in tracking arrhythmias. Magnetic resonance imaging may also be used. Nuclear angiography may be employed to evaluate ventricular function. If either surgery for obstructive disease or heart transplantation is an option, physicians may employ such invasive techniques as heart catheterization or angiography.

Treatment includes medical and surgical therapy. Physicians treat patients with obstructive hypertrophic cardiomyopathy with beta-blockers, calcium antagonists, or disopyramide, to counter obstruction and to ameliorate the obstruction's effect. When medical therapy fails, myectomy—the surgical widening of the outflow tract and the trimming of the ventricular septum—is used by some centers. Another approach to widen the outflow tract and relieve the obstruction is to use a pacemaker, which has proved highly successful in some cases. In some cases with arrhythmias, single therapies or combination therapies incorporating antiarrhythmic drugs, an automatic implantable cardiac defibrillator, and/or a pacemaker have proved successful.

For nonobstructive cardiomyopathy, physicians may prescribe calcium antagonists as long as systolic function is intact, and beta-blockers when patients find calcium antagonists difficult to take. Other drug therapy might include a medication to manage arrhythmia. Researchers are finding in experiments with rats that ACE inhibitors produce beneficial regression of hypertrophy. Electrophysiologic testing and thallium stress testing can, in some cases, help refine a patient's pharmacologic therapy.

Restrictive Cardiomyopathy

In the least common of the cardiomyopathies, restrictive cardiomyopathy, a rigid heart wall allows rapid initial filling during the diastolic phase but hinders midphase and late-phase filling with its constricting, inflexible shell. Like other cardiomyopathies, restrictive cardiomyopathy is characterized by impairment caused by factors other than coronary artery disease, hypertension, or valvular disease.

Many cases are caused by eosinophilic endomyocardial disease (responsible for obliterative restrictive cardiomyopathy), cardiac amyloidosis, or hemochromatosis (related to the nonobliterative type). Characteristics of both the obliterative and nonobliterative types include dilatation of the left and right atria and clots within the heart, but normal left ventricle size and pumping (systolic) function. Another, less common, cause is sarcoidosis, a chronic condition characterized by the formation of nodules. Sarcoidosis can involve almost any organ or tissue in the body, including the heart, and less often the pericardium. Arrhythmia or conduction disturbances may result from cardiac involvement.

Differentiating restrictive cardiomyopathy from constrictive pericarditis, in which an inflamed pericardium becomes stiff and tightly compresses the ventricles and prevents filling, is of paramount importance because of the tragic consequences of treating the condition as if it were inoperable when it is operable. In restrictive cardiomyopathy, the heart wall thickens and fibrosis occurs. The chambers become stiff and rigid. The valves then malfunction, and regurgitation results. The atria dilate in response. When the cellular disorganization affects conduction of the heart's electrical impulses or causes the sinoatrial node to malfunction, heart block can ensue. In the obliterative form, endocardial fibrosis obliterates the heart wall lining, thinning it. Compensatory hypertrophy stiffens it and restricts the diastolic function.

Restrictive cardiomyopathy occurs throughout the world, but its epidemiologic character varies by locale. Those with eosinophilic endomyocardial disease in the United Kingdom were found to be typically male, older, and victims of a systemic illness. Those with the same disease in the tropics were found in equal numbers in both sexes, were younger than their European counterparts, and had most often been afflicted with parasitic infection.

Eosinophilic endomyocardial fibrosis, which can cause the obliterative form of restrictive cardiomyopathy, is characterized by infiltration of the endocardium by bizarre eosinophils (white blood cells). One form of this condition is called Löffler's disease. Fibrosis follows, as well as scarring and clotting.

When amyloidosis, a protein metabolism disorder, causes restrictive cardiomyopathy, amyloid protein is found between the cells. The deposits may be dramatic and infiltrate small vessels as well. This condition may occur in isolation, or it may be linked with inflammatory diseases (tuberculosis or others) or neoplastic disease (non-Hodgkin's lymphoma, multiple myeloma, malignant B-lymphocyte lymphoma, for example). The myocardium becomes rubbery; the wall, atria, and ventricular septum enlarge; and valves thicken.

In hemochromatosis, excessive iron is interlaced in the myocardium, primarily in the ventricles. This metabolic disorder may be genetically transferred; it may be of unknown cause; or it may be related to excessive oral iron intake, to liver disease, or to receiving many blood transfusions without iron loss. The effects are the same: the heart wall hardens, restricting diastolic function. But unlike primary amyloidosis and amyloidosis associated with multiple myeloma, which have poor prognoses (progressive heart failure with death), hemochromatosis may be reversed. (Amyloidosis caused by tuberculosis, bronchiectasis, or osteomyelitis, for example, may be reversed if the primary disease is controlled.)

Other disorders that can cause restrictive cardiomyopathy are pseudoxanthoma elasticum, Pompe's disease (an acid maltase deficiency) or other glycogen metabolism abnormalities, and radiation-induced heart disease.

Patients with restrictive cardiomyopathy experience arrhythmias and heart block. Overall, experts estimate that about 30 percent survive five years after diagnosis. When the underlying condition can be identified, such as hemochromatosis, therapy can be instituted to combat it. Without identification, and sometimes even with it, as can be the case with amyloidosis, the outlook is guarded. For most of those cases, no therapy has proved useful. Some physicians use diuretics for the congestion that accompanies these conditions, digoxin for late-stage development of pumping failure (avoided in amyloidosis), and vasodilators to improve circulation.

Pericardial Diseases

Pericarditis, pericardial effusion, cardiac tamponade, and pericardial constriction are the major disorders of the pericardium.

Pericarditis

Pericarditis, or inflammation of the pericardium, may be caused by a viral or bacterial infection, tuberculosis, other infections, a heart attack, or a neoplastic disease. Myriad other causes exist as well. In the patient with acquired immunodeficiency syndrome (AIDS), it may appear in relation to any of these factors or Kaposi's sarcoma. Mild to severe chest pain, fever, and shortness of breath may accompany pericarditis. Leaning forward in a sitting position may relieve the pain; lying down may increase it. Physicians will use the physical examination and electrocardiog-

raphy to diagnose pericarditis, and may rely on tuberculin skin tests and other blood tests to identify underlying disease. Aspirin and other drugs are used to reduce the inflammation and pain; other therapeutic approaches are discussed in Chapter 22.

Pericardial Effusion and Cardiac Tamponade

The collection of excess fluid within the pericardial space (pericardial effusion) and the adverse compression of the heart that results when that condition persists and intensifies (cardiac tamponade) can range from well tolerated to life-threatening. While mild pericardial effusion may cause little or no discomfort, cardiac tamponade (Figure 21.3) always requires immediate pericardiocentesis (the surgical draining of the fluid, often blood) to relieve the progressively limiting effect of compression on ventricular filling, on the amount of blood pumped per heartbeat (stroke volume), and on the cumulative amount pumped in a minute (cardiac output).

Pericardial Constriction

Like restrictive cardiomyopathy, pericardial constriction (Figure 21.3) is characterized by fibrin (and sometimes calcium) deposits, scarring, and thinning followed by hypertrophy, and stiffening and thickening of the tissue layers. Though

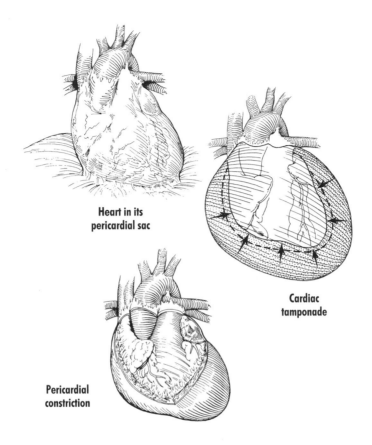

Heart in its
pericardial sac

Cardiac
tamponade

Pericardial
constriction

Figure 21.3. The normal pericardial sac (top) gently encloses and protects the heart. When fluid fills the sac, cardiac tamponade (right) can result, dangerously compressing the heart and impairing its function. Pericardiocentesis is a method for relieving the pressure of the fluid retention. In pericardial constriction (bottom), the layers of tissue making up the pericardium abnormally thicken and adhere to one another. This stiff pericardium may prevent efficient heart function and require removal of the pericardium.

its cause is usually unknown, it may follow an instance of pericarditis. Factors initiating the process may be cancer, trauma, tuberculosis, heart surgery, or radiation exposure. Patients experience vague abdominal symptoms, and their condition progressively worsens. Treatment is surgical removal of the pericardium (pericardiectomy).

CHAPTER TWENTY-TWO

Surgical Treatment of Acquired Heart Diseases Affecting the Pericardium, Myocardium, and Valves

In contrast to congenital heart disease, acquired heart disease is caused by conditions that occur after birth; atherosclerosis and coronary artery disease are typical examples. This chapter is devoted to acquired heart disease other than that affecting the coronary arteries. These diseases may affect the pericardium (the covering of the heart), the myocardium itself, or the valves of the heart and their associated structures.

Pericarditis

Inflammation of the pericardial sac may be acute or chronic. Acute pericarditis is associated with accumulation of fluid in the pericardial cavity around the heart. If the condition persists or is associated with subsequent deposition of fibrotic tissue, it becomes a long-term illness referred to as *chronic pericarditis.* Acute pericarditis

may occur as a complication of a myocardial infarction or cardiac surgery; it can be secondary to a virus, bacterial infection, or metabolic disturbance such as uremia, which occurs in kidney failure. Acute pericarditis usually does not interfere with the functioning of the heart, but may cause severe pain. It usually accompanies an acute illness with fever and chills.

On listening to the heartbeat with a stethoscope, the examiner may hear a "rub" due to friction between the pericardial sac and the epicardial surface of the heart during contraction. In chronic pericarditis, a constriction may interfere with the blood flow and thus produce back pressure. Fluid may also accumulate in the legs, and the liver may become congested. This condition is referred to as *right-sided heart failure.*

The treatment of pericarditis depends on the cause. Before the advent of antibiotic therapy, the most common infectious cause of pericarditis was tuberculosis. If a bacterial agent is the cause, antibiotic treatment and bed rest are indicated. Pericarditis associated with a myocardial infarction or after heart surgery may require only bed rest and control of fever and pain. But chronic constrictive pericarditis may call for more than treatment of the heart with medication. A surgical procedure consisting in stripping off a section of the pericardial covering (called a *pericardiectomy*) can relieve not only the back pressure on the right side of the heart but also many symptoms.

Postpericardotomy syndrome occurs sometimes after any injury and in patients undergoing cardiac surgery. It is characterized by chest pain, fever, pericardial effusion, a friction rub, and even pleurisy. Usually the condition is mild and self-limiting. Treatment with rest and mild pain-relieving drugs such as aspirin is sufficient. In more severe cases steroids may be used.

Myocardial Disease

Although coronary artery disease may result in damage to the myocardium, it is not primarily a disease of the myocardial muscle itself. The term "myocardial disease" describes a heterogeneous collection of disorders that include inflammatory processes, called myocarditis; infiltrative

processes in which the myocardium becomes filled with substances such as amyloid; and fibrotic diseases in which the heart muscle is replaced by fibrous connective tissue. Various infectious agents may cause myocarditis; among these the most common cause is Coxsackie B virus. In South and Central America, especially the rural areas, Chagas' disease caused by an infection with Trypanosoma cruzi is one of the most common causes of heart failure.

Dysfunction of the heart muscle can result in a condition called *cardiomyopathy*. This is a syndrome or a group of diseases in which the heart is enlarged and failing, and the heart muscle is not functioning adequately. If an underlying cause is identifiable, the cardiomyopathy (for example, due to ischemia or coronary artery disease) is said to be secondary, and treatment depends upon the cause. Agents such as alcohol may cause cardiomyopathy in susceptible patients. If no underlying cause can be detected, the cardiomyopathy is called primary. If an underlying cause is identified, it should be directly treated. Cardiomyopathy is sometimes divided into dilated and non-dilated types. The latter may be caused by an infiltrative process, which results in a stiff myocardium. An effort should be made to control associated heart failure and arrhythmias. Primary cardiomyopathy may require long periods of bed rest, and there is no satisfactory or generally accepted treatment at the present time. Heart transplantation may be required in some patients. A more detailed consideration of cardiomyopathy is presented in Chapter 24.

Acute Rheumatic Fever and Rheumatic Heart Disease

A streptococcal organism, Group A beta-hemolytic streptococcus, is the cause of rheumatic fever. Acute attacks of rheumatic fever occur most commonly in children between 7 and 14 years of age during the winter months, and the disease is associated with low socio-economic conditions. The advent of penicillin, which provides effective treatment for this variety of streptococcal infection, greatly reduced the incidence of rheumatic fever and its complications in the United States. An attack of acute rheumatic fever usually begins two or three weeks after the infection of the throat or tonsils. The patient does not always have history of a sore throat, however. Rheumatic fever is thought to be a hypersensitive reaction to the beta-streptococcal organism. In this sense, it represents a type of allergic reaction to the beta-streptococcus, but the exact pathogenic mechanism is undetermined. The most frequent manifestation is inflammation of the large joints of the body, called *migratory polyarthritis,* which

occurs in about 85 percent of all cases. Inflammation of the heart, seen about 65 percent of the time, may be manifested by increased heart rate, first-degree heart block, or the presence of a murmur, and about 30 percent of all patients develop a condition called *chorea,* which is a disorder of the central nervous system, named St. Vitus Dance. Chorea is characterized by spastic twitching of the muscles and occurs most commonly in prepubertal girls. Thus, during an attack of acute rheumatic fever, the patient may have inflammation of the joints, the pericardium, the myocardium, and the heart valves.

Of the utmost importance is proper early diagnosis and treatment with penicillin during the acute attacks in an attempt to prevent subsequent valvular disease. Bed rest and aspirin also help to relieve the pain in the joints. During the acute phase of the disease, the valves of the heart may become inflamed and filled with edema fluid. A pathologic condition characteristic of rheumatic fever is seen through the microscope on the endocardial, or interior surface, of the heart. Called the Aschoff nodule, it is a collection of several types of cells around a center of dead tissue. A long period of recovery is required after an attack of rheumatic fever. Once the acute illness has occurred, penicillin has relatively little effect on the course of the infection.

Rheumatic heart disease occurs years after acute rheumatic fever, and although it usually affects the mitral and aortic valves, it can also damage the tricuspid valve. It is important to distinguish whether valve damage is caused by bacterial endocarditis or rheumatic heart disease. In bacterial endocarditis, the damage to the heart valve is actually a result of bacterial infection on the valve itself. By contrast, in rheumatic heart disease the major damage to the valve does not occur at the time of the acute infection. Once an individual has had an attack of acute rheumatic fever, the heart valves may sustain severe damage from further attacks. In such persons, it is imperative to recognize the recurrence of a streptococcal infection very early so that it may be vigorously treated with antibiotics.

Endocarditis

Endocarditis is a condition in which the endocardium of the heart is inflamed. Usually this condition is caused by bacteria that affect the valves. Often, a heart valve previously damaged by rheumatic heart disease or damaged from birth will be the site affected by bacterial endocarditis. The disease may be classified as acute and subacute. The acute type usually arises as a complication of severe bacterial infections of the blood stream called *septicemia*. Parenteral drug abusers are at high risk for this type of endocarditis. In recent years, drug abuse has become a major cause of bacterial endocarditis affecting the valves of the right side of the heart.

A patient with acute bacterial endocarditis is extremely ill with fever and chills. The heartbeat is rapid, and congestive heart failure may occur. Arterial emboli are sometimes released from the damaged heart valves. The valves themselves may be practically destroyed in a relatively short time. An infected embolus may lodge in an artery and produce a type of aneurysm called *mycotic aneurysm*. Successful treatment requires identification of the infectious organism and an immediate and vigorous program of appropriate antibiotics.

Subacute bacterial endocarditis often is caused by organisms found in the otopharyngeal, pulmonary, and gastrointestinal tracts, mostly strains of streptococci, which are noninfectious under ordinary circumstances. A heart valve damaged from rheumatic heart disease or a congenital defect is more susceptible to attack by this insidious disease than a normal valve. An attack may follow oral surgery or dental work in which bacteria get into the blood stream. Whereas acute bacterial endocarditis results in large deposits forming on the surface of the heart valves, the subacute type produces smaller deposits. Damage to the valve may occur with either variety of the disease. Treatment for both acute and subacute bacterial endocarditis is aimed at identifying the causative agent and effectively treating it with antibiotics. Intravenous antibiotic treatment is often administered, sometimes for prolonged periods of time. Prophylactic steps should be subsequently taken, such as the use of antibiotics at the time dental work is to be done.

Mitral Valve Disease

Damage to the mitral valve produces progressive thickening and loss of pliability of the valve leaflets, with fusion to the edges, contraction of the *chordae tendineae,* and *calcium deposition* (Figure 22.1). These changes may produce

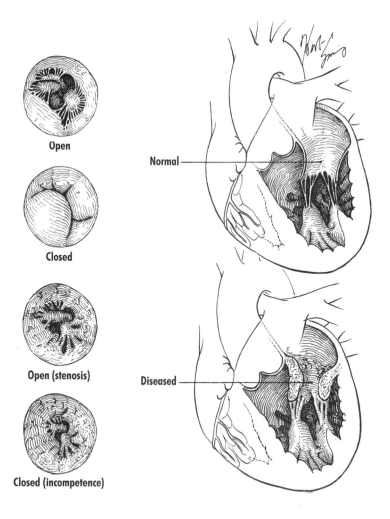

Open

Closed

Open (stenosis)

Closed (incompetence)

Normal

Diseased

Figure 22.1. A diseased mitral valve (below) as contrasted with a normal mitral valve (above).

narrowing of the valve opening, called *mitral stenosis,* in which blood flow between the left atrium and left ventricle is obstructed. The mitral orifice area in normal adults is about 4 to 6 cm. Mitral stenosis produces a decrease in this area, and when the orifice is reduced to 1.5 to 1 cm, it thus produces a significant pressure gradient across the valve, increasing the pressure in the left atrium and in the pulmonary vasculature and leading to right ventricular failure.

Alternatively, the valve may be incompetent; that is, the valve leaflets are unable to close (called *mitral insufficiency*). This may be the result of a number of causes, including particularly coronary artery disease, producing papillary dysfunction, rheumatic fever, congenital or inherited disorders, and left ventricular dilatation.

With the introduction of the echocardiogram, a condition called *mitral valve prolapse* has been diagnosed with increasing frequency, especially in women. In this condition, the valve leaflets balloon backward like a parachute instead of closing normally. There is an abnormal sound called a *click* and occasionally a murmur. The condition is usually a benign one, although if actual mitral insufficiency is present, there may be an increased risk of endocarditis. Also, some individuals with mitral valve prolapse have an increased frequency of atrial arrhythmias.

Although either stenosis or incompetence of the valve is the predominant dysfunction, there often is an element of both. When narrowing of the valve is the major change, the pressure in the left atrium increases, and thus produces elevation in pulmonary venous pressure, which increases the work of the right ventricle and ultimately results in heart failure. Along with this sequence of events, *atrial fibrillation* may produce irregular, poor contractions of the left atrium and potential thrombus formation with the danger of embolization. Irregular contraction of the left ventricle may develop, to further aggravate the problem. When the predominant valve dysfunction is incompetence, blood is shunted back and forth between the left and right ventricles (*mitral regurgitation*); this increases the work load on the heart and ultimately results in pulmonary congestion and heart failure. This disease occurs about four times more often in women than in men.

The effect on the heart varies with the degree of pathologic change in the mitral valve. In mild forms of the disease, the heart may compensate adequately, and the patient may have little disability. Most patients, however, suffer gradual and progressive disability over a period of years. Studies have shown that about 1 in 5 patients with mitral stenosis will die within one year after first seeking help from a physician, and about 60 percent of patients will die in 10 years. Treatment of mitral valve disease may be medical or surgical, depending upon the degree of disability and certain findings during a careful and precise examination, including particularly echocardiography and cardiac catheterization (Figure 22.2).

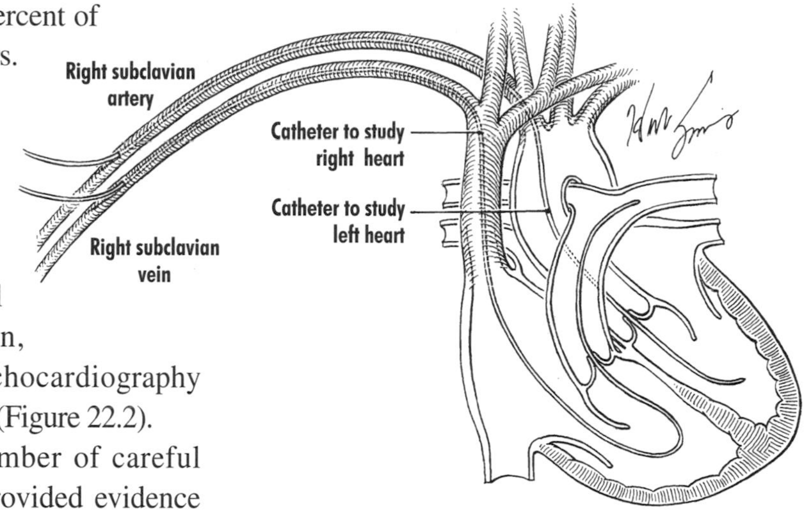

In recent years, a number of careful follow-up studies have provided evidence for general agreement that surgical treatment should be recommended at an earlier stage in the disease than was previously considered, namely, when symptoms develop. The risk of cerebral embolism with crippling stroke and deteriorating left ventricular function, along with progressive changes in the valve making repair difficult or impossible, have all directed attention to the concept of early operation based on certain hemodynamic abnormalities, such as reduction in cross-sectional area of mitral stenosis to 1.0 to 1.5 cm or significant mitral valve insufficiency as indicated by echocardiography.

Operations for mitral valve disease are directed toward repair or replacement of the valve, depending on the extent of the damage. In certain types of mitral regurgitation in which the valve leaflets are not significantly damaged, repair is usually

Figure 22.2. Catheters are passed into the left and right sides of the heart to obtain the information necessary for precise diagnosis and degree of dysfunction of valvular disease.

possible. This is also an advantage of early operation. In pure mitral stenosis, in which the valve leaflets are not badly damaged and are still pliable, it is also usually possible to repair the valve by separating or dividing the fused edges. These procedures are performed with use of the heart-lung machine, which allows the heart to be opened through an incision in the left atrium to permit direct vision of the mitral valve. This enables a more accurate assessment of the damage and a more precise technique for dividing or separating the fused edges of the valve or for repair of incompetent valves. In some patients, however, it may not be possible to open

A

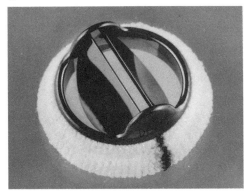
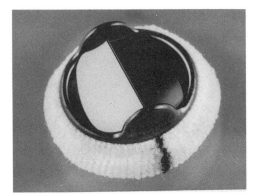

B

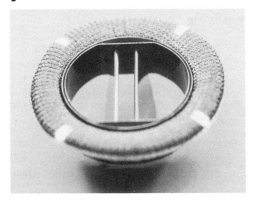
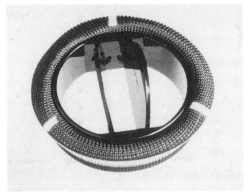

C

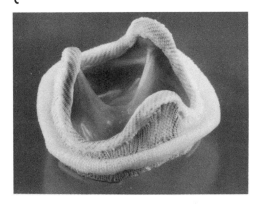
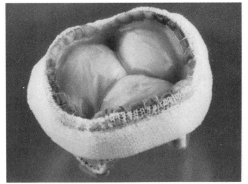

Figure 22.3. A. St. Jude Mechanical Valve Prosthesis.
B. Carbomedic Mechanical Valve Prosthesis.
C. Bioprosthetic Valve.

the narrowed valve adequately without inducing incompetence, or the valve may be so badly damaged with calcification and scarring that repair is impossible. Under these circumstances, valve replacement may be necessary and can be performed immediately.

In patients in whom valve replacement is required, either a bioprosthetic (porcine or pericardial) or mechanical prosthesis may be used. Virtually all prostheses currently being used are disk type with satisfactory valvular function, as exemplified by the St. Jude and the Carbomedic prostheses (Figures 22.3 and 22.4). The decision in choosing a bioprosthetic or mechanical prosthesis should be made by the surgeon and the patient. In this connection, an important consideration is that anticoagulant therapy must be used with all mechanical prostheses and, therefore, in patients in whom there is some contraindication to the use of anticoagulants, the bioprosthetic valve is preferable. Another consideration is the fact that bioprosthetic valves tend to deteriorate and require replacement after 10 to 15 years. Moreover, these valves deteriorate more rapidly in children. In many centers, bioprosthetic valves are now being used mostly in elderly patients.

The operation is performed following standard cardiopulmonary bypass and cardioplegic cardiac arrest. The mitral

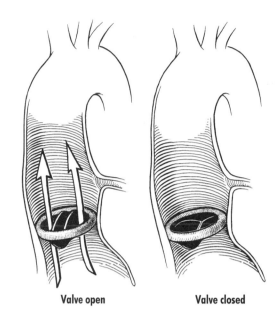

Valve open   Valve closed

Figure 22.4. The function of a prosthetic valve (St. Jude). The leaflets open (left) to permit blood flow into the aorta from the contraction of the left ventricle and close (right) to prevent blood from returning into the ventricle.

valve is then exposed by a vertical incision in the left atrium just below the overlying right atrium. Depending on the findings, the mitral valve is repaired or replaced (Figure 22.5).

The results of operation are generally highly satisfactory, with an operative mortality rate between 2.5 and 5 percent. The operative mortality rate is slightly less after repair than after replacement. Long-term results are also good, with a 15-year survival rate of about 75 percent. In an analysis of our experience with the St. Jude mitral valve prosthesis (Figure 22.3),

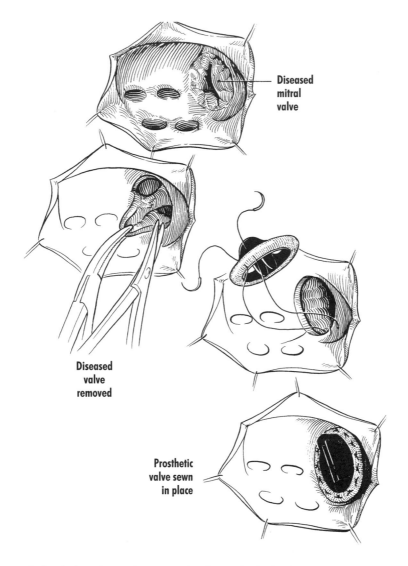

Diseased
mitral
valve

Diseased
valve
removed

Prosthetic
valve sewn
in place

Figure 22.5. Surgical technique for replacement of a diseased mitral valve.

which is a bileaflet, low-profile mechanical prosthesis made of pyrolytic carbon, the risk of operation was about 5 percent (ranging between 1 and 10 percent depending on the severity of disease, ventricular function, and associated conditions). In patients with a mechanical prosthesis, continuous anticoagulant therapy (warfarin or coumarin) must be employed. In our experience with the St. Jude valve, the incidence of moderate to severe non-fatal anticoagulant hemorrhage was 5.4 percent per patient year. Survival expectancy is excellent, with 5-year survival of about 80 percent and 10-year survival of about 75 percent. We have a number of patients leading normal lives 20 years after operation. Thromboembolism is relatively uncommon if the patient's conditions are properly monitored, with an occurrence rate of about 1 to 2 percent per patient year.

These patients require careful monitoring during the rest of their lives to detect and prevent complications such as hemorrhage, thromboembolism, arrhythmia, and infection. Endocarditis of the valve, for example, is a very serious complication, which may occur after such procedures as dental extraction, cystoscopic examinations, and trauma. The patient should be cautioned to take antibiotic medication before such procedures. Arrhythmia is another important complication, which may be associated with sudden death 5 to 10 years after operation. It is more common in patients with preoperative left ventricular dysfunction.

Aortic Valve Disease

Damage to the aortic valve may result in narrowing of the opening caused by thickening, distortion, and fusion of the valve cusps, as well as by *calcification* (Figure 22.6). Damage to the aortic valve may also result in valve incompetence. In stenosis, the flow of blood from the left ventricle is obstructed, and this increases the total work required by the heart, thereby causing progressive hypertrophy and failure, as well as arrhythmia. It may be caused by congenital bicuspid valve, rheumatic fever, or degenerative calcification, especially in the elderly. The development of aortic stenosis before the age of 30 years strongly suggests congenital stenosis. After that age to about 60 to 70 years, rheumatic disease or a calcification of a congenital bicuspid valve is more common. In patients over 70 years of age, degenerative calcification is the most common cause.

Ultimately, symptoms of failure develop in these patients, with attacks of shortness of breath, passing out, and chest pain. About one-fifth of the patients die suddenly without pre-existing symptoms. Aortic stenosis may mimic or worsen the symptoms of coronary artery disease.

Aortic incompetence or insufficiency was caused most frequently by rheumatic fever and syphilis in the past, but with the use of effective antimicrobial treatment, they are now less frequent causes. At present, diseases of the connective tissue and anatomic abnormalities of the ascending aorta have become more common causes. They include dissecting aneurysms, Marfan's syndrome, myxomatous changes in the valves, bacterial endocarditis, and calcific changes. As a consequence of

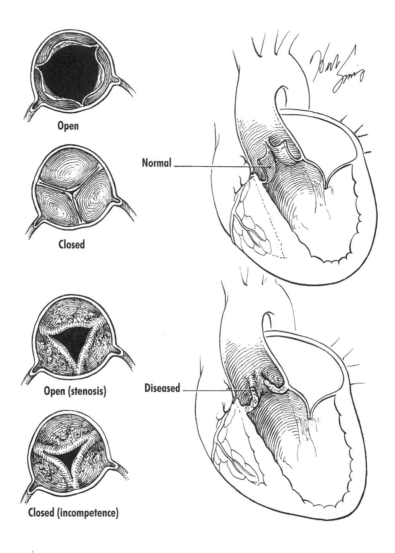

Open

Closed

Open (stenosis)

Closed (incompetence)

Normal

Diseased

Figure 22.6. Diseased aortic valve (below) as contrasted with a normal aortic valve (above).

valve incompetence, blood flowing out of the left ventricle during systole is partially regurgitated back into the ventricle during diastole. This produces an increased workload on the heart that causes it to enlarge and ultimately fail. Once symptoms of shortness of breath or pain in the chest develop, the prognosis is extremely poor, and life expectancy is reduced to possibly one to three years.

Surgical treatment is suggested for all patients with symptoms, as well as for those who are asymptomatic whose examination indicates progressive disease and a strain developing on the left ventricle. These determinations are best made by echocardiography and cardiac catheterization. Surgical treatment should not be delayed until severe symptoms develop unless there are significant contraindications to operation. Studies have shown that after onset of symptoms in aortic stenosis, survival expectancy at 1 year is 50 percent, and at 3 years it is 20 percent. It is generally recommended that operation be performed in asymptomatic patients when a mean aortic valve gradient is 50 mm Hg or when the aortic valve area becomes 0.8 cm or less.

Patients with aortic regurgitation may remain relatively asymptomatic for many years because of the compensatory mechanisms of the left ventricle. When the patient begins to have symptoms, they usually represent left ventricular failure, including particularly easy fatigability, shortness of breath, and swelling of the lower legs. The patient may also experience some chest discomfort.

The diagnosis can be established by physical signs, echocardiography, and cardiac catheterization. Patients with aortic regurgitation may remain relatively free of symptoms for long periods before development of heart failure, even up to 10 years in mild to moderate forms of the disease. Once failure occurs, however, there is usually rapid deterioration, with a survival rate of less than 2 years.

Since impairment of both ventricular and myocardial performance is associated with poor outcome after surgical treatment, operation is recommended before this occurs. In general, surgical treatment is recommended in the presence of early symptoms, significant elevation of left ventricular end–diastolic pressure, or any evidence of impairment of left ventricular function. Thus, if exercise testing yields evidence of decreased left ventricular function by scintigraphy or echocardiography, or development of hypertension or arrhythmia, operation is indicated. In patients with acute aortic regurgitation, however, regardless of the cause, such as bacterial endocarditis, trauma, or aortic dissection, operation is urgently recommended.

At operation, the heart is exposed through a vertical incision in the breastbone. The patient is placed on the heart-lung machine, and the ascending aorta is occluded (Figure 22.7). The valve is then exposed by an incision in the aorta. After the diseased valve is excised, the sutures are placed around the remaining annulus and then through the sewing ring of the valve. The valve is seated into the annulus and firmly attached by tying the sutures. Air in the heart is removed; the incision in the aorta is closed; and heart function is restored.

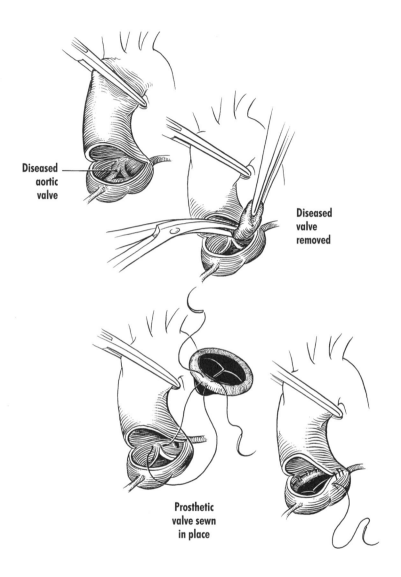

Diseased
aortic
valve

Diseased
valve
removed

Prosthetic
valve sewn
in place

Figure 22.7. Surgical technique for replacement of a diseased aortic valve.

A variety of valvular prostheses are available for aortic valve replacement. They may be considered in two groups, namely mechanical prostheses and biologic prostheses. The advantage of biologic prostheses lies in the fact that they do not require anticoagulation, but they have the disadvantage that they tend to deteriorate after 10 to 12 years, and in younger patients they have an even shorter span.

Young women during pregnancy may wish to have a bioprosthetic valve to avoid the danger of anticoagulation. Mechanical prostheses of various types are generally satisfactory and have a long life span of more than 20 years, but they do require anticoagulation. Choice of a particular valve in a patient depends on several factors, including medical factors and the ability to comply with the continuous maintenance of anticoagulation. The decision should be made jointly by the physician and the patient.

Results after aortic valve replacement are excellent, and the operative risk ranges between 2 and 5 percent. This risk is increased in patients older than 80 years, in those requiring associated coronary bypass or other associated corrective procedures, and in those with decreased preoperative left ventricular function. Long-term results are good, with most patients resuming relatively normal lives. The 10-year-survival expectancy is about 60 to 70 percent. In our own experience with the use of the St. Jude valve, survival expectancy was almost 90 percent at 5 years and about 70 percent at 10 years. Some of our patients are leading normal lives 20 to 30 years after operation.

Combined Valvular Disease

Some patients have significant disease of both the mitral valve and the aortic valve

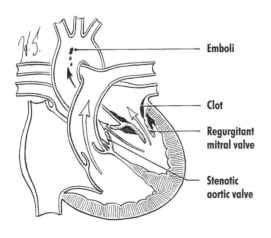

Figure 22.8. Disease in both the aortic and mitral valves. Clot forming around the base of the diseased mitral valve and in the left atrium may break off and form emboli that pass out of the aorta to lodge in an artery in another part of the body.

Emboli

Clot

Regurgitant mitral valve

Stenotic aortic valve

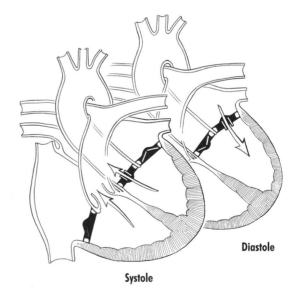

Diastole

Systole

Figure 22.9. Diagram of heart function when all three valves are replaced with prostheses.

347

(Figure 22.8). Under these circumstances, it may be necessary to replace both valves. This is done in the same manner as described for each valve separately. The risk of this combined procedure is about 5 to 10 percent, and the results are very satisfactory.

A small proportion of patients may have significant damage of the tricuspid valve associated with mitral valve disease or with mitral and aortic valve disease. It is often possible to repair the tricuspid valve, but occasionally it may be necessary to replace all three valves (Figure 22.9).

CHAPTER TWENTY-THREE

Aneurysms

The term *aneurysm* is derived from the Greek word that means to widen or dilate. This disease has been known for centuries and long recognized as a threat to life. It develops from a weakness or destruction of the medial layer of the aorta or a major artery. Once this occurs, the weakened part of the arterial wall gives way to the pounding pulse pressure within the artery and enlarges (Figure 23.1). Ultimately, lethal complications develop, either because of compression of surrounding structures or rupture of the aneurysm and exsanguination.

No effective treatment for aneurysms was available until relatively recently. Beginning in the early 1950s, effective methods for surgical treatment of

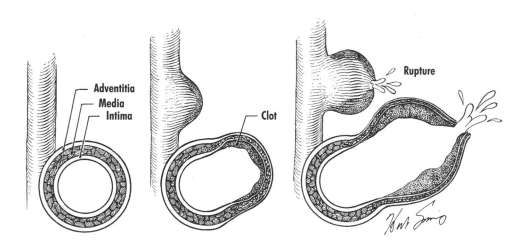

Figure 23.1. A normal artery (left) is weakened by arteriosclerosis or some other disease, and gradually balloons out, forming an aneurysm, which may be partially lined with a blood clot (center). Eventually the aneurysm may rupture (right).

aneurysms were developed and refined. From a technical standpoint, virtually all patients with aneurysms of the aorta and major arteries can be effectively treated with a high rate of success.

Aneurysms are classified according to cause, location, and morphology. By far, the most common cause is arteriosclerosis. It is not known why arteriosclerosis in some patients affects the medial layer of an artery leading to aneurysmal formation, and in others, affects the intima leading to obstruction of the lumen. Indeed, in some patients both types of arterial disease are present in different parts of the arterial tree. Less frequently, aneurysms are caused by specific infections, particularly syphilis, which was one of the most common causes in earlier years before effective treatment for the disease was available; blunt injuries to the chest, often resulting from automobile accident or from a fall; congenital lesions; and a special form of disease of the media.

Morphologically, aneurysms may be classified into two types: 1) *fusiform,* characterized by involvement of the entire circumference of the aorta with a tendency to assume a spindle shape; and 2) *sacciform,* characterized by a pouch-like protrusion with a narrow neck from the arterial wall (Figure 23.2).

Aneurysms tend to assume distinctive localized patterns regarding their extent and location, with relatively normal seg-

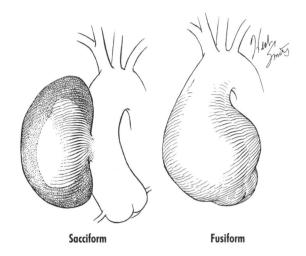

Sacciform   Fusiform

Figure 23.2. Types of aneurysms.

ments above and below the diseased segment. The most common pattern is a fusiform aneurysm of the abdominal aorta, which arises just below the renal arteries and extends down to encompass the common iliac arteries (Figure 23.3). Next in frequency are aneurysms of the descending thoracic aorta, which arise just distal to the left subclavian artery and extend to the middle or lower third of the descending thoracic aorta and sometimes to the diaphragm. Next are the aneurysms of the ascending aorta, the aortic arch, and the thoracoabdominal aorta. Aneurysms of the major arteries most often involve the common femoral artery in the groin, the popliteal artery behind the knee, the carotid artery in the neck, and the subclavian arteries. Occasionally, aneurysms occur in the renal arteries, the splenic artery, and the superior mesenteric artery.

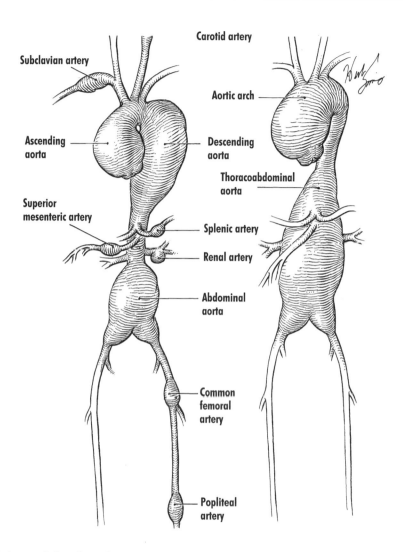

Carotid artery

Subclavian artery

Aortic arch

Ascending aorta

Descending aorta

Thoracoabdominal aorta

Superior mesenteric artery

Splenic artery

Renal artery

Abdominal aorta

Common femoral artery

Popliteal artery

Figure 23.3. Anatomic locations of aneurysms.

Aneurysms of the Abdominal Aorta

This is the most common type of aneurysm of the aorta and is caused by arteriosclerosis in most cases. It is one of the most lethal, causing death from rupture in a high percentage of patients. Studies of the natural history of the disease showed that about 50 percent of the patients died within one year after diagnosis, and less than 10 percent survived for 5 years. The disease may occur in patients ranging in age from the teens to the nineties, but the highest incidence occurs in people in their 60s and 70s. Men are affected in a ratio of

9 to 1 over women. About one-third of the patients have associated hypertension and occlusive disease in the carotid arteries or coronary arteries.

Patients may have no symptoms, and the disease often is found during a routine physical examination or by a routine abdominal x-ray, which reveals an outline of the aneurysm by the calcification in its wall. Sometimes the patient himself becomes aware of a prominent pulsation in the abdomen. Pain is an ominous signal, since it usually indicates progressive expansion with an imminent danger of leakage or rupture. The location and severity of pain depends on the nature and extent of the aneurysm. It may be located in the back, or it may extend into the flanks, groin, testicles, or legs. If leakage takes place, the pain may become more intense, and the patient will have a rapid heartbeat, sweating, and shock. If sudden rupture occurs, the patient may die within a few minutes.

The diagnosis can usually be made by a physical examination and x-rays of the

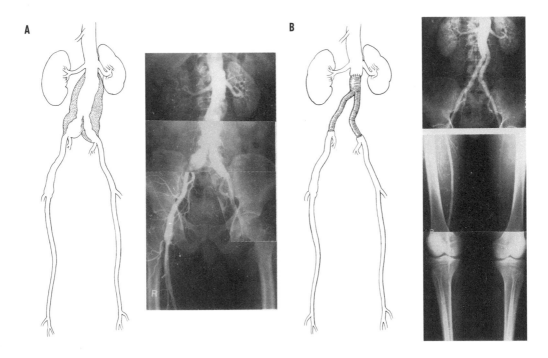

Figure 23.4. A. Drawing and preoperative aortogram of a 56-year-old man in whom routine physical examination uncovered a large fusiform aneurysm of the abdominal aorta involving both common iliac arteries.
B. Drawing showing method of surgical treatment, consisting in resection of aneurysm of abdominal aorta and both common iliac arteries and replacement with albumin-coated DeBakey Dacron® bifurcation graft, and aortogram made 10 years after operation, showing restoration of normal circulation through the graft. Patient remains asymptomatic 13 years after operation.

abdomen. Imaging with ultrasound, computed radiographic tomography, and magnetic resonance imaging (MRI) provide confirmation and precise measurements of the aneurysm. Aortography may be necessary in patients if additional information is needed concerning the presence of possible occlusive disease in the vascular bed (Figure 23.4).

Once the diagnosis is made, surgical treatment is recommended, particularly in patients whose aneurysm measures 5 cm or greater in diameter, since aneurysms of this size or larger have a greater tendency to rupture. The operation consists in applying occluding clamps above and below the aneurysm, opening the aneurysm by a vertical incision, removing the layered thrombus and detritus from the lumen, oversewing the bleeding lumbar arteries in the posterior wall, sewing an albumin-coated Dacron® graft from the inside of the sac to the proximal opening by continuous suture anastomosis, attaching the graft to the distal opening of the abdominal aorta in a similar fashion, and finally covering the graft with the outer wall of the aneurysm. In patients whose aneurysm involves the common iliac arteries, a Y-shaped Dacron® graft is used (Figure 23.4).

Results of the operation are good, with an operative risk of only about 2 or 3 percent and excellent long-term results. Some of our patients are leading normal lives 20 to more than 30 years after the operation. Contraindications to elective operation may include severe debilitating disease such as cancer, emphysema, and heart failure. Age itself is not a negative factor, since we have successfully operated on patients in their 80s and even 90s.

Aneurysms of the Descending Thoracic Aorta

Aneurysms of the descending thoracic aorta are usually fusiform in type and arteriosclerotic in origin (Figure 23.5). They may also be caused by severe trauma, especially the type produced by sudden deceleration, such as falling from a height of several stories (construction worker) or by an automobile accident (Figure 23.6). The tear in the aorta caused by such trauma occurs just distal to the origin of the left subclavian artery. Most patients who have this type of accident also have multiple injuries and fractures that are often fatal. Those who recover and have a small tear in the aorta will develop a "false aneurysm" produced by encapsulation of the clot that forms around the tear and prevents exsanguination (Figure 23.6). They are most common in men and may occur at any age, but most often develop between the ages of 50 and 80. Symptoms may not be present, but when they do occur, they usually are due to the compression of surrounding

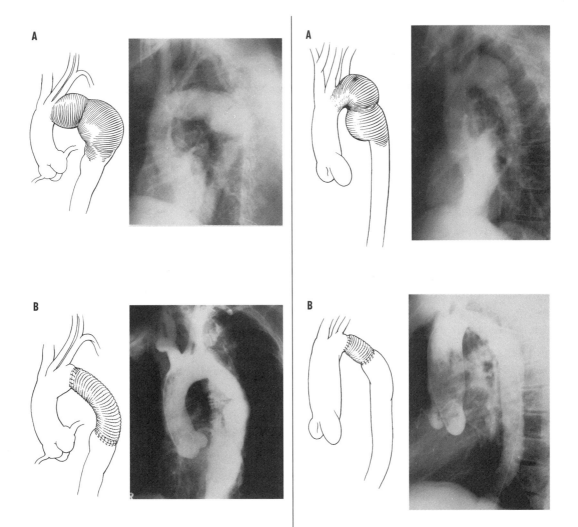

Figure 23.5. A. Drawing and preoperative aortogram of a 48-year-old man complaining of aching chest pain extending to the left shoulder and back, showing a large fusiform aneurysm of the descending thoracic aorta.
B. Drawing showing method of surgical treatment, consisting in resection of the aneurysm between occluding clamps and replacement with a Dacron® graft, and aortogram made 25 years after operation showing graft functioning normally. Patient remained well for approximately 30 years after operation.

Figure 23.6. A. Drawing and preoperative aortogram of a 26-year-old man who sustained severe multiple injuries after an automobile accident five years previously, showing well-localized aneurysm in upper portion of descending thoracic aorta just below origin of left subclavian artery.
B. Drawing showing method of surgical treatment, consisting in resection of aneurysm and replacement with Dacron® graft, and aortogram made 33 years after operation showing graft functioning normally. Patient remains well almost 35 years since operation.

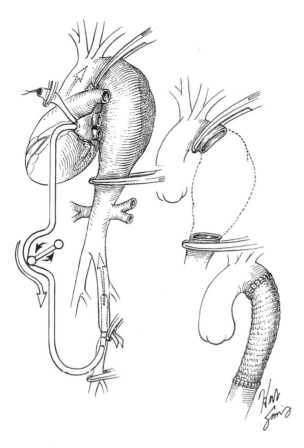

Figure 23.7. Surgical technique for an aneurysm of the descending thoracic aorta.

operation is performed by opening the left side of the chest through an incision between the ribs. The aneurysm is excised between occluding clamps on the aorta, and the defect is replaced with an albumin-coated Dacron® graft (Figure 23.7).

Results of the operation are excellent, with an operative risk between 5 and 10 percent. There is a low incidence (4 to 7 percent) of paraparesis or even paraplegia (weakness or paralysis) secondary to lack of blood supply to the spinal cord after the operation. Although various methods have been used to prevent this complication, none has proved completely effective. Left atria–to–femoral artery bypass during the time that the aorta is occluded is believed to reduce the incidence of this complication, as illustrated in Figure 23.7. In our experience, the survival expectancy following operation is quite good, with some of our patients leading normal lives for 20 to more than 30 years after operation (Figure 23.6).

structures, which results in pain in the chest or back and may radiate to the neck, shoulders, or abdomen. When the aneurysm compresses the trachea, it may cause a hacking cough. Increasing pain is an ominous sign of progressive enlargement and impending rupture.

Surgical treatment is suggested except in patients with conditions such as severe debilitating disease or heart failure. The

Aneurysms of the Ascending Aorta

These aneurysms may occur at any age, even during the first 10 years of life, when they are usually of congenital origin (Figure 23.8). Most occur in persons between the ages of 40 and 80 years and are of arteriosclerotic origin. Some are of undetermined cause and resemble aneurysms of the sinus of Valsalva, especially in younger patients. Others may be associated with aortic valve insufficiency. Symptoms may or may not be present, and the condition usually is discovered during a routine physical examination or on chest x-ray. Pain in the chest is one of the most common symptoms, and if aortic valve insufficiency is present, early heart failure may occur. The diagnosis can be made by imaging with ultrasound, computed radiographic tomography, magnetic resonance, and aortography (described in Chapter 5).

Surgical treatment is recommended for all patients except those with severe associated disease that would make the surgical risk prohibitive. The operation is performed with use of the heart-lung machine; the aorta is occluded just above the aneurysm, the aneurysm opened by a vertical incision, and an albumin-coated Dacron® graft attached proximally and distally (Figure 23.9). The aneurysmal sac is then tailored to fit over the graft and is sutured. If aortic valve insufficiency is present, an artificial valve is used to replace the diseased one. Results of this operation are excellent, with a risk of about 5 percent or less (Figure 23.8).

A

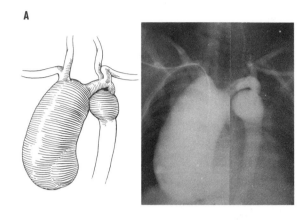

B

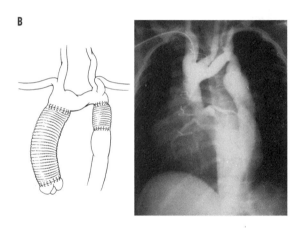

Figure 23.8. A. Drawing and preoperative aortogram of a 9-year-old boy, showing a large probably congenital, aneurysm of the ascending aorta and coarctation of the descending thoracic aorta with an aneurysm just below it.
B. Drawing showing method of surgical treatment, consisting in a two-stage operation, resection of the coarctation and aneurysm and replacement with a Dacron® graft, and three weeks later, resection of the aneurysm of the ascending aorta and replacement with a Dacron® graft. The postoperative aortogram shows restoration of normal aortic function. Patient remained well for more than 15 years after operation.

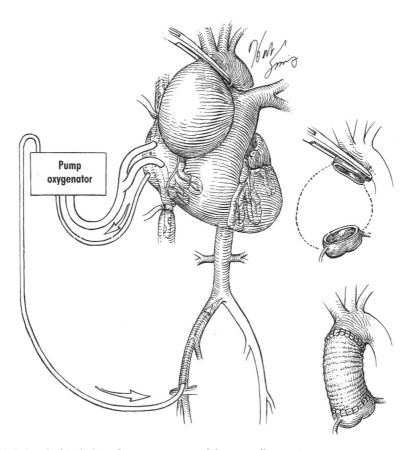

Figure 23.9. Surgical technique for an aneurysm of the ascending aorta.

Aneurysms of the Aortic Arch

This is one of the most serious and most difficult forms of aortic aneurysm to treat because it involves the major arteries supplying blood to the brain. It occurs predominately in men between the ages of 50 and 70 years. Symptoms are produced by compression of surrounding structures, particularly the trachea and esophagus. Pain in the chest or at the base of the neck is common; other symptoms may be a hacking cough or difficulty in swallowing. The diagnosis is made by aortography (described in Chapter 6).

Surgical correction is recommended unless there is associated disease that would create a prohibitive risk. The procedure is performed with use of the heart-

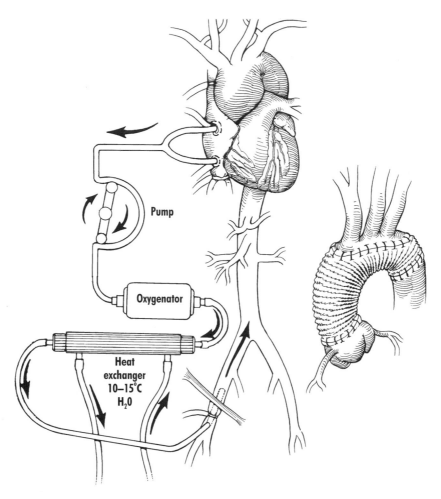

Figure 23.10. Surgical technique for an aneurysm of the entire aortic arch.

lung machine and profound hypothermia, the body temperature being reduced to about 15° to 16°C by means of the heart-lung machine (Figure 23.10). In addition to the profound hypothermia, retrograde perfusion of the brain through the superior vena cava is believed to add further cerebral protection. When the body temperature reaches 15° to 16°C, perfusion with the heart-lung machine may be temporarily stopped and only used intermittently during the graft replacement. The aneurysm is opened, and an albumin-coated Dacron® graft is sutured to the relatively normal aorta proximally and distally from within the aneurysm, and the large vessels arising from the arch are anastomosed to an appropriate opening in the

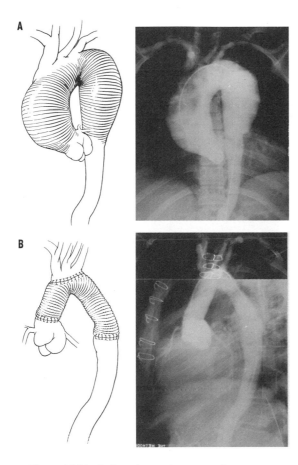

Figure 23.11. A. Drawing and preoperative aortogram of a 30-year-old woman, showing a large aneurysm of the ascending aorta and aortic arch.
B. Drawing showing technique of operation, consisting in resection of the aneurysm and replacement with an albumin-coated Dacron® graft, and postoperative aortogram showing restoration of normal aortic function.

graft. The wall of the aneurysm is then tailored to be sutured over the graft. The patient is then rewarmed using the heart-lung machine. Results of this operation are excellent, with an operative risk of about 10 to 15 percent (Figure 23.11).

Thoracoabdominal Aneurysms

These aneurysms are fusiform in type and usually occur in the lower descending thoracic aorta, with extension into the abdominal aorta for varying distances, to the bifurcation, and even into the common iliac arteries. They are most common in men between the ages of 50 and 70 years of age. Symptoms are similar to those associated with aneurysm of the abdominal aorta, except that the pain may be higher in the abdomen and in the chest or back. These aneurysms assume special significance because the arteries supplying blood to the organs of the abdomen arise from this portion of the aorta.

Our first successful method of treatment of this type of aneurysm consisted in first applying a bypass graft from the aorta above the aneurysm in the chest to the segment below the aneurysm in the abdomen and then attaching, sequentially, grafts to the renal, superior mesenteric, and celiac arteries, after which the aneurysm was excised. More recently, the technical procedure has been simplified. It consists in attaching an albumin-coated Dacron® graft by end-to-end anastomosis to the descending thoracic aorta above the origin of the aneurysm and then anastomosing an opening in the graft to the portion of aorta from which the celiac, superior mesenteric, and renal arteries arise (Figure 23.12). The

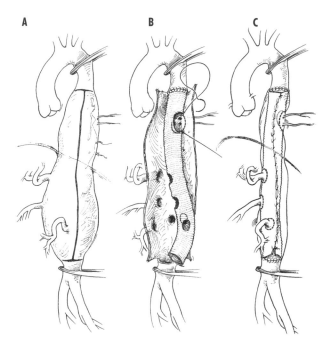

Figure 23.12. Technique of operation for thoracoabdominal aneurysm. A. The aneurysm is opened between occluding clamps on the aorta; B. an albumin-coated Dacron® graft is attached to the proximal opening in the descending thoracic aorta; large intercostal vessels are attached to an appropriate opening in the graft; and the celiac, superior mesenteric, and renal arteries are similarly attached to appropriate openings in the graft; C. after the distal anastomosis to the graft has been performed, the wall of the aneurysm is tailored to be sutured over the graft.

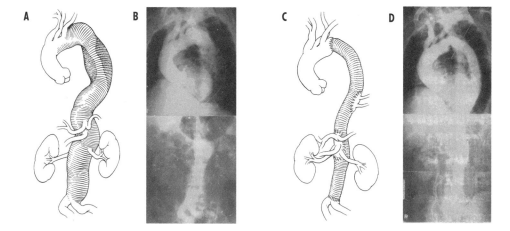

Figure 23.13. A. Drawing showing extent of thoracoabdominal aneurysm in a 58-year-old man with increased fatigability and dull aching pain in abdomen and back of chest; B. preoperative aortogram showing extensive thoracoabdominal aneurysm; C. drawing showing technique of operation; and D. postoperative aortogram showing restoration of normal aortic function.

terminal end of the graft is then anastomosed to the distal end of the abdominal aorta, or if the common iliac arteries are involved, a Dacron® bifurcation graft is interposed for this purpose. The outer wall of the aneurysmal sac is usually sutured over the graft.

Results of this operation are excellent, with an operative mortality rate of 5 to 10 percent (Figure 23.13). Survival expectancy is good, with some patients leading a relatively normal life after operation for 20 to 25 years. As in aneurysm of the descending thoracic aorta, paraparesis or paraplegia is a potential complication, occurring with about the same frequency previously cited.

Dissection and Dissecting Aneurysms of the Aorta

This is one of the most serious forms of aortic disease. Studies of the natural history of the disease have shown that about 35 percent of patients die within the initial 24 hours, 50 percent within 48 hours, 70 percent within one week, and 80 percent within two weeks, with few patients surviving 1 to 2 years. This disease occurs predominately in men between 40 and 70 years of age. About 80 percent of patients have severe hypertension. Certain conditions are associated with increased frequency of dissection.

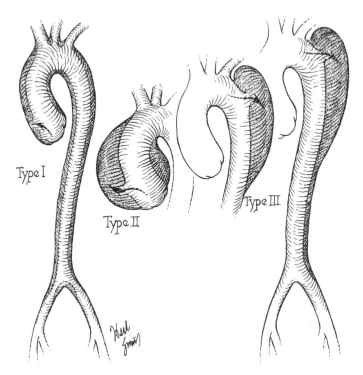

Figure 23.14. Types of dissection and dissecting aneurysms of the aorta.

These include congenital lesions, such as coarctation of the aorta and bicuspid aortic valve, aortic stenosis, and Marfan's and Turner syndromes.

The initial symptom is sudden onset of pain in the chest radiating to the back, shoulders, neck, abdomen, or legs. It is sometimes described as "crushing," "tearing," or "ripping." The condition is sometimes confused with an acute heart attack. A "marching" nature of pain is common, as it radiates upward or downward. Transitory numbness in the face or legs and arms and even paraplegia may occur.

The basic lesion of this disease of the aorta seems to be degeneration of the media of the aorta, termed cystic medial necrosis, not related to arteriosclerosis. A tear in the intimal layer, most often in the ascending aorta just above the aortic valve and the descending thoracic aorta just beyond the origin of the left subclavian artery, allows blood to enter the diseased media, and the force of blood pressure with each heartbeat causes a separation between these layers. This dissecting process occurs in only part of the circumference of the aorta, but depending on the type of separation, may extend throughout the aorta and even into the arteries of the legs.

On the basis of extensive experience, DeBakey classified dissections into three types (Figure 23.14). In Type I, the dissecting process extends throughout the aorta and sometimes beyond the bifurcation of the abdominal aorta, with the tear in the intima usually in the ascending aorta; Type II is similar but is limited to the ascending aorta, with aortic valve insufficiency often present. In Type III, the dissecting process begins in the upper portion of the descending thoracic aorta and extends downward for varying distances, sometimes even into the abdominal aorta and its bifurcation.

The diagnosis may be confirmed by computed tomography after intravenous administration of contrast material, by transesophageal echocardiography, or by magnetic resonance imaging (MRI). In acutely ill patients, computed tomography, or preferably in our experience, aortography provides preoperatively the precise type of dissection information more expeditiously.

The first successful surgical treatment of a dissecting aneurysm was performed by DeBakey in 1954.[1] Surgical treatment depends on the type of dissection and the condition of the patient (Figure 23.15). In most patients with Type I and Type II dissection, surgical treatment is indicated as soon as the diagnosis can be confirmed. Preoperatively, these patients should be

---

[1] Michael E. DeBakey, Denton A. Cooley, and Oscar Creech, Jr. "Surgical Considerations of Dissecting Aneurysm of the Aorta." *American Surgeon*, 142:586–612 (1955).

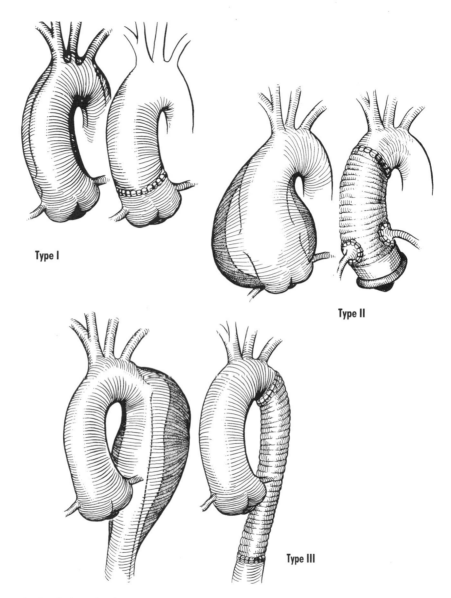

Type I

Type II

Type III

Figure 23.15. Surgical technique for the three types of dissection.

admitted to the intensive care unit for careful and continuous monitoring of vital signs and control of blood pressure.

In Type I dissection, the surgical procedure consists in excision of the dissected segment of the ascending aorta, obliteration of the false lumen by suture approximation of the inner and outer walls of the dissecting process, and replacement with an albumin-coated Dacron® graft with use of the heart-lung machine (Figure 23.16). The aortic incompetence that may be present can be corrected in some patients by resuspension of the valves. In others, however, it may be necessary to replace the valve with an aortic valve prosthesis.

In Type II dissection, the surgical procedure is similar to that described for Type I except that it is usually not necessary to obliterate the false lumen, since the dissecting process is limited to the ascending aorta. In most of these patients, however, it is usually necessary to replace the aortic valve. For this purpose, a composite Dacron® aortic graft and aortic valve prosthesis is used. In such cases, the ostia (openings of the coronary arteries) are attached to comparable openings in the Dacron® aortic graft as illustrated in Figures 23.15 and 23.16.

In Type III dissection, surgical treatment may not be as urgent as in Types I and II in most patients. Some physicians prefer medical treatment with particular emphasis on control of blood pressure, whereas others recommend surgical treatment. Even in those treated medically, surgical treatment is indicated if there is evidence of progression of the dissecting process, leakage of blood, continued thoracic pain, or occlusion of a major artery distally. In our experience, surgical treatment is preferable in the absence of serious associated disease, such as cancer, severe heart disease, or pulmonary or renal

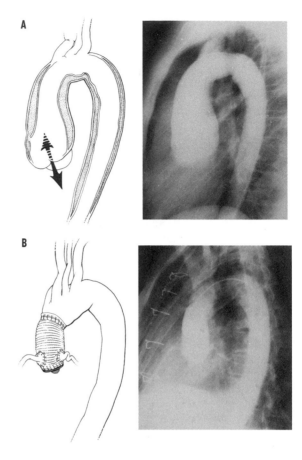

Figure 23.16. A. Drawing and preoperative aortogram of a 35-year-old woman with Marfan's syndrome complaining of acute left chest pain, palpitation, shortness of breath, and nausea, showing Type I dissection of aorta.
B. Drawing showing surgical treatment, consisting in replacement of ascending aorta and aortic valve with composite Dacron® graft and St. Jude aortic prosthesis with anastomosis of both coronary arteries to appropriate opening in graft; and postoperative aortogram showing function of graft and coronary circulation. Patient has remained well for almost 10 years after operation.

disease. The surgical procedure (Figure 23.15) consists in excision of the false lumen up to the level of the dissecting

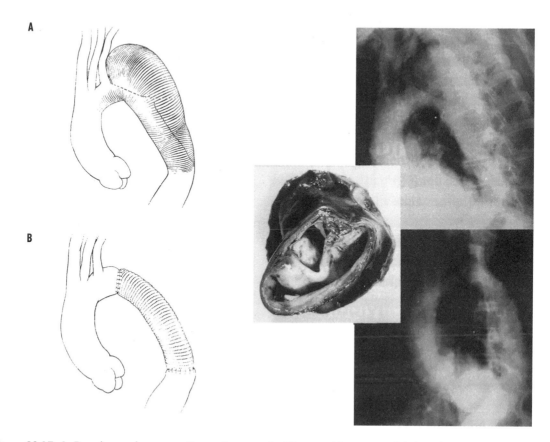

Figure 23.17. A. Drawing and preoperative aortogram of a 54-year-old man complaining of severe chest pain extending to midscapular region occurring two months previously, showing Type III dissecting aneurysm of descending thoracic aorta with small normal lumen and large false lumen, which is also illustrated in insert showing cross-section of excised aneurysm.
B. Drawing showing operative procedure, consisting in resection of dissecting process and replacement with Dacron® graft, and postoperative aortogram showing restoration of normal aortic function.

process, usually just below the origin of the left subclavian artery; obliteration of the false lumen distally by suture closure of the inner and outer layers; and replacement with an albumin-coated aortic Dacron® graft (Figure 23.17). In patients whose dissection extends into the abdominal aorta, it may be necessary to use a thoracoabdominal approach.

Results of these operations in our experience with over 1,000 patients, have been excellent, with an overall risk of approximately 10 to 12 percent. The highest risk is with the Type I dissection, which has a mortality rate of about 15 percent, and the lowest is with Type II, which is about 5 percent. Long-term results are excellent, with some patients surviving up to 25 years after operation. The 10-year-survival rate in Type II is about 50 percent, and the overall 10-year-survival rate is about 35 percent.

Aneurysms of Major Peripheral Arteries

These aneurysms are usually localized and fusiform in type. They most often involve the femoral, popliteal, carotid, and subclavian arteries. They may also occur in the major arteries to the abdominal viscera, such as the renal, superior mesenteric, celiac, and splenic arteries. They are found most often in men between 50 and 70 years of age. Surgical treatment is suggested for most of these aneurysms and consists in resection and Dacron® graft replacement (Figure 23.18). Results are excellent, with a low risk of about 1 percent or less (Figure 23.19).

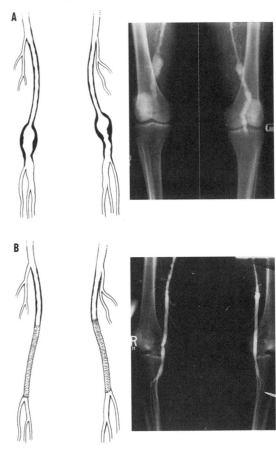

Figure 23.19. A. Drawing and preoperative arteriogram of a 71-year-old man complaining of tiredness in legs on walking, showing aneurysms of both popliteal arteries behind the knees.
B. Drawing showing method of surgical treatment, consisting in resection of popliteal aneurysms and replacement with Dacron® graft, and postoperative arteriogram showing restoration of normal circulation in legs.

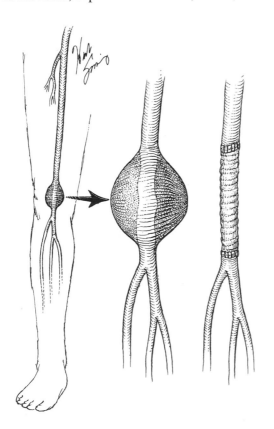

Figure 23.18. Surgical technique for the repair of an aneurysm of the popliteal artery.

Endovascular Surgery

In recent years, considerable interest and clinical investigations have been directed toward the use of endovascular prostheses or transluminally placed grafts for the treatment of both aneurysmal and occlusive disease. Various types of prostheses have been developed for this purpose, and undoubtedly, newer ones will be forthcoming from currently intensive research.

In general, the prosthesis consists of a compressible-expandable stent of a fine, mesh-like, springy, metallic material covered by a Dacron® or polytetrafluoreth-

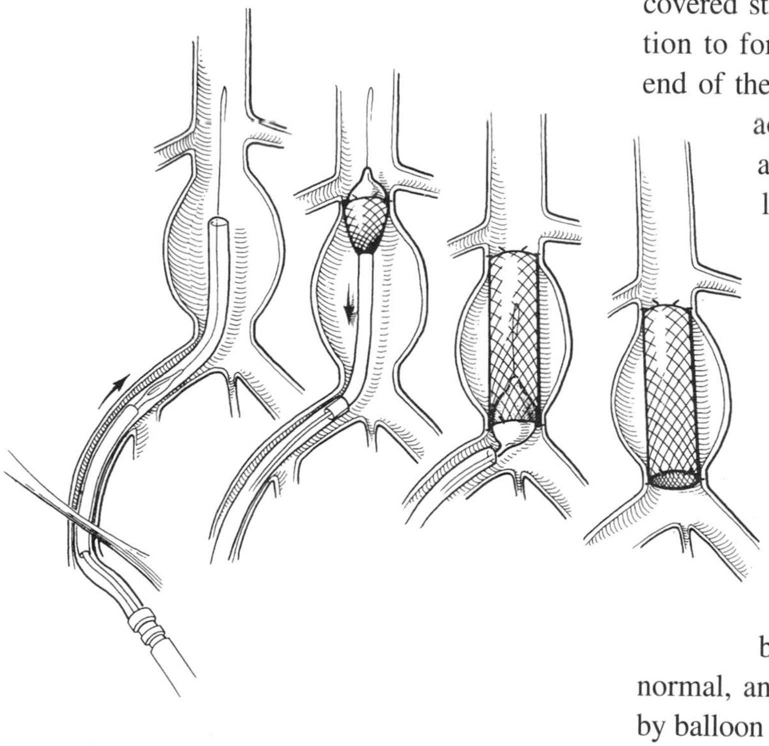

Figure 23.20. Technique for performance of transluminal endovascular prosthesis for treatment of aneurysm of the abdominal aorta.

ylene (PTFE), or even an autologous vein. Because of its compressibility, it can be loaded into a balloon catheter about the size of a No. 12 French catheter, a tube with a diameter of about one-fourth inch or about one-half centimeter, or possibly a little larger. This graft-loaded catheter can then be inserted into the common femoral artery in the groin. With a previously introduced guide wire, the loaded balloon catheter is advanced over the guide wire with fluoroscopic guidance to the proper proximal site in the aorta immediately above the diseased segment, and the graft-covered stint is expanded by balloon dilation to force attachment of the proximal end of the graft to the inner lining of the aortic wall. In aneurysms of the abdominal aorta, for example, the loaded catheter would be guided to the relatively normal aortic segment or neck of the aneurysm just below the renal arteries and would be balloon-dilated to ensure firm attachment of the proximal opening of the graft to the aortic wall. The distal end of the graft would be similarly guided to just above the bifurcation, if this is relatively normal, and attached in a similar fashion by balloon dilation, after which the catheter and guide wire would be withdrawn and removed from the groin site opening

(Figure 23.20). This method of endovascular stent grafting has also been used for some forms of occlusive disease in the legs and even in the carotid arteries.

The proponents of these procedures proclaim a number of advantages over conventional surgical procedures. Since they are much less invasive than open surgical procedures, they may be employed in some patients whose associated conditions, particularly disturbances of the heart, lung, and kidneys, make the conventional surgical procedures too risky. Another advantage is a shorter hospital stay and recovery period. The proponents of this method of therapy also report reasonably good early results, with a relatively small number of complications and immediate failures requiring conventional surgery. In occlusive disease, there seems to be a higher incidence of recurrence, about 30 percent, in the first one or two years afterwards, as compared with conventional surgical treatment, in which it is less than 5 percent. Long-term follow-up observations are needed to evaluate this form of therapy in aneurysmal disease. There is reason, however, to be cautiously optimistic, in light of the intensive research and investigations now being conducted in this field of endeavor.

CHAPTER TWENTY-FOUR

Cardiac Transplantation and Other Surgical Treatment of Advanced Heart Failure

BY JAMES B. YOUNG, M.D.

The Concept of Heart Failure

Considerable attention is being paid to heart failure today because of its epidemic nature. Despite the fact that mortality rates in the United States are declining for coronary heart disease and stroke, hospitalization for heart failure has increased dramatically. One explanation for this is that the prevalence of symptomatic heart failure rises as populations age, and the United States' population is aging rapidly. Furthermore, better treatments for atherosclerotic cardiovascular disease, valvular heart disease, and hypertension have delayed some aspects of heart damage so that patients with heart failure oftentimes consult physicians later than in prior eras.

Although these treatments for many heart conditions have reduced the mortality rate, patients are often still left with damaged hearts that develop functional deterioration later. Because of the large at-risk group in the aging United States, the economic and personal impact of heart failure is dramatic and will clearly worsen during the next decade. Indeed, it has been estimated that the prevalence of congestive heart failure is as high as four million people, with approximately 400,000 new cases diagnosed annually.

Congestive heart failure is the only cardiovascular disease with an increasing prevalence, and its incidence doubles in the general population with each decade over age 45. Additionally, heart failure is the third leading cause for hospitalization in all patients and the principal cause of hospital admission in those over 65 years of age. Furthermore, approximately 35 percent of the diagnosed pool of heart failure patients are hospitalized annually. Multiple hospitalizations over time are common, particularly in the elderly. Readmission rates after an index congestive heart failure hospitalization approaches 50 percent of patients within three months. Many factors are related to the high rates of hospitalization for heart failure, including the progression of underlying diseases such as hypertension and atherosclerosis.

It is intuitive that the heart, as a central force controlling cardiovascular pump dynamics, can precipitate substantive difficulties when diseases impair its proper function. Cardiac muscle injury severe enough to alter normal blood flow to vital organs and keep up with the body's metabolic demands is termed *heart failure*. The current perception of heart failure is somewhat different from that of past decades, and this is important to consider. Although the clinical syndrome of *dropsy*, or edematous states due to cardiac dysfunction, has been recognized for well over a century, recent observations indicate that a variety of pathogenic, neurologic, and hormonal changes develop in response to cardiac injury and heart failure. These secondary effects are largely responsible for precipitating and perpetuating the condition. Indeed, heart failure is not a specific disease, but rather a syndrome comprised of many molecular genetic, cell organelle, contractile protein, and neurohumoral abnormalities provoked by a spectrum of specific diseases that damage the cardiac and circulatory system. Obviously, the remarkably complex symphonic interaction of myocyte (muscle cell) contractile elements is susceptible to injury in the presence of many different diseases, such as hypertension, atherosclerosis, myocardial infarction, and valvular insufficiency or stenosis, among others.

Because cardiac muscle cells will not multiply and replace themselves after injury or cell death, as will the liver, spleen, or skin cells, when a myocyte is injured or dies, its ordinary workload must shift to a reduced volume of more normally functioning cells. Individual myocytes must work as a team to produce the normal pumping function of the heart. Cell injury or death is akin to a football team placing one of its critical players on "injured reserve." Others must assume the injured teammate's workload. Interestingly, myocyte proteins responsible for contractility turn over every 30 to 60 days in a normal cell. A variety of genetic programs can, therefore, be stimulated in an attempt to "beef up" remaining uninjured cells so that they may carry greater loads and better meet peripheral metabolic demands.

It is, after all, the rhythmic contraction of the heart that ultimately is responsible for peripheral organ perfusion with oxygenated blood. Carrying oxygen and nutrients to cells and organs distant from the heart and delivering the waste products of cellular respiration to the lungs, kidney, and liver for metabolism and elimination is the cardiovascular system's raison d'être. Thus, the inability to perform this task adequately, with resultant complications, has been termed heart failure.

Often it is a syndrome in which fluid retention (edematous or dropsical conditions) dominates, for reasons that will be explained, and short-windedness develops because of fluid accumulation in the lungs and in the leg secondary to fluid deposition there, as well as loss of appetite, early satiety, or abdominal bloating and discomfort when fluid builds up in the gastrointestinal organs (liver, spleen, intestines). Low output from the heart, with failure to meet metabolic demands of exercise, causes weakness and fatigue. Although patients with these congestive and low-output states generally have heart failure, this syndrome can also be present in essentially asymptomatic persons.

The beginnings of heart failure are obviously rooted in myocardial injury, which ultimately impairs individual muscle cell contractility. The extent of damage and number of myocytes injured generally dictate the syndrome's severity. As pump function deteriorates, the heart's ability to eject adequate quantities of blood during contraction (*systole*) decreases. Problems can also be caused by impairment to the filling (rather than decreased blood ejection) of the heart's main pumping chamber, the left ventricle, during the portion of the cardiac cycle termed *diastole*. Patients with this difficulty are said to have diastolic dysfunction, and those with decreased ejection capabilities, systolic dysfunction. More commonly, combinations of systolic and diastolic dysfunction (in varying degrees of severity) are present in any given case. The terms systole and diastole arbitrarily define the active and more passive electromechanical portions of the cardiac cycle. Difficulty filling the heart will obviously result in problems with emptying, and diastolic dysfunction is therefore as important as reduced systolic performance.

Two general types of difficulties ensue when heart failure develops (Figure 24.1). First, the decrement in forward cardiac flow, or output, results in more blood volume retained in the left ventricle. This causes cardiac chamber enlargement. This enlargement results from the inability of the heart to empty adequately with each contraction. As volume rises, pressure

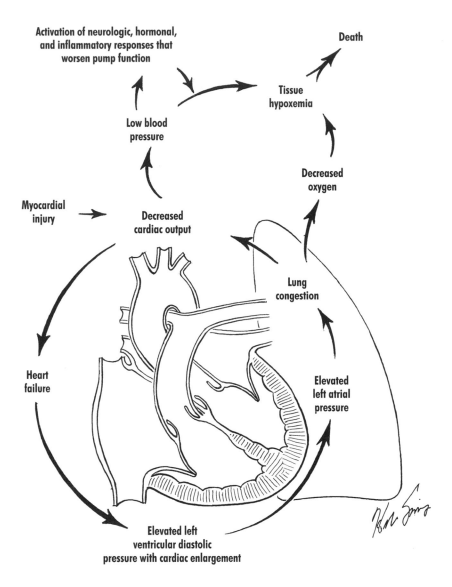

Figure 24.1. The vicious cycle of heart failure.

increases, and this pressure is transmitted backwards into the vasculature of the lungs, ultimately contributing to exudation of fluid into the alveolar sacs, where oxygen exchange occurs. This creates difficulty breathing. Because lungs with excess fluid are heavier than normal, the workload required to adequately aerate blood passing by the alveolar sacs increases; this causes patients with heart failure to perceive great difficulty breathing. Secondly, the decrement in forward cardiac output causes a state of hypoperfusion of peripheral organs such as the kidney, liver, central nervous system, and skeletal musculature. The kidney is an important regulator of fluid and salt balance in the body. When it perceives that perfusion is diminished, a variety of hormonal reflexes are triggered designed to increase intravascular volume and salt levels. Essentially, the kidneys are reacting as if the patient has had significant blood loss from trauma. Indeed, from an evolutionary standpoint, man is still using the compensatory mechanisms designed to be effective in cavemen suffering trauma that was likely to produce blood loss with subsequent hypovolemia! The kidney in heart failure patients, because of alterations in normal blood flow patterns to this organ, believes blood loss has occurred when, in fact, it has not. The subsequent salt and water retention further contributes to volume overload with worsening pulmonary congestion or edema, and subsequent symptoms of short-windedness. Because blood flow to other essential organs (particularly skeletal muscles) is reduced, exercise capacity is limited not only by short-windedness but also by decreased systemic skeletal muscle performance. Other reactions occur, including neurologic effected changes that theoretically also evolved to stimulate heart activity, raise blood pressure, and improve peripheral organ perfusion. These effects, however, ultimately increase the workload of the heart and eventually cause further decrement in efficient pump function.

Although heart failure patients often have fluid retention, many patients can be asymptomatic. The term *failure* simply means that parts, systems, or persons as a whole are not meeting certain standards of performance. Because of the compensatory mechanisms described, the circulatory system may fail to function normally, but compensation by factors such as those described initially attenuates difficulties so that symptoms will arise only with extreme demands, and the serious underlying difficulty is masked.

It is not inappropriate today to consider a molecular or cellular definition of heart failure, as much as we use clinical definitions that focus on fluid retention or exercise limitation. This is important because preventing further deterioration in patients with evidence of pump dysfunction is a high priority to attenuate the likelihood of development of more advanced heart failure, which can be treated only by radical and aggressive measures, such as cardiac transplantation, ventricular assist device insertion, mechanical total artificial heart implantation, or other unusual surgical procedures like cardiomyoplasty or reduction ventricular remodeling. Treatments for heart failure range from medication to these sophisticated and dramatic surgical procedures. Identification of the underlying disease that caused the heart failure in the first place is also important.

The diagnosis of heart failure is made after synthesis of a patient's medical history with information obtained during physical examination and data gathered from a variety of tests used to evaluate and quantify cardiovascular system performance. Evaluation of the patient's condition generally includes electrocardiography, echocardiography, various x-ray studies, and laboratory tests designed to provide the physicians with insight into cardiac integrity and diseases that can cause heart failure. Results of data integration will gauge the severity, allow appropriate diagnosis, and dictate treatment strategies for heart failure.

Treatments vary depending on many factors, with emphasis on the etiology and stage of difficulties. A variety of drugs and drug combinations are prescribed, and they often ameliorate the symptoms and attenuate heart failure pathophysiology. Occasionally, more routine cardiac operations, such as coronary artery bypass and heart valve replacement or repair, can be done to treat these patients. A great deal of skill and experience is required to design optimal therapeutic programs for these patients, but fortunately, much guidance is available.

With advanced heart failure, patients have severe dyspnea (short-windedness),
particularly on exertion. Difficulty sleeping because of short-windedness, inability to lie flat at night, and paroxysms of smothering sensations can also occur. In some patients with advanced heart failure, the downward spiral of symptoms can be attenuated with cardiac transplantation or other highly sophisticated surgical procedures that should be reviewed.

Cardiac Transplantation

Transplantation of the heart is a dramatic means of treating carefully selected patients with profoundly severe heart failure. It is impressive when patients with advanced heart failure or cardiogenic shock (extremely low blood pressure with dangerous organ hypoperfusion) exhibit profound functional improvement after a successful heart transplant. For many, transplantation is the only approach that can ameliorate the severe symptoms of heart failure and attenuate high mortality risk. This operation has been proved an important option time and again over the past decade. Although still filled with challenges, the procedure is now well accepted and is being performed more often. Unfortunately, the greatest limiting factor remains organ donor availability. Cardiac transplantation can be placed in better perspective by a review of the data regarding the procedure that is published by the United Network of Organ Sharing

(UNOS), the organization charged with donor organ distribution. In their experience, 14 percent of more than 100,000 solid organ transplants, or almost 15,000 operations since the late 1980s, have been cardiac transplants. Kidney transplantation represents about 19 percent of organ transplants done over the past decade.

Unfortunately, a plateau has been reached in the annual number of heart transplant procedures done in the United States, with only about 2,500 operations now being performed each year. More kidney transplants can be performed because of the duality of this organ in most donors and the ability to employ living related kidney donation (removal of one kidney from a family member of a patient, for example) with a high degree of success. Despite the plateau in number of cardiac transplants performed every year, the number of patients placed on the waiting list outweighs significantly the number transplanted. Indeed, the overall United Network of Organ Sharing waiting list is rapidly approaching 50,000 patients awaiting solid organ allocation, with approximately 8 to 10 percent of patients awaiting cardiac allocation. Still, when the procedure is performed, dramatic benefit generally ensues. It is worthwhile to review the remarkable history of the development of cardiac transplantation. It parallels the development of solid organ transplantation in general and is intimately related to progress made in cardiovascular surgery.

Historical Perspectives on Cardiac Transplantation

Many can remember the astonishment, excitement, and controversy that the first well-publicized human cardiac transplant operation caused. How was that point reached? Although there are many parallels between the development of solid organ transplantation in general and cardiac transplantation, several important distinctions should be noted. Probably most important is that the history of cardiac transplantation and artificial circulatory assist device development is intermingled. Their mutual interdependence was spawned by the need for developing cardiopulmonary bypass techniques that allowed support of extrathoracic vital organ circulation while diseased hearts were stopped and removed prior to replacement.

The concept of replacing a diseased heart to cure ailments thought to be cardiac in origin is not particularly new. Abstract reference to receiving "a new heart" is found in the Old Testament when the prophet Ezekiel proclaimed in the sixth century B.C., "A new heart also I will give you, and a new spirit I will put within you; and I will take away the stoney heart out of your flesh, and I give you a heart of flesh." In the fourth century B.C., the legendary Chinese physician, Pien Chiao, exchanged the hearts of two men in an attempt to cure an unfavorable disequilibrium in their respective "energies." The operation seemingly restored a proper balance of Yin and Yang.

Many chimeric Eastern and Western mythologic creatures demonstrate rather unusual combinations of organs and parts from man and beast. The xenotransplantation of an elephant's head onto a human child by the Hindu god Shiva produced the Indian god Ganesha. Western mythologic beasts, such as centaurs and the Minotaur, are additional examples.

Possibly the first well-documented description of a diseased part being replaced by a healthy one from a recently dead donor is reflected in the legend of St. Cosmas and St. Damian. A sacristan in the Basilica dedicated to these saints underwent a miraculous replacement of a gangrenous leg with a healthy one taken from an Ethiopian gladiator slain in exhibitory combat. Sometime in the first few centuries A.D., the legendary physician saints performed the transplant during a euphoric dream of the sacristan. This operation has been the subject of numerous historic artworks and has set the stage for modern concepts of organ donation, which focus on the retrieval, resuscitation, and use of formerly functioning parts and organs from recently deceased people for whom the tissues are no longer essential.

Whereas the thought of solid organ transplantation is not particularly new, it was only after detailed anatomic insight became available and organ-specific diseases were clarified that these operations could emerge in truly rational fashion. Indeed, it has been only about 100 years since the earliest direct cardiac operations were performed. In 1896, the German surgeon Ludwig Rehn became the first to successfully suture a cardiac stab wound. That set the stage for consideration of direct cardiac operation and, indeed, replacement of the heart. Experimental heart transplantation was performed shortly after that time when Alexis Carrel and Charles Guthrie, working at the University of Chicago in 1905, transplanted the heart of a small puppy into the neck of a larger dog. Carrel had a long-standing interest in perfecting arterial and venous hemostatic anastomosis technique in order to allow reestablishment of circulatory integrity after traumatic or surgical vascular injury. Not only did the model of heterotopic heart transplant (placing the organ in other than its normal position) allow demonstration of the feasibility of vascular anastomoses, but the transplanted heart was also observed to beat spontaneously for a period of time. Eventually, the heart stopped beating, and this was due to what we know today is rejection. Carrel also performed experimental kidney, ovarian, and testicular transplants with varying degrees of success.

Models of orthotopic cardiac transplants (placing the heart in its normal anatomic position) were used to study the nuances of cardiac and circulatory physiology. Mann and associates, performing cardiophysiologic experiments in 1933, suggested that orthotopic cardiac transplantation, as a therapeutic modality, was limited only by unknown biologic effects that always ultimately destroyed heart activity. Challenges of the operation in Mann's dog experiments were surmountable and secondary. The biologic effects limiting Mann's experiments were the same that caused Carrel's heterotopic dog transplants to end as well. We now know that these effects are caused by inflammatory defense systems that are present to ward off noxious attack by foreign organisms. This response is rooted in man's ability to recognize his own tissue without mounting destructive inflammatory attack.

Early insight into what we call humoral (antibody-mediated) and cellular (white blood cell–mediated) rejection was rudimentary, but the power of self-recognition was well understood. Rudimentary insight into this awesome phenomenon can actually be traced to observations made in the late sixteenth century. The great renaissance Italian surgeon Gasparo Tagliacozzi, described with extraordinary accuracy transplant tissue rejection in a detailed accounting of failed nose transplants. Tagliacozzi had attempted to engraft the noses of slaves serving as organ donors onto the faces of a few noblemen who had lost their proboscises for various ignominious reasons. Unfortunately, the tissue swapping, although at first seemingly successful, was subsequently characterized by a necrotizing inflammatory event that was dramatically speeded up if the recipient had undergone a previous attempt at nose transplant. Ultimately, it was understood that the power of self-recognition was at work.

Many centuries were required to explain how this all worked. It was subsequently demonstrated that utilization of a patient's own tissue, rotating a tissue flap from the forehead to fashion a nose, for example, could be successful. However, it was work done during and shortly after World War II that really set the stage for understanding immunologic mechanisms responsible for organ and tissue rejection. In an attempt to treat the devastating blitzkrieg bomb burns Londoners were suffering, skin grafts from unrelated tissue donors were sometimes used. Although successful for short periods of time, cell-mediated and humoral rejection ultimately caused failure of these grafts.

Luminaries, such as Nobel laureate Peter Medawar, performed experiments that ultimately gave great insight into the immunologic properties accounting for Tagliacozzi's failed operations. Medawar's experiments led directly to further studies that provide today's extensive but still incomplete understanding of antigenic signals and alloimmune responses during organ and tissue transplantation. Current gaps in our knowledge of this response are what prevent, for example, successful organ transplants from animal to man.

Parallel developments were occurring with respect to cardiovascular surgery in general. Obviously, refinement of the surgical approach to a direct cardiac operation was critical to the success of cardiac transplantation. The use of extracorporeal circulation (circulating the blood outside of the cardiovascular system and body to keep it adequately oxygenated while the ordinarily beating heart is stopped) became the focus of much research. Any mechanical device accomplishing this feat must do so without damaging the cells and blood components required to deliver oxygen and remove metabolic waste products. Very early proposals considered pumping blood through a donor lung removed from an animal and oxygenated with the use of artificial respiration. Creating adequate blood flow through the circulation of the patient with a suitable pump would still be problematic.

Serious development of the heart-lung bypass machine was the goal of John Gibbon who, in the mid 1930s, began animal experiments designed to demonstrate the feasibility of completely bypassing feline hearts and lungs with a rudimentary pump and blood oxygenator system. Ultimately, the roller pump, created

by Michael E. DeBakey to facilitate direct transfusions of blood from donor to patient, was incorporated into Gibbon's device, and with better oxygenating systems, success in animal models in the latter 1940s was obtained. This led to demonstration repeatedly in the latter 1950s that circulatory arrest with surgical correction of intracardiac abnormalities was possible. This development set the stage for sophisticated and dramatic cardiovascular operations.

In the 1960s, enthusiasm began to build with respect to complete replacement of diseased hearts with healthy donor hearts. During the early part of that decade, surgical investigators, principally Norman Shumway and Richard Lower at Stanford University, demonstrated that animal cardiac transplant models could survive for many months. Few are aware that it was actually in 1964 that the first patient to undergo well-documented cardiac transplantation received a primate heart rather than a human allograft. James Hardy in Jackson, Mississippi, transplanted the heart of a chimpanzee into a 68-year-old gentleman with diabetes mellitus, severe coronary artery disease, diffuse peripheral vascular disease, and a terribly unstable cardiovascular state. Shock syndrome had developed because of severe coronary ischemia, and emergency coronary artery bypass grafting was attempted. When the patient could not be weaned from the heart-lung machine because of severe native heart dysfunction, cardiac transplantation, a procedure that had been contemplated by Hardy for some time, was attempted with the primate heart. Although the graft was successfully implanted and the patient was partially off cardiopulmonary bypass, the xenoheart did not seem large enough to support circulation adequately, and the patient subsequently died in the operating room.

Hardy's decision to use a primate heart is both interesting and important because of the controversy surrounding definition of death with respect to organ donation. Concepts of brain death had not yet been completely developed or accepted. Consideration of these issues was, however, driven by the urgencies of more successful treatment of end-stage renal disease with kidney transplantation. A subsequent landmark in cardiac transplantation occurred in 1966 when Richard Lower, who had moved to the Medical College of Virginia, transplanted a human cadaveric heart that was still beating after the kidneys had been removed, into a chimpanzee. Lower demonstrated that the organ was quite capable of maintaining adequate circulatory support for the animal over several hours.

Based on the promising observations made by Shumway and Lower, human-to-human cardiac transplantation was being seriously considered as a clinical option in the late 1960s. It was, however, Christian Barnard who performed the first relatively successful human-to-human heart transplantation December 3, 1967, at the Groote Schuur Hospital in Cape Town, South Africa. The patient survived only 18 days, dying of pneumonia and systemic infection. The operation shocked the public, stirred controversy in the medical professional community, and fueled debate regarding definition of an appropriate heart donor with respect to the concept of brain death. Nonetheless, an initial rush to heart transplantation began. Three days after the Cape Town procedure, Adrian Kantrowitz, in New York, transplanted the heart of an anencephalic infant into an 18-day-old child with a life-threatening congenital cardiac abnormality. The infant survived for only a few hours. During the next 12 months, 102 heart transplants were performed in 17 nations, with more than half of them in the United States. Setbacks were repeatedly observed, with only a few long-term survivors. The main difficulties seemed to be rejection and overwhelming infection caused by the relatively crude immunosuppressive techniques.

Unrealistic expectations had been fostered, and because only 21 of the first 165 heart transplant patients between 1967 and 1971 were alive, most transplant surgeons ceased performing these operations. Indeed, early studies suggested that only 35 percent of heart transplant recipients lived more than three months, and only 10 percent survived two years. Still, those long-term survivors were impressive. They demonstrated remarkable functional rehabilitation when compared to their devastating preoperative condition.

With dogged persistence, primarily by the Stanford and University of Virginia programs, characterization of rather successfully immunosuppressive protocols, especially the ability to diagnose acute rejection by endomyocardial biopsy specimens from a percutaneous intravenous approach, emerged and provided a dramatic boon to treating cardiac transplant patients. Particularly important was the development of new immunosuppressive drugs. Specifically, the introduction of the potent and somewhat more selective agent cyclosporine in the early 1980s gave impetus to restart cardiac transplantation with new vigor throughout the world. This drug, particularly when used in combination with azathioprine and prednisone (traditional agents proving effective in kidney transplants), coupled with greater understanding of the allograft rejection process and improvements in cardiovascular surgical technique, set the stage for cardiac transplant programs to explode in number and dramatically improve postoperative survival. This occurred in the setting of an already burgeoning renal transplant experience and emerging reports of successful liver, lung, intestine, and pancreas transplantation.

The Cardiac Transplant Operation

Figures 24.2 and 24.3 demonstrate the surgical techniques for cardiac transplantation. Two approaches can be taken. Orthotopic cardiac transplantation is the most commonly performed (Figure 24.2). In this operation, the diseased native heart is completely removed and replaced. After sternotomy and establishment of cardiopulmonary bypass, the connections at the aorta, pulmonary artery, and left and right atrium of the native heart are severed. Attachments to the inferior and superior venae cavae are also severed. The operative field is then prepared for insertion of the new heart.

Donor hearts are usually procured during multiorgan retrieval in suitable organ donors. Several transplant teams are usually present, focusing on liver, kidney, lung, and pancreas explantation. Donor hearts are exposed after a median sternotomy is made, and the chest is opened in a fashion similar to that used in most cardiac operations. The heart is visually inspected and then palpated to ensure that it is free from disease of its own. The donor heart is removed after it has been stopped (cardiopleged) by infusion of a cold solution containing a variety of salts (particularly potassium), which causes cessation of cardiac contraction. The donor heart is completely removed with incisions

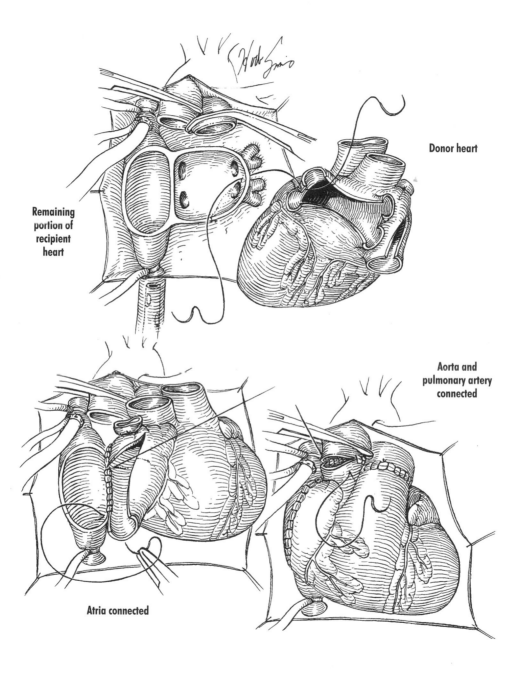

Figure 24.2. Technique for orthotopic cardiac transplantation.

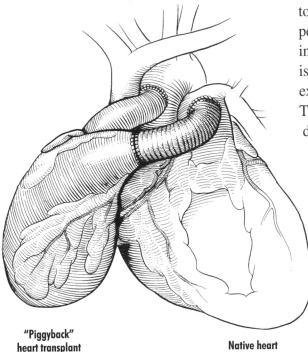

"Piggyback" heart transplant

Native heart

Figure 24.3. Technique for heterotopic or "piggyback" cardiac transplantation.

made in the inferior and superior venae cavae, pulmonary artery, aorta, and at the level of the posterior left and right atria, in the same fashion as is done during native heart removal.

Adequate preservation of the organ is important so that muscle cell damage does not develop during the several hours that the heart is outside of both the donor's and recipient's bodies. During this time, no nutritive blood flow is occurring. Donor hearts preserved in this fashion generally work satisfactorily after reimplantation if the cold ischemic duration is less than four

to six hours. The likelihood of substantive permanent muscle cell damage appears to increase significantly after six hours. That is why every effort is made to reimplant an excised donor heart as quickly as possible. This is one reason that prompts cardiac donor allocation schemes to focus on local distribution patterns rather than disseminating organs over wide geographic distances. This is also why harvesting teams must often travel by jets and helicopters to shorten operation time as much as possible. Unfortunately, our inability today to achieve adequate cardiac function after prolonged extracorporeal storage precludes prospective tissue matching of cardiac donors and recipients, such as that performed during kidney transplantation.

The donor heart is reimplanted by connection of the cuff of native atrial tissue to the appropriate left and right atrial portions of the donor heart. The aorta and pulmonary artery of the donor are anastomosed to those of the recipient. Obviously, size matching of donor hearts to recipients is of some importance, and fashioning appropriately proportioned atrial chambers is critical. Large recipients will not fare well with very small donor hearts. Likewise, cardiac output demands often are not well met by undersized organs. These facts emphasize several important issues with respect to matching donor hearts with recipients. Blood type, size, severity of heart failure, and distance of donor from recipient are juxtaposed to waiting times to determine organ allocation priorities.

Heterotopic transplantation ("piggyback") may have a therapeutic niche but is still infrequently performed. In this operation (graphically presented in Figure 24.3) the native heart is left in place, and the donor heart is implanted in parallel fashion to the circulation. End-to-side donor-to-native aortic and pulmonary artery connections are fashioned. Right atrial anastomoses allow admixture of blood into this "piggyback" type of transplant. Variable degrees of contribution to pulmonary and systemic circulation occur in this procedure, and it should be considered a type of biologic ventricular assist device.

The mortality rate after piggyback transplantation seems higher than that after orthotopic transplantation. Nevertheless, some advantages do exist. First, the native heart is not removed. Should recovery of function be observed, the piggyback donor heart can be removed. Moreover, when a donor heart is small in relation to a given recipient, heterotopic transplantation might present an alternative by adding partial, but not complete, support to the cardiovascular system. The native heart would still be relied on to contribute to global cardiac output. The possibility of using xenographic transplants (animal donor hearts) in heterotopic positions for short periods of time presents an intriguing futuristic option for patients requiring short-term hemodynamic cardiac support.

Postoperative care of the heterotopic transplant patient is largely the same as for those receiving orthotopic donor implants, except that anticoagulants must be given to ensure that blood clots do not form in the weakened native heart, which remains behind in this operation and occasionally becomes so weak that it eventually fails to contract at all. In these patients, the donor heart slowly takes over the circulatory demands, but risk of thrombosis of the native heart remains.

The Cardiac Donor

As indicated, the major rate-limiting factor to cardiac transplantation is donor organ availability. The first successful transplantation of a solid organ from one person to another actually occurred in 1954 when Joseph Merrill transplanted a normal kidney from one identical twin to the second twin who had end-stage and chronic renal failure. This successful kidney transplant between identical twins demonstrated that if problems of organ harvesting and preservation coupled with rejection could be solved, widespread organ transplantation would be possible.

The opportunity for a healthy, living, perfectly matched twin as a donor obviously is extremely rare. With pressure rising to perform more kidney transplants because of the lack of hemodialysis opportunities, use of cadaveric organ donors was considered. Initially, such kidneys used for transplantation in the early 1950s came from cadavers. The heavy reliance on living related organ donors initially addressed the issue of rejection. As immunosuppressive drugs such as azathioprine and steroids became available in the 1960s, however, even more donor organs were necessary. Furthermore, since living kidney donors were used almost exclusively in the early era of kidney transplantation, concern arose about potential coercion of donors and commercialization of organ donation.

A rare source of donors was the patient dying in the operating room during open heart surgical procedures. Although they could not survive the removal of cardiopulmonary bypass, viable kidneys could be procured from these patients before discontinuation of circulatory support and pronouncement of death. Kidneys obtained in such a circumstance were first used in 1962. Although these donors were certain to die when cardiopulmonary bypass was stopped, they were not dead before kidney removal, and therefore, brain-death criteria were not employed.

Organ procurement from persons with beating hearts and stable circulation (not in cardiopulmonary bypass) but cessation of significant brain function began in Sweden in 1964. A kidney was removed from a donor on mechanical ventilation in the neurosurgical intensive care unit at the Karolinska Hospital. The donor had massive intercerebral bleeding and was unresponsive, paralyzed, and not breathing. Importantly, at that time, the concept of brain death had not been well defined or accepted. Consent for donor kidney removal was obtained from the family and only one kidney was harvested. This allowed some renal function for a period of time because the second kidney remained behind. This particular donor was subsequently pronounced dead two days later after suffering cardiac arrest, an expected outcome. As can be imagined, a ferocious medical-legal debate ensued, but the ultimate result was the formulation of the concept of cerebral death. This characterized patients with major central nervous system injury precipitating profound swelling of brain tissue with subsequent increased intracranial pressure and concomitant decreased cerebral blood flow. Cerebral activity on electroencephalography (EEG) would be absent and cessation of heart function with, ultimately, cardiac death likely in a short period of time. Initially, the concept was poorly received. Indeed, it was not until more than two decades later that several Western countries formally established brain-death criteria and legislation.

With respect to the 1967 Cape Town heart transplant, the donor, a young woman, had suffered lethal traumatic injury in an automobile-pedestrian accident and was pronounced brain dead by a neurosurgeon. Christian Barnard pointed out subsequently that this was possible because the definition of death in South Africa was imprecise and suggested that if "a doctor so deemed, death of the brain was legally acceptable as evidence of death." Despite this, the first heart transplant donor was taken to the operating room on mechanical ventilatory support, which was then removed by Barnard, with subsequent donor heart procurement occurring only after the heartbeat ceased. Barnard stated that he waited for the heart to stop beating only to avoid any controversy that might arise because the concept of brain death was not well understood.

Obviously, this thinking was new and controversial with great public concern expressed regarding organ harvesting in persons having a chance for survival. This dilemma had to be juxtaposed to concern regarding the removal of organs for transplantation from perfectly healthy living donors, such as was occurring during kidney transplantation. Furthermore, for unmatched organs, such as the heart and liver, organ donations from living donors was completely impossible.

In 1966, shortly before the first human cardiac transplant and driven by the dilemma of kidney transplantation, a symposium was sponsored by the CIBA Foundation, at which the concept of brain death was formally presented and generally endorsed. The issue of patient or cadaver treatment thus became clarified with specific definitions of death. Brain death was considered equal to more traditional definitions of death that were rooted in cessation of heartbeat and cardiovascular flow. In brain-dead patients, the heart would most surely stop beating in a short time. Brain-death criteria today, as well as in the late 1960s, focused on cessation of total brain function. Cerebral, cerebellar, and brain stem function had to be completely absent to meet brain-death criteria.

The so-called Harvard brain-death criteria emerged from a second consensus committee statement in 1968. The Harvard Committee on brain death indicated that its purpose in defining neurologic criteria for death was to decrease inevitable burdens placed on family and society by continued care of brain-dead persons whose hearts would eventually stop beating and to update the obsolete criteria for death (permanent cessation of cardiac function) that had led to controversy and difficulties in obtaining solid organs for transplantation. Creating situations whereby solid organs would become available for transplantation was not the prime purpose of the committee. This group also was not seeking, necessarily, to define death, but rather to develop acceptable criteria for its determination. They indicated that ventilator-bound patients who met neurologic criteria for death could be pronounced dead before the ventilator was turned off so that attending physicians would not be criminally charged with causing the patient's death by removing life-support systems. This enabled physicians to consider removal of nondamaged solid organs for transplantation after declaring patients brain dead.

Many states subsequently enacted brain-death criteria, beginning with the state of Kansas in 1970. These individual state acts ultimately led to broadly applicable guidelines and coalesced into the Uniform Anatomical Gift Act (UAGA). Great controversy still ensued, fueled primarily by factions concerned that brain death would be a sham excuse to simply withhold necessary medical care and life support from persons incapable of defending themselves, or in situations where solid organs were coveted for transplantation. Ultimately, however, the concept of total brain death came to be well accepted in most Western nations.

Some cultures, however, still do not recognize that a person meeting brain-death criteria is, actually, dead. As late as 1985, surgeons in Japan were indicted on murder charges for the removal of solid organs for transplant from a person they had declared brain dead. Transplantation in Japan is still hampered because of the lack of public acceptance of brain-death definitions, with cadaver organ donation in Japan occurring only in situations where organs are harvested from cadavers or persons pronounced dead by permanent cessation of cardiac function.

Requirements for a diagnosis of brain death today are no evidence of cerebral cortex function with complete absence of brain stem activity. Patients must be in a deep coma (totally unresponsive) without evidence of cerebral receptivity. Absence of brain stem activity is apparent when no pupillary light reflexes or other cranial nerve responses are noted after appropriate stimulation. The cause of death must be known, and there are no significant concomitant hypothermia, hypotension, metabolic perturbation, drug intoxication, or significant use of pharmacologic central nervous system depressants. Clinical findings should persist over time without change, and if appropriate, confirmatory tests, such as electroencephalography, radionuclide cerebral blood flow imaging, or cerebral angiography can be used to help clarify confusing situations. These tests should not substitute for bedside acumen, however.

Most situations in which brain death occurs and spontaneous heartbeat persists happen in tragic and unexpected circumstances. Young people suffering spontaneous intracranial hemorrhage or blunt head trauma represent a large cohort. Obviously, the unanticipated nature of these tragedies places great stress on the family, friends, and loved ones. It is in this difficult environment in which a request must be made for organ donation. It is a remarkable testament to the generally humane nature of mankind that permission for organ donation is frequently given after persons responsible for the patient understand the implications of brain death.

The so-called gift of life is made in a totally unselfish and unconditional fashion. Families of organ donors do not (with rare exception) know where or in whom donated organs will ultimately be used. Particularly important is the fact that this true act of love, unconditional organ donation, is something endorsed and encouraged by all major religions. Cultural constraints, on the other hand, such as those noted in Japan, may influence some populations not to embrace the concept of brain death and organ donation enthusiastically. That is unfortunate because death of a potential donor is unrelated to retrieval of organs for transplantation. The tragedy will remain, and indeed, will be compounded in the opinion of some, if organs that could otherwise have been used to help devastatingly ill patients are buried.

Present hospital management regulations dictate that the next of kin be asked permission for organ and tissue donation in appropriate situations. Everyone is urged to consider this noble act and indicate or confirm the desire to be an organ donor by endorsing an organ donor card. Many states have made arrangements for drivers' licenses to be signed as an organ donor card. In Texas, this act is akin to creating a will.

Allocation of specific organs to patients on cardiac transplant waiting lists is based primarily on the severity of a given patient's heart failure syndrome, blood type, size, and proximity of the patient to the donor. Another important factor is the length of time patients have been waiting. Guidelines for acceptance of cardiac donors focus on a relatively young age (although cardiac donors older than 50 and even 60 years have sometimes been successfully used). Furthermore, donor hearts should be reasonably healthy and free of coronary atherosclerosis or effects of hypertension.

Function of the Transplanted Heart

Irrespective of the degree of increased survival cardiac transplantation offers, the transplant recipient generally shows dramatic rehabilitation when substantive symptoms have been present before transplantation. Still, transplanted hearts do not function entirely normally, and exercise tolerance, though generally excellent, may be slightly limited when compared to age-matched controls without heart disease. Because nerves regulating certain aspects of cardiac function are severed during organ retrieval and not reattached during implantation, heart rate response to exercise is slower. In addition, this denervation precipitates several subtle changes in the overall cardiovascular system signaling circuits that lead to high blood pressure and fluid retention. These difficulties are usually easily managed with medication.

Certain complications after cardiac transplantation can lead to some impairment of function as well. Rejection is the difficulty that causes most concern and can occur soon after transplantation (acute rejection); it is related primarily to white blood cell infiltration and antibody-mediated damage to the myocardium. Chronic rejection is the term used to describe development of coronary artery disease in the transplanted heart. In contradistinction to atherosclerosis developing in nontransplant patients, this process can sometimes occur quickly (within several months or a few short years). It appears to be related primarily to inflammatory injury of the donor-heart vascular lining. The endothelial cells

lining the blood vessel walls are exquisitely sensitive to immune-mediated injury or inflammation. Damage to the myocardium will obviously cause a decrease in the ability of the transplanted heart to function. Fortunately, immunotherapeutic medicine can control most rejection episodes. Additional difficulties, such as hypertension, decreased kidney function, and infections, are related more to the immunosuppressive medications used to control rejection than to anything else.

In contradistinction to the experience after cardiac transplantation in the late 1960s and early 1970s, survival after cardiac transplantation is now a reasonable expectation. This is especially notable when postoperative survival is contrasted with the natural history of patients with advanced heart failure. Indeed, in the 1995 Annual Report of the United States Scientific Registry for Organ Transplantation, which included patients undergoing cardiac transplantation between October 1987 and December 1995, one-year survival was 82 percent and three years, 75 percent. Generally speaking, most cardiac transplants are done in persons with a no better than 50 percent chance of surviving one year, and indeed, many cardiac transplant surgeons try to select patients with only a 10 or 20 percent chance of living six months. Data from the International Society for Heart and Lung Transplantation Registry, which now contains observations made on more than 30,000 heart transplants performed worldwide since the mid-1980s, suggests that 10-year survival is between 50 and 60 percent. Again, this represents a rather dramatic improvement over the national history of advanced heart failure, since similar patients not undergoing cardiac transplants would not have been expected to survive that long.

It is difficult to predict what the realistic long-term survival rate of cardiac allografts will be; however, several patients have now passed the 20-year follow-up mark. Given today's technology and understanding of rejection, it is reasonable to assume that the transplanted heart will likely function adequately for at least 15 to 20 years, provided rejection and complications of chronic immunosuppressive drug therapy can be managed. Of course, the patient has the great responsibility to compulsively take medications, optimize body weight, eat healthy diets, and maintain reasonable aerobic physical conditioning.

All things considered, cardiac transplantation represents an extraordinary option for patients with advanced heart failure, in view of the fact that most patients today do quite well. Indeed, rehabilitation generally is to a degree that enables remarkable levels of physical activity and function. Again, the rate-limiting factor of organ donor availability can be frustrating, and for that reason, alternative strategies using mechanical pump support systems have been aggressively pursued.

Ventricular Assist Devices and Total Artificial Heart Implantation

Development of mechanical circulatory assist devices, specifically the ability to perform extracorporeal circulatory support with oxygenation and vital organ perfusion, allowed cardiac surgery to develop and progress. Cardiac transplantation could not be performed without these remarkable machines. Their development paralleled and comingled with progress in cardiovascular surgery in general. Furthermore, the obvious shortage of donor organs pressed urgently the need for alternative treatment strategies in patients with advanced heart failure. Strategies emerged to completely replace the heart with a mechanical system (total artificial heart) or to temporarily or permanently sustain left and/or right heart circulation (ventricular assist devices). Particularly attractive were methods designed to stabilize advanced heart failure in patients with partial left heart bypass pump systems while awaiting donor heart allocation and cardiac transplantation.

The number of patients with advanced heart failure in the United States alone who might benefit from some form of mechanical circulatory assistance is estimated to be as high as 60,000 (granted, a debatable figure). Many people require support of this sort. Even if one only focuses on the 4,000 patients currently awaiting cardiac transplantation, with only about 2,500 donors becoming available annually, the need for such circulatory support machines is emphasized. Furthermore, many patients suffering from acute myocardial infarction or undergoing valve replacement or coronary artery bypass grafting require temporary support pumps to tide them through periods of time when cardiac function is depressed, but adequate heart pump recovery is ultimately possible. Concepts have included both large and small devices; totally implantable artificial hearts; extracorporeal devices; devices which bypass the right, left, or both ventricles; and heart pumps that can be inserted but subsequently removed. Because of this need, research and development of ventricular assist pumps for augmenting function of the failing left ventricle and circulation have received a high priority by the National Heart, Lung, and Blood Institute for the past several decades.

Sporadic attempts at experimental extracorporeal solid-organ perfusion and support began in the 1930s (Alexis Carrel again being the pioneer when he teamed with aviator Charles Lindbergh to pursue development of a tissue-oxygenating device). It was, however, John Gibbon who ultimately showed the feasibility of a heart-lung bypass pump and oxygenation system for total body perfusion that made successful open heart surgery possible and gave impetus to further exploration of a variety of ventricular assist devices.

Interestingly, along a somewhat different line of research, in 1961, S. D. Moulopoulos and Wilhelm Kolff developed an intra-aortic balloon pump counterpulsation device. Wilhelm Kolff was the innovator who first experimented with renal dialysis machinery. Figure 24.4 shows placement and use of an intra-aortic balloon pump assist device. This approach to supporting the failing circulation, although not dependent in the strictest of terms on direct mechanical flow augmentation, remains the most common form of mechanical assistance used in patients with left ventricular failure. The balloon in the aorta is alternatively inflated and deflated. Deflation occurs during systole and decreases resistance against which the heart has to pump to empty its contents. During diastole the balloon is inflated, and this causes forward displacement of blood that has been pumped from the heart during systole. Furthermore, balloon inflation results in higher diastolic pressure in the circulatory system, particularly in the proximal ascending aorta, which causes increased blood flow to the brain, coronary arteries, and kidneys.

This novel device can increase oxygen delivery to the heart and reduce overall

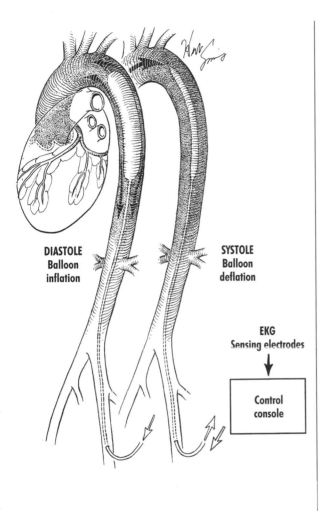

Figure 24.4. Use of intra-aortic balloon pump to assist the heart.

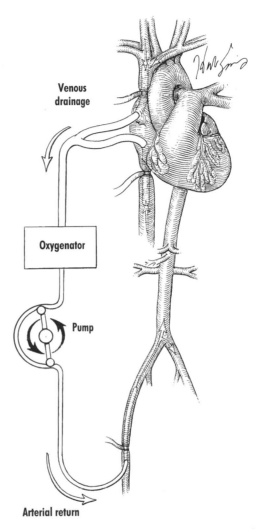

Figure 24.5. Total cardiopulmonary bypass with use of a roller pump and extracorporeal oxygenating system.

ventricular workload, making the heart much more efficient. Its advantages lie in the relatively simple and low risk insertion technique. The most common use is in patients with severe heart failure or shock after a myocardial infarction or cardiac surgery. Unfortunately, the device can be left in for only several days, or a few weeks at the most, and requires patients to

be immobilized in bed. This technique does not dramatically augment cardiac output. Moreover, problems might occur with arterial injury at the femoral access site.

Temporary mechanical cardiac assistance can also be accomplished for short periods of time with a type of heart-lung bypass machine. This is called Extra-corporeal Membrane Oxygenation (ECMO). Figure 24.5 is a diagrammatic illustration of total cardiopulmonary bypass, which is the essence of pump oxygenator systems used during any cardiac operation that requires the heart to be stopped. When it is used for more long-term support, care must be taken to avoid damage to the blood cells and plasma protein components. As with the intra-aortic balloon pump, the duration of device application is limited. Long-term extracorporeal membrane oxygenating pump systems are rarely successful if used for more than a few days.

As opposed to the intra-aortic balloon counterpulsation pump or other left ventricular assist devices, an important advantage of this system is its ability to adequately oxygenate the blood. As Figure 24.5 demonstrates, unoxygenated venous blood returned to the right atrium is removed with suction, passed through an oxygenating system, and ultimately returned to the arterial circulation by either a roller pump or a spinning centri-fugal flow pump device (described subse-quently). As with the intra-aortic balloon counterpulsation device, use of ECMO is usually limited to those patients with

cardiogenic shock believed to have, at least for the most part, reversible left ventricular dysfunction.

Both of these techniques may be used as a bridge to other operations, such as cardiac transplantation or more permanent ventricular assist device insertion. Because donor organ allocation cannot be anticipated with any certainty, this short-term device is most often removed when native heart pump function will adequately (if not optimally) support the circulation. Otherwise, it serves as a bridge to permanent ventricular assist device implantation.

The first isolated extracorporeal left ventricular assist device was implanted by Michael E. DeBakey in 1963. The device pumped blood from the left atrium into the descending thoracic aorta, and although the patient subsequently succumbed to anoxic cerebral injury, evidence indicated that the bypass pump functioned ade-quately to assist left ventricular perfor-mance for some time. Further development of this machine resulted in successful implantation in 1966, when a 37-year-old woman with severe heart failure from aortic and mitral valve disease required surgical replacement of both valves and could not be weaned from the standard heart-lung bypass machine.[1] The left

[1] Michael E. DeBakey, "Left Ventricular Bypass Pump for Cardiac Assistance." *American Journal of Cardiology,* 27:3–11 (1971).

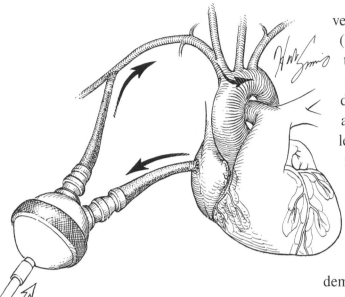

Figure 24.6. The DeBakey left ventricular assist device first used as a temporary extracorporeal pump system.

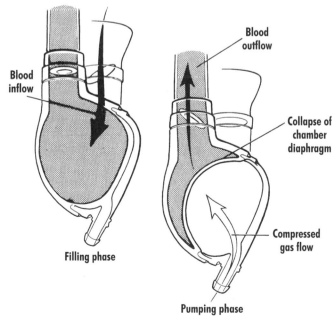

Figure 24.7. Diagram of a pneumatic-powered ventricular assist device.

ventricular assist device was implanted (Figure 24.6) by connection of tubes to the left atrium and right axillary artery. This made it possible to discontinue cardiopulmonary bypass, and after 10 days of support by the left ventricular assist device, the heart recovered enough to allow removal of the pump system. The patient recovered completely and resumed a normal life, but was tragically killed six years later in an automobile accident. This was the first demonstration that such a device could contribute substantially to the support of cardiovascular circulation for prolonged periods of time and provide an opportunity for native heart function to return.

Because the left ventricular bypass pump takes blood oxygenated by the patient's lungs from the left atrium and pumps it directly into the arterial circulation, it does not require an extracorporeal oxygenating system. Such devices will not adequately function if significant pulmonary difficulties are present. Because the pump lowers left atrial pressure and pressure in the left ventricle at the end of diastole, pulmonary congestion is reduced, and therefore oxygenation is generally improved. Also in contrast to the cardiopulmonary bypass machines, the left ventricular assist pump allows much more blood to flow per minute, is less damaging to blood components, and provides pulsatile flow that more closely resembles native heart action.

The bypass pump initially used three decades ago by DeBakey bears a remarkable resemblance to many of the systems implanted today. It was a hemispherically shaped, rigid, plastic pump with two inner chambers separated by a flexible plastic membrane, or diaphragm. One chamber filled with blood, and the other filled intermittently with gas. The chamber accommodating blood flow had entry and exit conduits with one-way valves directing blood flow appropriately from the left atrium into the pump chamber and then out to the systemic arterial network. When pressurized carbon dioxide gas was pulsed into the gas chamber at the appropriate systolic time point (gauged according to electrocardiographic activity), the flexible diaphragm collapsed the blood chamber, forcing blood through the exit valve and into the axillary artery. When the pressure in the gas chamber was released or vented, blood refilled the fluid chamber once again. The regular, continuous repetition of this process pumps blood in a manner much like the pulsatile left ventricle. Figure 24.7 graphically demonstrates the interior workings of this type of pneumatic, pulsatile, extracorporeal ventricular assist device. All pneumatic devices currently used today operate on this same basic principle.

Centrifugal pump systems work quite differently. They operate by spinning blood as a solid body vortex within an inner chamber. Nonpulsatile pressure develops as kinetic energy and is created by the spinning motion of the pump device. Inflow of blood occurs through a central inlet port. Anticoagulation is required because of problems with clot formation in the spin chamber. These devices have also been used primarily for myocardial failure after cardiac surgery or as a short-term bridge to cardiac transplantation. Because the device produces nonpulsatile circulatory flow and implantation is associated with challenging postoperative problems of bleeding, hemolysis, and thromboembolic events, its use is limited to several days. Additionally, flow rates are only about half of those generated by other types of mechanical ventricular assist devices.

Several commercially available pulsatile flow systems based on the previously described pneumatic principle are currently used as temporary support systems. Figure 24.8 is a diagram of the ABIOMED BVS 5000 extracorporeal pulsatile ventricular assist device system. As the figure shows, it can be used for left heart, right heart, or combined left and right heart bypass ventricular support. Use of this device is hampered by the extracorporeal nature of the pump and by the large complicated console required to accommodate the pneumatic and control components of the pump.

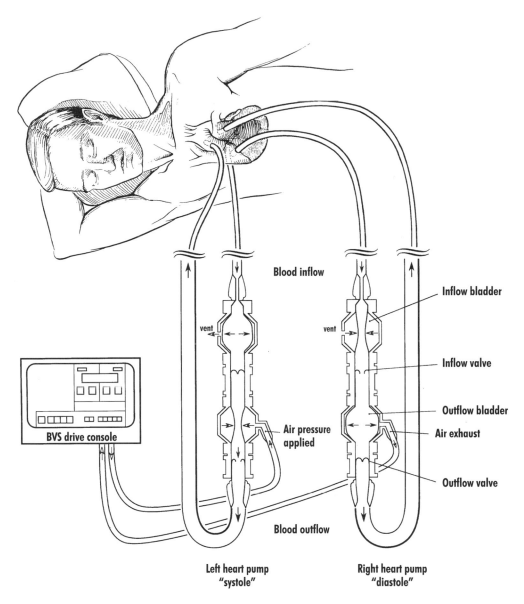

Figure 24.8. Diagram of the ABIOMED BVS 5000 ventricular assist device, demonstrating chamber and bladder apposition during systole and diastole. Positioning of the device in the patient is also depicted.

Devices that can be totally implanted include the Novacor and HeartMate left ventricular assist systems. Both of these devices can be implanted in a patient's abdomen with blood removed from the apex of the left ventricle, pumped into the pumping chamber, and then back out into the systemic arterial circulation via the ascending aorta. Inflow and outflow conduits can be fashioned to pass through the diaphragm, with the actual pump buried in the abdomen. Both pneumatic and electrically driven devices are being developed. Now commercially available, the pneumatic HeartMate left ventricular assist device is used as a bridge to cardiac transplantation.

Whereas all these devices require connection via tubes and cables exiting the abdominal wall to a console, remarkable progress has been made with the development of portable and user-friendly systems. Figure 24.9 represents one configuration of the electric HeartMate left ventricular assist device, showing how the battery pack components can be carried in a small, portable vest. Patients are surprisingly active and ambulatory with this device. Furthermore, patients have been supported by this system for as long as one year. Observations in such patients lend credence to the concept that mechanical circulatory machines can be a permanent option in some patients with advanced heart failure.

In the electrically driven systems, rather than the pneumatically induced membrane collapse sucking blood into and driving it back out of the device, an electric motor turns cogwheels that then drive pusher plates or pistons to effect directional flow. Advantages of any of these systems are the relatively high flow rates that can be achieved (10 or 11 L/min) and the pulsatile nature of the blood flow that allow a reasonable degree of exercise.

A variety of techniques and methods have been used to limit development of thrombus in the systems. Any time blood comes in contact with foreign elements, thrombi can be generated. Moreover, there is a possibility of subsequent liberation into the arterial circulation, which may

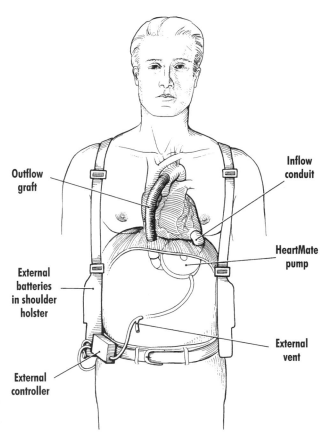

Figure 24.9. The electric-powered HeartMate ventricular assist system with portable vest, demonstrating compact nature of this device.

produce devastating complications such as stroke. Newer devices have a variety of chamber linings that allow more natural tissue growth over surfaces, with subsequent reduction in risk of blood clot formation and thromboembolism. Other challenges and difficulties relate to damage of blood components as they pass through the pump, as well as infection.

Total artificial hearts have presented a different challenge. Tetsuo Akutsu and Wilhelm Kolff reported the first experimental implantation of a total artificial heart in an animal model in 1958. However, all animals survived less then 24 hours, and it took some time before more reasonable success could be demonstrated. The total cardiac prosthesis must consist of two heart bypass pump systems set up in parallel to replace the function of both native right and left ventricles.

This artificial heart, developed under a grant from the National Institute of Health, in which Michael E. DeBakey was the principal investigator, was surreptitiously removed from his experimental laboratory and used without his knowledge and without approval by the Baylor College of Medicine Committee on Research Involving Human Beings or by the National Institute of Health.[2] It was implanted in 1969 and, as with the first heart transplant,

generated a great deal of controversy. The system was used in a patient with advanced cardiac failure caused by ischemic heart disease and a large left ventricular aneurysm. After failure of an attempt to resect the aneurysm and the inability to wean the patient from cardiopulmonary bypass, the total artificial heart was inserted in an attempt to create time for organ donor identification and subsequent cardiac transplant. The device supported the patient's circulation for 64 hours, at which time cardiac transplantation was performed. The patient died of pneumonia 32 hours after the transplant procedure.

Controversy again arose in December 1982, when William DeVries implanted the so-called Jarvik 7 pneumatic artificial heart into Barney Clark at the University of Utah without any intention of bridging the patient to cardiac transplant. He survived for 112 days but ultimately succumbed to multiorgan failure and did not appear to have reasonable rehabilitation during any period of his postoperative recovery. Between 1984 and early 1985, three subsequent Jarvik 7 model implants were performed at Humana Hospital in Louisville, Kentucky, with one patient surviving 620 days. A handful of additional permanent total artificial heart implants have been attempted worldwide,

---

[2] Michael E. DeBakey, et al., "Orthotopic Cardiac Prosthesis. Preliminary Experiments in Animals with Biventricular Artificial Heart" in *The Year Book of General Surgery* (Chicago: Year, Book, 1970), 69–72.

but all patients eventually died of device-related complications including thrombosis, thromboembolism, and infection.

In general, cardiovascular surgeons implanted the total artificial heart as a bridge to cardiac transplant. Indeed, about half of the 100 or so machine devices inserted as bridges to cardiac transplantation between 1986 and 1989 were total artificial heart pumps. Because of greater success with isolated ventricular assist devices, as contrasted with the problems and failure of total artificial heart systems, virtually no total artificial hearts were used as bridges to cardiac transplantation between 1990 and 1993. Newer total artificial heart systems are emerging and are occasionally used in experimental fashion today to bridge patients to transplantation. Fortunately, most patients requiring mechanical support only need left ventricular bypass systems. The total artificial heart may be required when patients have substantive failure of the right side of the heart or elevated pressures in the lung circuits that are particularly difficult to treat with medications. Left ventricular assist systems assume that the right side of the heart can adequately pump blood through the lungs for oxygenation.

The Combined Registry for the clinical use of mechanical ventricular assist pumps and the total artificial heart, in conjunction with cardiac transplantation, supported by the International Society for Heart and Lung Transplantation, now has more than 2,000 patients in the database that covers the period 1985 through January 1994. A substantial increase in the number of implants inserted as bridge systems to cardiac transplant has been noted, with about half of the implantations in 1988 being total artificial heart devices, in contrast with none being used in 1992 and 1993. Nearly 70 percent of the entire group in the Registry ultimately underwent cardiac transplantation, with 69 percent surviving to hospital discharge. Statistics would suggest that devices used as isolated left ventricular support systems are more successful than devices used to bypass the right side of the heart only or combinations of devices to bypass both the right and the left sides.

Within the grouping of left ventricular assist devices, no individual mode of support proved particularly advantageous over another, with respect to rates of transplantation or hospital discharge. Newer and more sophisticated devices, however, are not included in this Registry project. The 30-day mortality rate for all patients with these devices was approximately 36 percent, which is higher than for patients undergoing orthotopic cardiac transplantation without bridging at similar time points of follow-up. However, none of the patients receiving mechanical circulatory

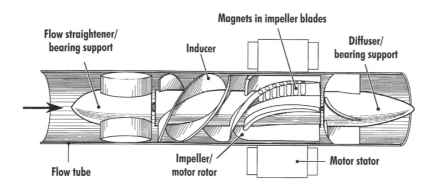

Figure 24.10. DeBakey/NASA Axial Flow Ventricular Assist Device currently being developed.

support as a bridge to transplant would have survived to receive organ allocation without application of this support technology.

As even greater insight is gained into adverse events including infection, thromboembolic complications, right ventricular dysfunction, and sustained ventricular arrhythmias after device insertion, better solutions will emerge, and patients will do even better. Whereas the systems presently used can produce dramatic results in carefully selected patients with advanced heart disease, unrealistic expectations should be avoided. Still, the long-term successes with respect to functional improvement noted in patients having the electric HeartMate and Novacor devices inserted generates a great deal of enthusiasm. Continued success with staged cardiac transplantation after mechanical device insertion appears to be driving enthusiasm and support for

the permanent implantation of these machines without cardiac transplant as an endpoint. This excitement is radically different from the disappointment that emerged after multiple failed attempts at permanent total artificial heart implantation over a decade ago.

Research continues on newer forms of pump systems that are small, easily inserted, and have low energy requirements. Another type of ventricular assist device recently receiving increasing attention by investigators is based on the principle of axial flow. This is illustrated by the *DeBakey/NASA Axial Flow Ventricular Assist Device.* During the past several years Michael DeBakey and his colleagues at Baylor College of Medicine, in collaboration with the NASA/Johnson Space Center, have developed such an axial flow VAD that is 7 cm long, and 2.67 cm at its largest diameter, and weighs 53 gm (Figure 24.10).[3] At approximately 10,000 rpm, the pump generates 100 mm Hg pressure providing an output of 5,000 to 6,000 cc per minute and requires less than 10 watts of power. Animal tests after one month of continuous function demonstrated no pump-related adverse effects, no evidence of thromboembolism, and an acceptable plasma-free hemoglobin level indicating minimal red blood cell destruction. The highly encouraging experimental data now being collected to ensure its safety and efficacy provide the basis for starting clinical trials within another year. If these trials validate the experimental observations, this type of pump could have wide clinical application in the treatment of patients with various forms of heart failure because of its small size, simple surgical application, and low energy requirement (Figure 24.11).

Dynamic Cardiomyoplasty

Dynamic cardiomyoplasty is an interesting operative procedure for patients with heart failure. The recent interest in this operation generated by several publications has resulted in the operation being performed more often. In the early 1980s, Ray Chiu of Montreal, Canada, developed the concept of muscle transformation to achieve assisted cardiac transplantation. This concept consists in converting skeletal muscle fibers from fatigable units to the fatigue-resistant fibers characteristic of myocardial cells by

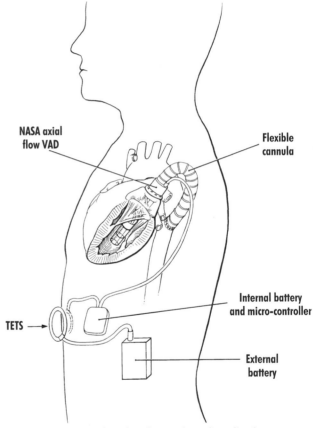

Figure 24.11. Drawing showing projected application of the DeBakey/NASA left ventricular assist device, completely implanted with internal battery recharged through the skin.

---

[3] Michael E. DeBakey and Robert Benkowski, "The DeBakey/NASA Axial Flow Ventricular Assist Device" (paper presented at the 6th International Symposium on Artificial Heart and Assist Devices, July 30–31, Tokyo, Japan, 1996).

applying low frequency, repetitive electrical stimulation to the skeletal muscle. It also includes mobilizing a large skeletal muscle whose normal function could be sacrificed, and adjusting the muscle in the chest such that it wraps around the heart and augments contraction during electrocardiographic systole. Alain Carpentier in Paris, France performed the first dynamic cardiomyoplasty procedure on a patient in 1985. At this writing, the patient is reported to be alive and doing well.

The patient's own latissimus dorsi (usually the left), a large muscle stretching across the back, is obtained, and after the muscle is mobilized in the chest, it wraps around the failing heart. Two intramuscular pacemaker leads are inserted into the latissimus dorsi close to the nerve supply. Myocardial pacemaker leads are also inserted to allow sensing of the contractile activity. When the electrical muscle stimulation of the latissimus dorsi is segued with the beginning of the native heart ventricular contraction, augmentation of contractile function should theoretically occur. The cardiomyostimulator system is then essentially a pacemaker type of device. The system senses and paces the heart, and during appropriate intervals, provides pulsed stimulation to the latissimus dorsi muscle synchronized with heart contraction. Figure 24.12 graphically demonstrates the concept of using the latissimus dorsi to augment systolic left ventricular function.

Obviously, critical to the success of this procedure is successful conversion of skeletal muscle performance from the fatiguable to fatigue-resistant muscle cells. Since skeletal muscle is accustomed to working intermittently rather than continuously, as the heart does, overcoming the fatigue factor was important if contractile power was to be translated from the latissimus dorsi's shortening. The demonstration that pulsed electrical stimulation of the skeletal muscle in regular fashion could induce or transform the latissimus dorsi into a fatigue-resisted muscle was the major breakthrough leading to increased interest in dynamic cardiomyoplasty.

Since the first clinical application of dynamic cardiomyoplasty in 1985, it has been estimated that more than 650 patients worldwide have undergone this procedure. Apparently, patients need to be carefully selected. First, adequate nutrition needs to have been ensured so that the skeletal muscle has enough integrity to perform as a contractile element. Previous cardiac or other surgical procedures on the chest make the operation more challenging because of scar tissue and the possibility of bleeding. It may be best that patients have had no prior thoracic surgical procedures. Moreover, although some select patients with coronary artery disease seem to benefit from this procedure, it theoretically may be better for patients with dilated cardiomyopathy and normal coronary

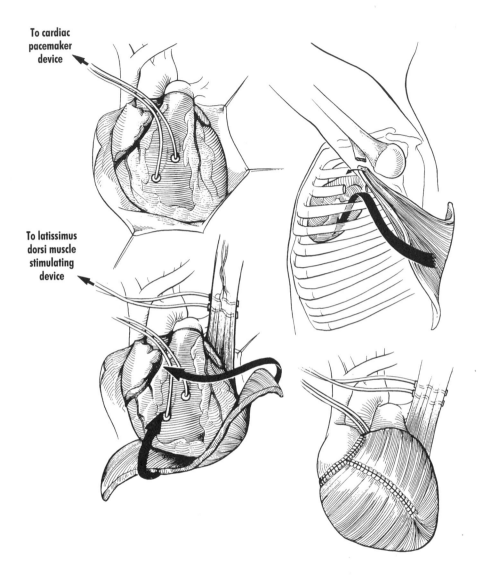

To cardiac
pacemaker
device

To latissimus
dorsi muscle
stimulating
device

Figure 24.12. Graphic demonstration of the cardiomyoplasty procedure, consisting in mobilization of the left latissimus dorsi muscle into the chest and pacemaker-induced sequencing to cardiac contractility.

anatomy. A tremendously enlarged heart and substantive mitral regurgitation also seem to create difficulties.

Clinical studies available to date suggest that dynamic cardiomyoplasty is less risky when performed in patients without severe advanced heart failure symptoms. Consensus is beginning to develop indicating that the operation should, in all likelihood, not be performed in patients considered candidates for cardiac transplantation. Additional factors making the operation unduly risky appear to be pulmonary hypertension, poor pulmonary function studies, severe fluid retention with failure of both right and left ventricles, and preoperative dependence on potent intravenous inotropic support medications. Older patients, prior sternotomy or thoracotomy, massive cardiomegaly, need for concomitant cardiac surgery (such as coronary artery bypass grafting), presence of atrial fibrillation, poor right ventricular performance, severe mitral regurgitation, and malignant ventricular arrhythmias (including those treated with implantable defibrillating devices), all seem to predict poor outcome and should be considered relative contraindications to this operation. Still, clinical studies suggest that quality-of-life improvement can be seen in more than 80 percent of patients surviving the operation, with a significant portion of patients showing substantive improvement in clinically relevant hemodynamic parameters.

In order to place cardiomyoplasty more definitively in the perspective of clinical heart failure therapeutic strategies, scientists have begun a large randomized clinical trial to compare outcomes after this procedure with aggressive medical treatment of heart failure patients. Overall mortality rate, as well as exercise endpoints, quality-of-life scores, and congestive heart failure symptoms, are being evaluated. It is hoped that clinical trials will give better insight into the impact of this operation and assist in determining characteristics of patients most likely to benefit from this procedure.

Left Ventricular Volume Reduction (Remodeling) Surgery

An innovative surgical procedure has been suggested recently as an additional alternative to treatment for patients with advanced heart failure. Randas J. Viela Batista, a Brazilian cardiovascular surgeon, described removal of portions of the left ventricle in heart failure patients, particularly those with severely dilated hearts due to cardiomyopathy. Ventricular remodeling involves removing a wedge from the enlarged heart to relieve wall stress, reshaping the pumping chamber, reducing mitral valve leakage, and improving global mechanical function. Batista has performed more than 300 such operations in Brazil, where long-term therapeutic options, particularly cardiac transplantation, for these patients are limited.

The operation is distinct from surgical procedures designed to remove scar tissue or aneurysm in patients with left ventricular aneurysm after myocardial infarction, in the sense that patients undergoing remodeling operations have myocardial tissue removed, rather than scar tissue. There are several theoretical advantages to having a smaller and more normally shaped left ventricle; however, complete characterization of expectations after this procedure are unavailable. Most patients undergoing this procedure have dilated cardiomyopathy as the cause of their disease, rather than ischemic heart disease. Observations suggest that patients have some immediate hemodynamic improvement, but whether this is translated into long-term benefit is unknown. As clinical and surgical experience grows, the proper utilization of this operation will also become clearer.

CHAPTER TWENTY-FIVE

Women and Heart Disease: Special Issues

John is a 45-year-old sales executive. His daily diet often consists of doughnuts and fast-food hamburgers eaten on the run between meetings. When he finally arrives home after work, he heads to his favorite chair to sleep or watch television.

Mary is a 55-year-old secretary who spends her days dealing with a demanding employer; she chain-smokes cigarettes as she handles the latest crisis. Her evening hours are devoted to catching up with routine chores at home.

Which person is likely to develop coronary heart disease? John and Mary are both prime candidates for coronary heart disorders.

Physicians and the public have tended to underestimate the incidence of coronary heart disease in women. We now know that coronary heart disease is not just a man's problem and that it is dangerous to believe that women are immune to cardiac disorders.

Coronary Heart Disease in Women

Coronary heart disease kills more women in the United States than any other single cause. Almost one-half of the nearly 500,000 heart attack victims each year are women, and each year more than 87,000 women die of stroke. Women also have higher mortality rates from their first heart attack than do men: 44 percent of women who have heart attacks will die within a year, compared with 27 percent of men. Furthermore, more girls than boys are born with some form of congenital heart defect (see Chapter 16), and valvular disease, especially mitral valve prolapse, is also more common in women than in men (pp. 338–343).

In the United States, all cardiovascular diseases combined kill more than 479,000 women annually. In comparison, all forms of cancer combined kill about 245,000 women. While age-adjusted death rates from cardiovascular disease have been decreasing since the 1960s, women's rates have been falling at a slower pace than those of men.

It is true that, overall, a woman's risk for developing coronary heart disease is not as great as a man's until after menopause; the hormones that regulate the menstrual cycle, especially estrogen, appear to protect most women (although not diabetic women) against coronary heart disease during their reproductive years. In the diabetic woman, there may be some protection by estrogen, but her relative risk is increased to approximately that of a man; thus, the relative protection is lost. Coronary heart disease is much less common in premenopausal women than in men of the same age, particularly between the ages of 35 and 44. But once a woman reaches the age of 50 and that protection disappears, her coronary heart disease risk rises dramatically. In just the first decade after menopause, women experience a fourfold increase in the incidence of coronary heart disease.

The difference between men and women in terms of coronary heart disease risk is not a question of *if* a woman will get heart disease, but *when* she will get it. Women will develop coronary heart disease: they will just develop it six to 10 years later than men.

The Perception Gap

Despite the dangers of coronary heart disease to postmenopausal women, most women still do not worry as much about their own coronary heart disease risk as they do about that of their husbands, sons, brothers, and fathers. Women are more likely than men to experience periodic episodes of angina pectoris, or chest pain, as the first symptom of coronary heart disease. But women are also more likely to ignore their own chest pain or other heart disease symptoms, to attribute their symptoms to another cause, and to postpone getting treatment even if they do suspect a problem. A woman may attribute her own chest pain to indigestion or a pulled muscle but will rush her husband to the doctor or the emergency room if he experiences similar symptoms. Consequently, when a woman finally does get medical attention for her heart problems, it may be too late.

Further complicating the evaluation and treatment of coronary heart disease in women is the fact that most of the available research data describe coronary heart disease in men. Coronary heart disease research traditionally has been conducted either exclusively or predominantly in men, in part because the research is somewhat easier and less expensive. To be affordable, a clinical trial needs a population with a high rate of the disease being studied (which allows a smaller trial) and preferably with the disease at a relatively young age (when confounding factors from other diseases are fewer). Coronary heart disease in men fits these criteria. Now, however, coronary heart disease research is being undertaken in many population subgroups, including women, the elderly, and various racial groups.

The Treatment Gap

Women also may be less likely than men to be prescribed certain cardiovascular diagnostic tests and treatments and to experience more complications than men when they do undergo these procedures. The treadmill stress test, which is commonly used to detect heart disease, has been found to have a higher number of false-positive results in women than in men for unknown reasons. Women also have been found to have higher mortality rates than men following coronary artery bypass surgery, and both short- and long-term mortality rates after heart attack (myocardial infarction) have been found to be higher in women than in men. These higher mortality rates may be attributed to a number of causes, including the fact that women tend to be older when they experience a myocardial infarction or undergo cardiac surgery, and, consequently, more likely to have developed other health problems, such as diabetes, hypertension, and obesity. Concern about the increased risk for complications may lead both a woman and her physician to postpone necessary surgical procedures; however,

such a delay can put the woman at even greater risk because she may have to undergo the procedures on an emergency basis. That women's coronary arteries are slightly smaller than men's may also contribute to women's heart disease risk.

The Research Gap

While women's cardiovascular health has been a neglected area in medicine, physicians are becoming more vigilant in looking at women's coronary heart disease risk factors, and, as noted above, research studies have started to focus specifically on coronary heart disease risk, prevention, and treatment in women. The Women's Health Initiative (WHI), initially funded in 1993 by the National Institutes of Health, is the first comprehensive study of women's health undertaken in the United States. The WHI will involve about 163,000 women of various racial and ethnic backgrounds at 40 centers across the country, including Baylor College of Medicine in Houston. The study will focus on the leading causes of death in postmenopausal women, ages 50 to 79, including breast cancer, colorectal cancer, and osteoporosis, as well as coronary heart disease. The results of the WHI and other clinical trials on women will be pivotal in shaping the future of the prevention of these conditions that so greatly affect the health of women.

Women's Coronary Heart Disease Risks

The risk factors correlated with the development of coronary heart disease (see Chapter 7) apply to both women and men, although some differences do exist between the sexes regarding the impact of these risk factors. Such coronary heart disease risk factors as diabetes, high-density lipoprotein (HDL) cholesterol level, and triglyceride level may be more important in women.

Age

Heart disease risk increases with age. While the rise in coronary heart disease incidence is fairly constant in men as they age, women experience an abrupt increase in coronary heart disease incidence between 50 and 59 years of age. By the time a woman is in her 70s, her coronary heart disease risk is nearly equal to a man's. One in eight women age 45 and over has had a heart attack or stroke, and this figure increases to one in three at age 65 and beyond, according to the American Heart Association.

Sex

A woman's coronary heart disease risk increases significantly after menopause. Women who experience early menopause (whether surgical or natural) and do not receive estrogen-replacement therapy have a higher risk for coronary heart disease than premenopausal women of the same age.

Women who take oral contraceptives were formerly thought to be at increased risk of heart attack. Early research studies found a strong association between the use of oral contraceptives, which at that time contained higher levels of estrogen, and cardiovascular disease and stroke. However, more recent studies suggest that newer, low-dose oral contraceptives are not linked with significant cardiovascular risk when used by healthy, nonsmoking women younger than 40 years of age who do not have other cardiovascular disease risk factors or a history of cardiovascular disease. There are subgroups of women in whom hypercoagulability (increased tendency toward blood clotting) occurs with the use of oral contraceptives.

Heredity

Both men and women are more likely to develop coronary heart disease if close blood relatives have had coronary heart disease.

Ethnicity

Death rates for coronary heart disease and for stroke are higher for black women than for white women. According to the American Heart Association, the death rate from heart attack between ages 35 and 74 is twofold higher in black women than in white, and threefold higher in black women than in women of other races. These higher death rates are due at least in part to the greater incidence of hypertension in black women.

Diabetes

Diabetes mellitus is a strong coronary heart disease risk factor for women, even for those women who have not yet undergone menopause. As mentioned above, diabetes abolishes the relative protection that premenopausal women have against coronary heart disease because of their sex. The incidence of coronary heart disease is three to four times greater in diabetic women than in nondiabetic women. The risk is even greater if a diabetic woman also has other coronary heart disease risk factors, such as obesity and hypertension. Diabetes has a differentially more severe effect as a coronary heart disease risk factor in women than in men, and age-adjusted cardiovascular death rates have been found to be higher in diabetic women than in diabetic men.

Cigarette Smoking

Smoking is the greatest single preventable cause of death in women or men. Not only are more young American women beginning to smoke than young men, but also fewer women than men are giving up smoking. Twenty-four million American women smoke today, and their risk for having a heart attack is more than twice that of nonsmoking women.

Stopping reduces risks. Smoking cessation has been found to reduce heart attack risk in women within months, and to lower risk within two to three years to a level similar to that of people who have never smoked. Research has shown that women smokers who use oral contraceptives may have a much higher risk for heart attack than women who neither smoke nor use oral contraceptives.

Lipid Profile

A woman's blood lipid profile (her cholesterol and triglyceride levels) is often different from a man's (see below), but, as in men, varies with age. (The interaction between hormone-replacement therapy and lipid profile is discussed below.)

Hypertension

Hypertension, or systemic high blood pressure, which is defined in adults as systolic pressure higher than 139 mm Hg or diastolic pressure higher than 89 mm Hg, increases risk for stroke, coronary heart disease, and kidney disease. (See Chapter 11 and pp. 89–90.) High blood pressure is more common in men than in women until early middle age; after that period, high blood pressure becomes more common in women than in men. Women with normal blood pressure sometimes develop high blood pressure during pregnancy, which may play a role in a woman's development of coronary heart disease in the future. A woman who takes oral contraceptives may be more likely to develop high blood pressure if she is overweight, has mild kidney disease, has a family history of high blood pressure, or developed high blood pressure when she was pregnant. The risks associated with hypertension are compounded if a woman has other risk factors, such as cigarette smoking or elevated blood cholesterol.

Obesity

Obesity has been linked with the development of coronary heart disease in both women and men. Some research evidence has found that body fat distribution, that is, where the body stores excess fat, may be an even more important influence on coronary heart disease risk than actual weight. The android pattern of body fat distribution, in which weight tends to concentrate in the upper body and abdominal area, has been linked with higher incidence of heart disease, hypertension, and diabetes than the gynoid pattern, in which excess weight tends to settle in the lower body area. People with excess upper body fat, who are sometimes described as apple shaped, tend to have lower HDL-cholesterol and higher triglyceride levels than those whose additional weight is concentrated in the lower body, who are often referred to as

pear shaped. While women tend to be pear shaped instead of apple shaped, some women do store excess weight in the upper body area. Women entering menopause sometimes experience a change in their area of fat accumulation, and shift from being pear shaped to being apple shaped. (See Chapter 7 for a discussion of coronary heart disease risk factors for both men and women.)

Physical Inactivity

The association between physical fitness and a more favorable coronary risk profile is more pronounced for women than for men.

Hormone-replacement Therapy and Cardiovascular Risk

Physicians often prescribe estrogen-replacement therapy for postmenopausal women, to help relieve menopausal symptoms, such as hot flashes, those brief instances of flushing and sensation of heat caused in menopausal women by endocrine imbalance. Estrogen is also prescribed to help delay the progression of osteoporosis, a common, sometimes debilitating, condition in postmenopausal women.

Increasingly, physicians also are recommending postmenopausal hormone-replacement therapy for its long-term benefits against coronary heart disease. Menopause seems to have such a detrimental effect on heart health because a woman no longer has the protective effects of reproductive hormones, especially estrogen. The increase in coronary heart disease incidence after menopause is due at least partially to changes in lipid levels, and postmenopausal hormone-replacement therapy has been found to have beneficial effects on a woman's blood lipid profile.

In women who undergo natural menopause, lipid levels have been found to change in a way that makes a woman more susceptible to developing atherosclerosis. Before women reach menopause, they tend to have lower low-density lipoprotein (LDL) cholesterol ("bad" cholesterol) and higher HDL-cholesterol ("good" cholesterol) than men of approximately the same age. At menopause, women's LDL-cholesterol levels begin to rise rapidly as they age, until the levels may actually be higher than LDL-cholesterol levels in men. Women's HDL-cholesterol levels may decrease moderately at menopause, although they do ordinarily remain higher than men's HDL-cholesterol levels from the time of puberty on, throughout the life span.

There is little difference in triglyceride levels between men and women at puberty. Triglyceride levels increase gradually in both men and women after puberty, although they increase at a slower pace in women. In middle age, while triglyceride levels may actually decrease in men, they continue to increase gradually in women, so that by age seventy, average triglyceride levels in women are equal to those of men. Data from the Framingham Heart Study have shown that an elevated triglyceride level appears to be an independent coronary heart disease risk factor for women, especially elderly women.

While researchers are unsure of the exact mechanism by which estrogen protects women from coronary heart disease, they do know that when estrogen is replaced in postmenopausal women, HDL-cholesterol levels typically rise and LDL-cholesterol levels typically fall, often to premenopausal levels. Data from large population studies support the benefits in coronary heart disease risk reduction of prescribing oral estrogen-replacement therapy after either natural or surgical menopause. Some research results indicate as much as a 50 percent decrease in coronary heart disease risk and a 50 percent decrease in death from any cardiovascular cause with estrogen use.

But in addition to raising HDL-cholesterol levels and lowering LDL-cholesterol levels, oral estrogen may increase triglyceride levels, especially in women who already have an elevated triglyceride level. For this reason, a physician may decide against prescribing oral estrogen for a woman whose level is elevated. When oral estrogen is prescribed, a physician should monitor the woman's triglyceride level. Transdermal estrogen (patch or cream) has less effect on lipid levels.

When given alone, estrogen also has been found to increase risk for cancer of the endometrium, the lining of the uterus. Women who have not had a hysterectomy should be given hormone-replacement therapy that includes both estrogen and progestin. The combination of estrogen plus progestin decreases, and in some cases even eliminates, the increased risk for uterine cancer that is found with administration of estrogen alone.

Taking high dosages of estrogen over a long time period has also been found in some studies to increase breast cancer risk, although this is very controversial and the role of replacement estrogen in breast cancer has not been clarified. Women should follow standard recommendations for breast cancer screening. In addition, estrogen increases risk for the development of gallbladder disease and can cause nausea and vomiting, breast tenderness or enlargement, and enlargement of benign uterine tumors.

Women should talk with their physicians about the potential benefits and risks of hormone therapy in the context of their own medical history and that of their immediate family members. For many postmenopausal women, cancer risk from hormone-replacement therapy will be less than for coronary heart disease, particularly if they have other coronary heart disease risk factors such as an elevated LDL-cholesterol level, a low HDL-cholesterol level, or a strong family history of premature coronary heart disease.

Taking Action Against Coronary Heart Disease

Much remains to be discovered about the mechanisms by which coronary heart disease develops in women, as well as the effectiveness of various medical and surgical treatment interventions. In the meantime, there are actions women can take to lower their heart disease risk. One of the most important things a woman can do is to become aware of her own coronary heart disease risk factors. Many risks can be prevented or altered by the individual, and even seemingly unchangeable coronary heart disease risk factors can be moderated by minimizing controllable risk factors and adopting healthy lifestyle habits. Coronary heart disease may be prevalent in close family members, for example, but regular exercise and a low-fat diet can greatly lower an individual's likelihood of developing heart problems. Likewise, losing weight can lead to improvements in blood pressure levels, diabetes control, and a decrease in overall risk. For both women and men, controlling risk factors by leading a healthy lifestyle is central to reducing risk for coronary heart disease.

Coronary heart disease represents a very real threat to women today. Therefore, all women should be sure that their coronary heart disease risk is evaluated by their physician as part of their regular health care regimen. A woman should familiarize herself with the early symptoms of coronary heart disease, and, in particular, with the symptoms of angina pectoris. A woman should immediately inform her physician if she experiences any suspicious symptoms, especially persistent chest pain. While chest pain can be related to other conditions, any unusual chest pain or pain in an adjacent area should be investigated by a physician. Angina can be expressed as pain in the neck and jaw, pain in one or both arms, pain in the back, or feelings of lightheadedness or nausea (see pp. 259–261). Women may experience bouts of angina over a longer period of time before having a heart attack. Heart attack symptoms are described on pp. 262–263.

Keeping up with new findings from cardiovascular research can also help women remain focused on those risk factors most important to preventing heart disease and to maintaining good health.

CHAPTER TWENTY-SIX

The Heart Healthy Lifestyle

Cardiovascular disease has an enormous impact on the nation, killing almost one million people per year, more than half of them women. That is almost as many people as claimed by all other causes of death combined. By itself, coronary heart disease—just one facet of cardiovascular disease—is responsible for one-half of all deaths due to cardiovascular causes, amounting to nearly as many deaths as attributed to all cancers combined. This threat may be omnipresent, but it is not an inevitability. Through aggressive medical and lifestyle management of the factors known to increase risk for heart disease, individuals can reduce their risk. Heart healthy lifestyle choices include eating a low-fat, low-cholesterol diet without over-stepping body weight limits or sodium intake boundaries, exercising regularly, and not smoking.

At stake is not just length of life, but quality of life. Advances in medication and life-saving interventions are making it possible for many people who have heart disease to live longer. For some of these patients, it means a revolution in lifestyle. A heart attack, for example, can be a dynamic motivator for changing personal behaviors to decrease the chances of another hospitalization. Many other people, though never having personally experienced a heart attack or symptom of heart disease such as chest pain, are also ready and willing to initiate action that will help prevent or delay the onset of cardiovascular disease. These "ready–willing–able" souls accept responsibility for those behaviors they can control and make changes, say, in diet or such personal habits as smoking, to work toward a healthier cardiovascular system.

What makes it possible for one person to make such lifestyle changes and what explains another's difficulty with such modifications cannot be answered except on a case-by-case basis. Some general observations, however, may be helpful. First, understanding why it is important to change—that is, understanding the risk from, say, smoking or inactivity—has proved to be a major motivating factor. Second, those who try and fail to achieve what may be unrealistic goals need to be easier on themselves. Accepting one step backward for every two steps forward may be necessary to achieve overall advancement. In other words, no one's perfect. Third, it helps to remember that improvement in one area will pay dividends in another; this may make maintaining the course easier.

Ten factors are recognized as major risk factors for coronary heart disease (see Table 7.2, p. 82). Three cannot be altered: age, a personal history of atherosclerotic disease, and a family history of early coronary heart disease. Fortunately, however, the other seven can be changed: smoking, high blood pressure, an elevated level of "bad" cholesterol, a low level of "good" cholesterol, diabetes mellitus, obesity, and physical inactivity. (You can estimate your risk from modifiable risk factors by using Table 7.1 on page 81.) Lifestyle changes to reduce risk from these seven factors are the focus of this chapter. Also discussed are ways to reduce triglyceride levels and stress.

Smoking

The advice health experts give about smoking is clear-cut: if you smoke, stop; if you don't smoke, don't start. Smoking is the most preventable cause of death in the United States. If you believe you have only enough energy to make one change in your lifestyle to improve your health and you are a smoker, stop smoking.

To stop smoking is difficult. For some it takes life-threatening disease to make them break the habit; for others, it takes the recognition of smoking's threats:

- Sudden cardiac death is two to four times more common in smokers than in nonsmokers, and smokers are almost twice as likely as nonsmokers to have a heart attack.
- Smoking is responsible for about 30 percent of all cancer deaths and for about 90 percent of all cases of lung cancer.
- Smoking is responsible for about 20 percent of all deaths from coronary heart disease.
- Smokers are also at increased risk for stroke, emphysema, chronic bronchitis, sexual impotence, and other disorders, even if they are considered "light" smokers.
- Smokers are practically the exclusive sufferers of one form of cardiovascular disease—peripheral vascular disease—in which the vessels carrying blood to the arms or legs are narrowed.

Does It Really Make a Difference?

- **20 MINUTES AFTER QUITTING:** Your blood pressure and pulse rate drop to normal. The temperature of your hands and feet increases to normal.

- **8 HOURS AFTER QUITTING:** The carbon monoxide level in your blood drops to normal. The oxygen level in your blood increases to normal.

- **24 HOURS AFTER QUITTING:** Your chance for heart attack decreases.

- **48 HOURS AFTER QUITTING:** Your ability to taste and smell is enhanced.

- **2 WEEKS TO 3 MONTHS AFTER QUITTING:** Your circulation improves. Walking becomes easier. Your lung function increases as much as 30 percent.

- **1 TO 9 MONTHS AFTER QUITTING:** Coughing, sinus congestion, fatigue, and shortness of breath decrease. Your lungs are cleaner and more resistant to infection.

- **1 YEAR AFTER QUITTING:** Excess risk for coronary heart disease is 50 percent that of a smoker's.

- **2 TO 3 YEARS AFTER QUITTING:** The risks for coronary heart disease and stroke decrease to those of people who have never smoked.

- **5 YEARS AFTER QUITTING:** The lung cancer death rate for the average former one-pack-per-day smoker decreases by almost half. The risks for cancer of the mouth, throat, and esophagus are half those of a smoker.

- **10 YEARS AFTER QUITTING:** The lung cancer death rate is similar to that of nonsmokers. Precancerous cells are replaced. Risks for cancer of the mouth, throat, esophagus, bladder, kidney, and pancreas decrease.

Figure 26.1. Chronologic benefits of quitting smoking.

Modified from the American Cancer Society and the Centers for Disease Control and Prevention. Reprinted with permission.

- Cigarette smoke harms not only smokers but also others who come in contact with it: coworkers in the office, relatives in the home (especially children), and the unborn child in the smoking mother's womb—all are adversely affected by secondhand smoke. During the first two years of life, children in the homes of smokers are more likely to have pneumonia or bronchitis, and they have more colds than children in the homes of nonsmokers.

- Smokers also harm those around them by passing on the habit as well as the smoke: teenagers who have smokers as parents are more likely to become smokers themselves than are their counterparts in homes with nonsmoking parents.

A study published in the *Journal of the American Medical Association* found that most smokers who want to quit smoking endeavor to stop on their own, and they are almost twice as likely to be successful at stopping as are others who seek help. But there is no one right way to quit smoking. Individual or group counseling may be right for you.

Patients who are encouraged by a doctor to quit are more likely to be successful at quitting. So if your doctor hasn't told you to quit, please take our advice to stop. Look at Figure 26.1, which lists a number of benefits. In a national survey, physicians and the clergy were found to have the lowest prevalence of smoking of any of the occupations surveyed. These are professionals who are aware of the economic and health costs of smoking and the burden it carries.

Whether you stop "cold turkey" (withdrawing from smoking all at once), gradually, or with nicotine replacement therapy, the important issue is *deciding to quit*.

Nicotine replacement therapy is available without a prescription, and is helpful for some people. In this approach, the nicotine of cigarettes is replaced by chewing gum or a skin patch, whose use or dosage is tapered off. The American Cancer Society recommends tailoring the replacement to the smoker. Carrying the gum is easy and leaves control of the dosage in the hands of the person trying to quit. Smokers wanting to quit who need something to chew or to occupy their hands, who want to control cravings when they occur, and who smoke at irregular intervals (or any two of these three) may find nicotine gum their best choice. On the other hand, those smokers who smoke steadily throughout the day, who prefer not to chew gum, and who want the convenience of once-a-day administration of therapy (or any two of these three) may find that skin patches may be a better choice than gum. Skin (transdermal) patches evenly administer a continuous dose of nicotine over as much as a 24-hour period. With either therapy choice, you are replacing cigarettes with something that will ease your cessation efforts, perhaps providing the bridge necessary to cross over completely to nonsmoking status. In the future, inhalants and nasal spray forms of nicotine replacement therapy are expected to be marketed.

Most smokers can use these nicotine replacement therapies without any adverse effects, although an allergy or hypersensitivity to nicotine could prevent successful use. Users of the gum have complained of jaw fatigue, hiccuping, burping, and nausea. Users of the patches have reported short-lived mild itching or swelling. These are only important insofar as they prevent patients from using the methods to achieve smoking cessation.

Quitting smoking will have implications for any drug therapy you may be receiving and for coffee-drinking habits. Researchers have found that the body may metabolize drugs differently after smoking cessation, so ask your doctor about any changes you detect. Dosages may need to be altered. In another study, researchers learned that caffeine concentrations in the blood increased more than 250 percent after cessation. The anxiety and sleep disturbances characteristic of nicotine withdrawal are similar to effects seen in caffeine overdosing.

Many people worry about weight gain with smoking cessation. About one-third of people gain weight when they quit, in part because their senses of taste and smell are improved and they enjoy food more. But the average weight gain is only 5 pounds. You can avoid weight gain by eating a healthy, low-fat diet, using carrot sticks, raisins, or apples for oral substitutes. Regular physical activity will help you stay busy and relax.

Do whatever works for you to quit smoking, and don't feel alone when you are discouraged. Each year about one-third of American smokers attempt to quit—that's about 19 million smokers—but only about 10 percent succeed. Many quit successfully only after several tries. Remember, too, that about 44 million Americans are former smokers who have quit. Don't let hard-nosed nonsmokers who are antagonistic poison your efforts to quit. They may have never smoked and may not understand how difficult it can be. The American Cancer Society recommends:

- Keeping busy
- Avoiding environments that encourage smoking
- Enlisting family and friends in the effort
- Rewarding yourself for every step forward

If you do lapse, don't give up. Just start again.

High Blood Pressure

Most cases of high blood pressure cannot be cured; however, the good news is that it can be controlled by lifestyle changes and, when necessary, medication. High blood pressure can often be prevented through exercise and control of weight, sodium intake, and alcohol intake. The following changes can be effective in lowering your blood pressure or in preventing high blood pressure:

- Reach and maintain a desirable body weight. Weight control is one of the most important factors in preventing and treating high blood pressure. Most people who are more than 10 percent above ideal body weight will lower their blood pressure with weight loss. In many cases, moderate weight loss of about 10 pounds or more lowers blood pressure. With weight loss comes the additional benefit of enhancing the effectiveness of medications prescribed to lower blood pressure.

- Reduce sodium intake to 2,400 mg or less per day (the equivalent of about $1^1/_8$ teaspoons of salt). Compare this level to the 4,000 to 5,800 mg that American adults typically consume daily. Eighty percent of the sodium in the American diet can be attributed to the salt and other sodium compounds added to food during processing. One review of research found patients with high blood pressure to be more "salt

sensitive" than those without. The review reported that about 60 percent of patients with high blood pressure respond to increased dietary sodium with increased blood pressure.

- Limit alcohol intake to no more than two drinks per day (see p. 105 for the definition of one alcoholic drink). Alcohol intake of three or more drinks per day has been cited as the cause for as many as 7 percent of all cases of high blood pressure. Reducing alcohol intake can lower blood pressure, whether high blood pressure is present or not. Furthermore, drinking excessively can interfere with the intended effect of medications used to treat high blood pressure. Therefore, people with high blood pressure who drink alcoholic beverages should drink in moderation.

- Exercise regularly. Being sedentary—inactive—can be dangerous to your health. People who are sedentary are 50 percent more likely than those who are not to develop high blood pressure. Those who become active typically experience a modest decrease in their blood pressure, whether or not they lose weight. In attempting to lower blood pressure, it is more important to exercise daily, if possible, than just three times per week. Low- to moderate-intensity exercise is as effective as high-intensity exercise in reducing blood pressure. But before beginning any exercise program, be sure to check with your physician.

Blood pressure risk changes by age. From young adulthood to early middle age, men are more likely to develop high blood pressure; from early middle age to old age, women are more likely to be its victims. Women who take oral contraceptives are at higher risk when they are over-weight, have a family history of high blood pressure, have had high blood pressure during pregnancy, or have mild kidney disease. Race is also a factor: blacks are more likely to have high blood pressure than whites.

Controlling blood pressure is an important way of maintaining or improving cardiovascular health. Don't let one high reading upset you. Reliable measures are those that are consistent over several readings. Work toward your goals, but if you are on medication, *never* drop it and rely on lifestyle changes alone without checking with your physician.

High blood pressure is also the subject of Chapter 11, and medications to lower blood pressure are discussed in Chapter 27.

Cholesterol Levels

In *The New Living Heart Diet,* a book we coauthored with colleagues, we present a comprehensive plan for eating and lifestyle designed to reduce risk for heart disease by lowering blood cholesterol and triglyceride levels, blood pressure, and body weight. The diet component is a well-balanced, nutritious diet that decreases saturated fat intake, decreases dietary cholesterol intake, and controls body weight, incorporating both weight loss and weight maintenance plans. (For an order form for *The New Living Heart Diet,* see the last page of this book.)

The Living Heart Diet© has three steps. Step I and Step II (Table 26.1) and a third step called the "very low fat diet." Each step is designed to achieve progressively greater blood cholesterol lowering. The Step I Diet is recommended for children 2 years of age and older and for adults who *do not have* heart disease. Adults who *do have* heart disease or other atherosclerotic disease should follow the Step II Diet, in which saturated fat and cholesterol are limited further. The Step I and II Diets are the same as the Step I and II Diets of the American Heart Association and the National Cholesterol Education Program. The very low fat diet is a plan suited to those who cannot achieve blood cholesterol lowering to an acceptable level with the other diet plans.

Table 26.1. The Living Heart Diet©—Step I and Step II

Element	Step I Diet	Step II Diet
Calories	A level to achieve or maintain desirable weight	Same
Total fat	30% or less of calories	Same
Saturated fat	8% to 10% of calories	Less than 7% of calories
Polyunsaturated fat	Up to 10% of calories	Same
Monounsaturated fat	Up to 15% of calories	Same
Carbohydrate	55% or more of calories	Same
Protein	About 15% of calories	Same
Cholesterol	Less than 300 mg per day	Less than 200 mg per day

NOTE: The very low fat diet is described on pages 424–425.

The Living Heart Diet—Step I

Saturated fat, dietary cholesterol, and calories are the three dietary components that significantly affect blood cholesterol.

Saturated fat, found in meats and certain plant oils, raises blood cholesterol. In the American diet, about two-thirds of the saturated fat consumed comes from animal fats. These include butterfat (in butter, whole milk, cheese, cream, sour cream, and ice cream) and fat from meat (beef, pork, lamb, and poultry). Plant oils that are high in saturated fat are palm, coconut, and palm kernel oils.

We all differ in the extent to which consuming *dietary cholesterol* raises our blood cholesterol levels. Cholesterol we consume in our diet may also contribute to saturated fat's ability to increase blood levels of cholesterol. Dietary cholesterol is found only in animal foods: egg yolk, meat, poultry, fish, and dairy products.

Egg yolk is the most concentrated source of dietary cholesterol.

Achieving weight control by controlling *calorie intake* is an important component of The Living Heart Diet. Obesity, which results from excessive calorie intake, can raise the levels of blood cholesterol, triglyceride, blood pressure, and blood glucose and can lower the level of high-density lipoprotein (HDL) cholesterol ("good" cholesterol). Weight reduction can significantly improve these conditions. Making the attack on weight with calorie reduction *and* regular physical activity is better than relying on either method alone. Individuals who exercise regularly are more likely to keep weight off after losing it than individuals who do not exercise.

The Living Heart Diet emphasizes selecting foods that are low in fat as a means of reducing saturated fat intake and controlling calories. Counting grams of fat

Table 26.2. Maximum Grams of Fat at Selected Calorie Levels

Calorie Level	Grams of Fat Equal to		
	30% of Calories	20% of Calories	10% of Calories
1,200	40	27	13
1,600	53	36	18
2,000	67	44	22
2,400	80	53	27
3,000	100	67	33

is an effective way to control fat intake. In Table 26.2, we list the grams of fat equal to 30, 20, and 10 percent of calories from fat at several calorie levels.

For The Living Heart Diet—Step I, use the column showing the grams of fat equal to 30 percent of calories and consume no more than the number of grams of fat listed. In the Step I Diet, less than 10 percent of calories come from saturated fat (not shown in table). It is usually not necessary to count grams of saturated fat on the Step I Diet because saturated fat is decreased as the fat is decreased. For packaged foods, the grams of fat per serving is shown on the label. To find the grams of fat in a food that does not have a label, refer to *The Living Heart Guide to Eating Out* and *The New Living Heart Diet,* both companion volumes to this book.

Success in losing weight by accounting for all the fat you consume depends on how many fat-free and low-fat foods you eat that are high in calories. Remember that the calories in fat-free desserts add up

quickly. Such foods may be very high in sugar (or other sweetener). Eating fat-free and low-fat foods in excess can prevent weight loss or even cause weight gain, even though the fat intake may be very low. *Fat free* does not mean *calorie free.* It is helpful for some people who need to lose weight to also count the calories they consume. The number of calories per serving is part of the nutrition label on packaged foods.

The Living Heart Diet—Step II

Patients with coronary heart disease or other atherosclerotic disease should begin with the Step II Diet. The Step II Diet is also designed for individuals who are not able to lower their blood cholesterol to the desired goal level by following the Step I Diet. The Step II Diet differs from the Step I Diet in only two ways: (1) saturated fat intake is reduced to less than 7 percent of calories, and (2) dietary cholesterol is reduced to less than 200 mg per day (Table 26.1). The additional decreases in saturated fat and cholesterol can be achieved by selecting leaner meats; by eating less meat, poultry, and fish; by substituting fat-free dairy products for low-fat dairy products; and by consuming no more than two egg yolks per week. Food choices for the Step I and Step II Diets by food group are shown in Table 26.3.

The Living Heart Diet—Very Low Fat

A very low fat diet is one in which total fat is reduced to 20 percent or even 10 percent of calories. Table 26.2 shows the grams of fat for each of these plans at several calorie levels. This more aggressive reduction in fat facilitates further reduction in saturated fat. The benefit of restricting fat to less than 20 percent of calories has been shown in several clinical studies.

Eating a diet with less than 20 percent of calories from fat requires careful planning to ensure adequate nutrition. Both the 20 percent and 10 percent fat levels can include small amounts (3 to 5 ounces cooked) of extra lean meat, poultry, and seafood. Some people prefer a vegetarian approach. A vegetarian diet can be adequate nutritionally and satisfying. Whether or not meat is included, special attention should be paid to each food group. (See

Table 26.3. Food Choices for The Living Heart Diet©—Step I or II

Food Group	Step I or II Diet Servings
Meat, poultry, fish (lean)	5 to 6 ounces (cooked) per day
Eggs	Step I: no more than 4 yolks per week
	Step II: no more than 2 yolks per week
	Egg whites may be consumed without limit.
Dairy products (low-fat, fat-free, or skim)	2 to 3 servings per day
Fats and oils (low in saturated fat)	No more than 8 teaspoons per day
Bread, cereal, pasta, and starchy vegetables	6 or more servings per day
Nonstarchy vegetables	3 to 5 servings per day
Fruits	2 to 4 servings per day
Sweets and alcohol*	No more than 2 alcoholic drinks per day (see Table 11.3, p. 175)
	Fat-free and low-fat sweets only in moderation (control calories)

NOTE: The very low fat diet is described in text above.

* For diabetics, sweets and alcohol are usually limited; check with your physician or dietitian.

The New Living Heart Diet for a broader discussion of this topic.) In addition to using the appropriate number of servings of food from each food group, counting grams of fat is an effective method for limiting fat intake (see Table 26.2). Food choices in the very low fat diet are described below.

Meat, Poultry, and Fish

On a diet with 20 percent of calories from fat, limit extra lean meat, poultry (white meat without skin), or low-fat fish to no more than 5 ounces (cooked). If meat containing more fat is eaten, the number of ounces needs to be reduced. On a diet with 10 percent of calories from fat, no more than 3 ounces of cooked poultry (white meat without skin) or low-fat fish may be included. It is usually helpful on the diet with 10 percent of calories from fat to combine the meat with other foods, such as pasta, rice, or vegetables. For both the diet with 10 percent of calories from fat and the diet with 20 percent of calories from fat, good sources of protein that may be substituted for meat include low-fat and fat-free cheese and cottage cheese, dried beans and peas, reduced-fat peanut butter, and egg whites.

Eggs and Dairy Products

One egg yolk per week is allowed on the very low fat diet that limits fat to 20 percent of calories, but no eggs are allowed on the diet limiting fat to 10 percent of calories. Egg whites may be eaten without limit. Dairy products should be fat free or skim, and two to four servings may be chosen per day.

Fats and Oils

Fats and oils used in the very low fat diet should be chosen with care. Select only oils with very low levels of saturated fat (for example, canola oil), and account for the grams of fat in your allowance for the day. (A tablespoon of canola oil has 13.6 grams of fat.) If a margarine is used, it should be fat free, "diet," or of a reduced-fat type. Check the label for grams of fat. Salad dressings and sandwich spreads should be fat free.

Grains, Fruits, and Vegetables

Six or more servings per day may be chosen of breads, cereals, pasta, and starchy vegetables (for example, potatoes or crackers). Two or more servings of fruit may be chosen, and three or more servings of all nonstarchy vegetables may also be included.

Sweets and Alcohol

All sweets should be fat free and must be eaten in moderation, keeping in mind the extra calories they provide. If you drink alcohol, servings should be limited to no more than two drinks per day (see Table 11.3, p. 175, for the amount of alcohol in one drink).

Expectations with The Living Heart Diet

The levels to which The Living Heart Diet—whether Step I, Step II, or very low fat—lowers blood cholesterol will vary according to an individual's "typical" diet, compliance with the diet, individual biologic responsiveness to diet, and, if overweight, the amount of weight loss. The Step I Diet usually lowers total cholesterol 3 to 14 percent; however, some people lower their cholesterol level as much as 25 percent. The Step II Diet should lower total cholesterol an additional 3 to 7 percent, depending on the extent to which saturated fat and dietary cholesterol are restricted. Weight reduction on a diet low in saturated fat improves blood cholesterol lowering. For example, obese individuals who have a very high intake of saturated fat can often lower their total cholesterol by 25 percent on diets having 10 to 20 percent of calories from fat and lose weight as well. Cholesterol lowering results on the very low fat diet can be comparable to those achieved with some lipid-lowering medications. (Lipid-lowering drugs are discussed in Chapter 27.)

• • •

Combining changes in diet with increased physical activity surpasses the simple addition of the parts. Besides reducing risk for coronary heart disease through lower blood cholesterol, the combination can

- Lower triglyceride levels
- Raise HDL-cholesterol
- Decrease high blood pressure through weight reduction and decreased sodium (salt) and alcohol intake
- Decrease angina pectoris (chest pain) on a very low fat diet
- Improve glucose tolerance as the result of weight reduction

In addition, a low intake of saturated fat has been shown to reduce risk for the sudden formation of a blood clot capable of clogging an artery. This effect may also be achieved by *regular* exercise.

Using The Living Heart Diet to Lower Triglyceride Levels

When the aim is lowering blood triglyceride levels, the emphasis is on the following methods:

- Controlling weight
- Restricting alcohol intake (in some patients)
- Eating a diet low in saturated fat and cholesterol
- Exercising regularly
- Decreasing simple carbohydrate intake (if intake is very high)
- Stopping smoking

Alcohol restriction is important in individuals who are sensitive to alcohol and in whom alcohol intake triggers an increase in triglyceride level. Avoiding all alcohol may be necessary. For those who are overweight and need to lower their triglyceride level, weight control should be the overriding concern. The triglyceride level usually falls as the weight is lost, often reaching a normal level. The weight loss program should be combined with regular exercise.

Using The Living Heart Diet to Raise HDL-Cholesterol Levels

No dietary changes are specifically geared to raising HDL-cholesterol levels, but usually The Living Heart Diet—Step I is recommended. The following lifestyle changes need special emphasis:

- Weight loss, if overweight
- Regular moderate exercise
- Smoking cessation

Low HDL-cholesterol levels are often associated with elevated triglyceride levels; therefore, the lifestyle changes recommended to increase the HDL-cholesterol level are similar to the recommendations for decreasing triglyceride level, which are listed just above.

Using The Living Heart Diet to Lower Blood Pressure

For blood pressure lowering, the lifestyle changes listed below are effective:

- Reaching and maintaining a desirable body weight
- Exercising regularly
- Limiting alcohol intake to no more than two drinks per day (see p. 105 for the amount in one drink)
- Reducing sodium to 2,400 mg or less per day

Weight loss (for overweight individuals) as part of The Living Heart Diet—Step I is one of the most important factors in treating high blood pressure. Most people who are more than 10 percent above their ideal weight will lower their blood pressure with weight loss. Losing weight also helps enhance the effectiveness of blood pressure medications. Another dietary effort—reducing sodium intake—can help, too. (For more information about a low-sodium diet, consult *The New Living Heart Diet*).

Using The Living Heart Diet to Decrease Angina

The Living Heart Diet—Very Low Fat, which restricts fat to 10 to 20 percent of total calories, can reduce the frequency, duration, and severity of angina pectoris (chest pain).

Using The Living Heart Diet to Improve Glucose Tolerance or Control Diabetes

Management of diabetes involves lifestyle changes (including diet, exercise, and weight control) and, if necessary, medication (oral medication or insulin). Diet is the cornerstone of treatment for diabetes. The Living Heart Diet—Step I is recommended for controlling blood glucose. Weight loss should play an important role if the patient is overweight. Diabetic individuals with known heart disease or other atherosclerotic disease should follow The Living Heart Diet—Step II.

The incidence of heart disease is at least doubled in diabetic men and at least quadrupled in diabetic women compared with their nondiabetic counterparts. Glucose levels must be carefully monitored in all diabetic individuals. When blood sugar is tested before eating breakfast, it should be between 80 and 120 mg/dl; at bedtime, it should be 100 to 140 mg/dl.

Physical Inactivity

Physical inactivity is a modifiable risk factor for coronary heart disease, and becoming active is important for preserving or improving health. The benefits associated with regular moderate physical activity probably cannot be overestimated. A powerful predictor of longevity, physical activity is indispensable as a method for achieving cardiovascular fitness.

Over time, much of the physical labor of employment has been eradicated. Research by Dr. Jeremy Morris found that evidence of coronary heart disease was four to five times more common in men

45 to 50 years old who did light work rather than heavy work. He expanded his work to studies of leisure time and his results were similar: men who regularly practiced aerobic exercise had a lower incidence of coronary heart disease than men who did lighter leisure work such as gardening. A colleague, Ralph Paffenbarger, Jr., who himself is a record-setting marathon runner, likewise investigated the hazards of a sedentary life by following college athletes out of college and into the workplace. He found that the athletes retained their low risk for heart disease only if they remained active. These studies helped lay the foundation for establishing physical inactivity as a risk factor for coronary heart disease, and the message to the workers who sit behind computer screens or have other sedentary jobs is that regular exercise is essential to achieving and maintaining cardiovascular fitness.

Regular exercise contributes to controlling blood pressure, helps prevent the development of non-insulin-dependent diabetes mellitus, and provides other important health benefits. Performing regular moderate aerobic endurance exercise has been shown to accomplish the following:

- Reduce death rates from all causes
- Reduce risk for heart attack and stroke
- Increase blood levels of HDL-cholesterol ("good" cholesterol) and,

in some people, decrease LDL-cholesterol ("bad" cholesterol)

- Decrease blood pressure
- Decrease triglyceride level
- Help with weight reduction
- Improve glucose tolerance
- Strengthen heart, lungs, bones, and muscles
- Increase strength and energy
- Help manage stress
- Improve sleep
- Improve body image and enhance self-esteem

These benefits are not hard to unlock: they begin to be realized at the first walk, the first jog, or the first exercise class.

Before beginning an exercise program, check with your physician. Especially if you have had a heart attack or suffered a stroke, you need to know what your physician thinks about the program you have selected. People who are at high risk for coronary heart disease or who have a history of coronary heart disease may be asked to undergo exercise electrocardiography (ECG) to establish a suitable level of exercise. This is intended to help ensure that your exercise program will do what it is supposed to: help you, not hurt you. If you plan to use heart rate to measure the intensity of your exercise, also talk with your physician about your recommended target heart rate during exercise (see Table 26.4).

Table 26.4. Target Exercise Heart Rate

Age	60% Maximum Heart Rate	70% Maximum Heart Rate	80% Maximum Heart Rate
20	120	140	160
25	117	137	156
30	114	133	152
35	111	130	148
40	108	126	144
45	105	123	140
50	102	119	136
55	99	116	132
60	96	112	128
65	93	109	124
70	90	105	120

SOURCE: Adapted from *The New Living Heart Diet* (New York: Simon & Schuster, 1996).

Types of Physical Activity

Another factor to consider before beginning your exercise program is your aim in exercising. Consider whether you want more endurance and stamina, more strength in your muscles, or more flexibility. You may want a combination. After determining what effect you want to achieve from the exercise you perform, begin your workout by warming up (by walking, for instance); exercise until you arrive at a level that requires just a little more effort than is comfortable; and then cool down. To ensure improvement, increase the number of times you exercise per week; exercise for a longer period each time; or increase the intensity of the exercise. Though you want to move ahead, never push yourself until you experience joint pain or chest pain.

Endurance Exercises

Endurance exercises build stamina and burn calories, both during the exercise and for a period of time after exercise is completed. These exercises employ large muscles such as those in the hips and legs in continuous motion at a moderate intensity for 20 to 60 minutes. Walking briskly outdoors or on a treadmill, hiking, jogging, outdoor or indoor cycling, swimming, rowing, using stair-step machines, taking aerobic dance or step classes, cross-country skiing, and performing various endurance

game activities all build endurance. Working out at a moderate intensity, you burn both oxygen and fuel (from the food you have eaten in the last three to eight hours and/or body fat) to produce energy for prolonged muscle contraction. Make sure you can pass the "talk test"—that at no time does the activity push you to breathlessness and an inability to talk while you exercise. Aerobic endurance exercises are especially useful in cardiovascular conditioning, that is, increasing the strength and efficiency of the heart.

Strength Training

Strength training includes activities such as weight lifting, sit-ups, push-ups, and other body-lifting exercises. Each exercise builds specific muscles by working them briefly but intensely. If your goal is to build muscle mass, use heavier weights and few repetitions. If your goal is to strengthen muscles, use lighter weights and more repetitions.

Flexibility Exercises

Yoga and other bending and flexing exercise programs enable your body's joints to move through a wider range of motion. The basic movement in these exercises is to extend the muscle, hold it in position until light to moderate tension develops, and then hold it for about 10 seconds. Flexibility exercises should be done slowly and evenly. Do not bounce or push too hard when the muscle is extended or you could cause small tears in muscles and ligaments.

Warm-up and Cool-down

Whatever routine you choose, remember to allow your body time to warm up beforehand and cool down afterward. Try walking or pacing as a warm-up, or gentle stretching (not bouncing). Warm-up exercises gradually introduce activity, allowing the entire body to get properly ready for physical effort. Cool-down exercises, which might also include walking or stretching, alert your body's circulation and metabolism to return to a less active state.

Targeting Your Heart Rate

Building aerobic fitness increases your cardiovascular fitness. The intensity of a workout is sometimes measured by comparing your heart rate (pulse count) during exercise with a target exercise heart rate. To determine your target exercise heart rate (1) subtract your age from 220 to get your maximum heart rate and then (2) multiply your maximum heart rate by an appropriate percentage, based on your level of fitness. Never attempt to reach your maximum heart rate. Beginners should aim to achieve 60 percent of their maximum heart rate. Suggested target

heart rates for different ages and levels of activity are shown in Table 26.4. For example, a 50-year-old who has not been physically active might calculate her target exercise heart rate at 60 percent of maximum heart rate, or 102 (220 − 50 = 170; 170 × 0.60 = 102).

Your heart rate can be measured by gently pressing the first two fingers of your hand on the inside of the opposite wrist. Or use these two fingers against an artery in your neck, which you can feel slightly to the side of your neck. Practice finding the best spot. You need not hold your wrist for a full minute to calculate your pulse. Simply hold your fingers there for 10 seconds and multiply by six to get your heart rate per minute. Be sure not to pause between stopping exercise and taking your heart rate, or the count will not be accurate. Another option is purchasing and using a heart rate monitor.

Stress

Though psychosocial stress has long been linked in the popular imagination with heart disease, evidence is only now being scientifically and systematically collected in a wide range of explorations of the relations between the two. Determining whether stress initiates cardiovascular disease or exacerbates it is part of the investigation. On a personal level, many of us have been aware of instances in which a stressful situation immediately preceded angina, heart attack, or sudden cardiac death. We expect with time to better understand how our thinking and emotions affect our cardiovascular health. Psychosocial stress as a potential risk factor is discussed in more detail in Chapter 7.

Identifying the stressors in your life and examining how you meet their challenges, and then acting on that information by reducing them and/or their effect, may play a part in improving overall cardiovascular health. The benefit may be indirect—for example, reduced stress may reduce overeating or smoking. At any rate, stress reduction improves overall sense of well-being, and has not been associated with any health hazards.

Deep breathing from the diaphragm, which increases the amount of oxygen in your lungs; muscle-relaxing exercises in which you systematically mentally relax sets of muscles throughout your body; and meditation, which focuses your mind on a positive thought and away from everyday worries, all help your body relax. Meditation and exercise are two techniques many people have found useful for managing stress.

Meditation is learning how to stop all you are doing and start paying attention to the present moment. It is learning how to make time for yourself, how to slow down and nurture calmness and self-acceptance, and how to observe what your mind is up to from moment to moment. It is simply being present—not living in the past or future, just paying attention to the present. The more regularly you practice meditation, the more it will work for you. A successful way to start meditating is to concentrate on your breathing—the air as it goes in and out of your nose. When learning to meditate, most students find it helpful to have a teacher.

Exercise also fulfills the requirements of focusing the mind outside everyday worries and relaxes the body by stretching muscles. Of course, with exercise you get the added benefits of improved physical condition, along with the peace of mind that you are doing something about your health. Exercise has also proved to be an antidote to depression and is a much-favored alternative to the alcohol or drug abuse that sometimes accompanies the negative feelings that are part of depression.

A Program That Teaches the Heart Healthy Lifestyle

A program begun at Baylor College of Medicine in Houston teaches individuals how to reduce their risk for coronary heart disease and the problems associated with it. It is called *Living Hearts!*[SM] Based on recent research showing that the progression of coronary heart disease can be slowed or in some instances reversed, the Living Hearts! program provides a medically managed regimen of dietary intervention, exercise, and stress management for individuals who need and want to reduce aggressively their risk for coronary heart disease. It is designed for people at risk of developing coronary heart disease, and for those who already have it and want to decrease their risk for future heart attack or heart surgery. The program is conducted by a team of health care professionals. Living Hearts! emphasizes aggressively lowering total and LDL-cholesterol levels, triglyceride level, high blood pressure, glucose level (for persons who are diabetic), and weight (for persons who are overweight); raising HDL-cholesterol level; and assisting in smoking cessation. Medications are prescribed to control selected factors if lifestyle changes (diet, exercise, smoking cessation, and stress management) do not achieve the desired results.

Individuals in the Living Hearts! program see a physician for an initial examination and for initial fasting blood tests for total cholesterol, triglyceride, HDL, LDL, and glucose levels. Regularly scheduled follow-up visits evaluate progress toward goal values. During the first two months, individuals attend three group meetings per week (two hours each), where they exercise and participate in diet and stress management classes. During the remainder of the year, they attend one-hour group meetings each week.

The goals of the Living Hearts! program for participants *with* heart disease are the following:

- Decrease risk for future heart attacks
- Decrease frequency, duration, and severity of angina
- Decrease the need for angioplasty and bypass surgery
- Lower LDL-cholesterol level
- Raise HDL-cholesterol level
- Lower triglyceride level
- Decrease blood pressure
- Improve control of blood sugar
- Help participants lose or control weight

For people *without known* heart disease, the goals are the following:

- Decrease risk for heart attack
- Lower LDL-cholesterol level
- Raise HDL-cholesterol level
- Lower triglyceride level
- Decrease blood pressure

- Improve control of blood sugar
- Help participants lose or control weight

The interdisciplinary staff work as a team to provide an individualized program meant to help participants make lifestyle changes that will address specific aspects of their cardiovascular profile. Physicians, dietitians, exercise physiologists, and a psychotherapist work collegially through multiple sessions with participants to personalize a program of diet, physical activity, and stress management.

Summary

The choices we make daily far away from the doctor's office have great implications for what is written in the medical chart kept there. What we eat, whether we choose to smoke, how we adapt to diabetes or diagnosed cardiovascular disease, whether we exercise regularly, and how we respond to stress all affect our well-being. Feeling better and living longer will depend on many factors, some of which we can control and others we cannot. Those lifestyle choices we can make to improve our health are ours alone to make.

CHAPTER TWENTY-SEVEN

Cardiac Medications

Lifestyle modifications are often primary therapy for disorders, such as high blood cholesterol and hypertension, that can lead to heart disease, as well as for some heart diseases themselves. In such cases, medication may not be started, if it is needed, until after lifestyle therapy. In other cases, medication may be started immediately, usually in conjunction with lifestyle changes. Medication typically is a first-line therapy for many cardiac arrhythmias, congestive heart failure, and angina. Many patients do well with medication and lifestyle changes and need no further intervention.

A cardiac medication may be used alone or, as is often the case, in combination with other agents. Finding the right medication—or achieving the right mix of agents—may require some trial and error. The goal is to balance benefit (effectiveness) and risk (including side effects), with consideration of cost as necessary.

Many side effects are mild, and some dissipate with time. If you continue to be troubled by the effects of a medication,

talk with your doctor. With all the therapeutic choices available today, you should aim to find a medication that is both effective and well tolerated. Never discontinue any drug without checking with your doctor. Abrupt discontinuation of some cardiac drugs can cause a dangerous rebound of risk levels or symptoms.

Thrombolytic agents ("clot busters") are discussed in Chapter 14.

Medications for Angina

Angina may be treated by medication and lifestyle changes alone, or it may indicate the need for invasive therapy such as angioplasty or bypass surgery. Whether to proceed to an invasive treatment is a decision that takes into account the extent, location, and severity of the arterial blockages. The patient's age and the presence of coexisting health problems also will influence the decision.

The squeezing pain of angina is a symptom—a warning that the heart is not receiving enough oxygen-rich blood.

Angina results from an imbalance between coronary oxygen supply and demand. Angina is classified as stable, unstable, or variant (also called Prinzmetal's angina).

With *stable* angina, the supply of oxygen to the heart is relatively constant. An imbalance occurs when demands on the heart increase, as happens during exercise or when a rhythm disturbance develops. *Unstable* angina, as the name implies, is less predictable. Attacks become more frequent and when uncontrolled by rest or medication require emergency intervention. This form of angina is believed to arise when plaque (the fatty material that can accumulate in arteries) ruptures or when platelets form unstable plugs on the surface of a plaque. The formation of clots or plugs that partially obstruct blood flow is believed to underlie episodes of unstable angina. In *variant angina* a spasm in a coronary vessel suddenly reduces the supply of oxygen to the heart.

Because several factors can contribute to the imbalance between oxygen supply and demand that characterizes angina, more than one type of medication may be needed. Following are descriptions of some of the most common medications used to control angina.

Nitrates

Nitrates, which include the well-known agent nitroglycerin, are among the oldest cardiac medications. Nitrates are vasodilators—agents that dilate blood vessels—and they remain an important therapy for angina today. Although they have effects on both arteries and veins, their primary effect is dilation of veins. This reduces the heart's work load by making it easier for blood to circulate. Nitrates also increase nitric oxide within the vessel wall.

Nitrates are available in several forms: sublingual nitroglycerin, long-acting oral medications, nitroglycerin ointment, transdermal nitroglycerin patches, and nitroglycerin spray. Sublingual nitroglycerin is the most familiar form—a tiny tablet that is placed under the tongue. The medication goes to work straightaway.

The most common side effect is headache. Rarely, hypotension and inappropriate bradycardia occur. Store the nitroglycerin in its original container and under the conditions specified on the label. Nitroglycerin tablets should ideally be stored under controlled room temperature. With proper use and storage, nitroglycerin tablets should maintain their potency through the expiration date indicated on the package. Replace your prescription when the expiration date nears. Traditionally, patients have judged whether a nitroglycerin tablet is potent by whether there is a tingling or burning sensation after the tablet is dissolved under the tongue. Such potency testing is less useful today, since the newer tablets containing stabilized nitroglycerin are less likely to produce these effects.

Tolerance (the body's becoming less responsive to the medication over time) can develop with long-acting nitrate preparations. As a result, your doctor may schedule your dosages to accommodate a 10- to 12-hour "off" period each day.

Long-acting oral agents include isosorbide dinitrate, isosorbide mononitrate, and oral sustained-release nitroglycerin. The topical 2 percent nitroglycerin ointment is an alternative for people who cannot take medication by mouth. The ointment is applied with a controlled-dose applicator to a small area of skin and then covered with an airtight material to ensure proper absorption. Topical nitroglycerin typically is applied every four to six hours and begins working in about 30 minutes. Sustained-release nitroglycerin can be delivered by transdermal patches. The patches, which adhere to the skin, typically remain on the skin for as many as 12 hours per day but are removed for 12 hours each day to prevent development of tolerance. The spray is used to place droplets onto or under the tongue and should not be inhaled.

Beta-Blockers

Known officially as *beta-adrenergic antagonists*, beta-blockers are used to treat a variety of cardiovascular ailments, including angina, hypertension, and cardiac arrhythmias. Beta-blockers act by decreasing oxygen demand through slowing the heart rate and creating a negative effect on muscular contraction. By occupying

Beta-Blockers: How They Work

Nerve impulses from the ends of certain nerve fibers stimulate the heart. These signals are carried by the chemical messenger norepinephrine to beta-receptors in heart muscle, blood vessels, and airways.

Receptors are structures on the surface of cells that are similar to a docking site, where specific chemicals lock into place. Beta-blockers occupy the beta-receptor sites, thereby preventing the chemical linkup and interfering with signal transmission.

By blocking the nerve impulses that stimulate the heart, beta-blockers slow heart rate and reduce the heart's work load. This ability makes beta-blockers useful in treating angina, hypertension, and cardiac arrhythmias. These medications also may be given after a heart attack to preserve heart muscle and prevent rhythm disturbances.

Beta-blockers are classified as either *cardioselective* or *noncardioselective*. Cardioselective drugs work primarily on beta-1 receptors, found predominantly in heart muscle. Noncardioselective drugs affect both beta-1 receptors and beta-2 receptors (located primarily in blood vessels and airways).

At lower dosages, cardioselective drugs may be less likely to cause or aggravate breathing difficulties and conditions related to reduced blood flow to the limbs.

receptor sites on the surface of cells in the heart and blood vessels (see "Beta-Blockers: How They Work" on p. 437), these agents block transmission of signals from the central nervous system: they block the effects of *catecholamines*, chemical messengers through which nerve cells communicate with one another. Interfering with these nerve impulses reduces the heart's reactivity to stress and exercise. Heart rate drops and oxygen demand declines, reducing the frequency and severity of angina attacks and improving exercise tolerance.

The two types of beta-blockers— cardioselective and noncardioselective— appear to be equally effective in relieving angina. Their differing side effect profiles may determine which type of drug works best for you. Breathing difficulties and a worsening of circulatory problems are two of the most worrisome side effects of beta-blocker therapy. Because cardioselective drugs target the heart more precisely— and have less affinity for receptors in the airways and blood vessels—they may be less likely to aggravate asthma, bronchitis, or poor circulation in the legs and feet. At higher dosages, however, cardioselective drugs become less "selective," losing their advantage. Certain beta-blockers can lower levels of high-density lipoprotein (HDL) cholesterol, referred to as "good" cholesterol, and raise triglyceride levels.

Selected Beta-Blockers

Cardioselective Agents	Noncardioselective Agents
acebutolol (Sectral)*	betaxolol (Kerlone)
atenolol (Tenormin)	carteolol (Cartrol)*
metoprolol (Lopressor, Toprol XL)	labetalol (Normodyne, Trandate)
	nadolol (Corgard)
	penbutolol (Levatol)*
	pindolol (Visken)*
	propranolol (Inderal, Inderal LA)
	sotalol (Betapace)
	timolol (Blocadren)

Capitalization indicates trade name.
* Has intrinsic sympathomimetic activity.

Beta-blockers in general have a wide range of other potential side effects. These include bradycardia, bronchospasm, cold hands and feet, impotence, fatigue, depression, nightmares, memory problems, mental "fogginess," low blood pressure, salt retention, and unrecognized low blood sugar in diabetics.

Some side effects will diminish with time. Nonetheless, if persistent side effects are compromising your quality of life, ask your doctor about switching to another medication. Side effects can be highly variable among the different beta-blockers, and with all the ones to choose from, you should be able to find one that works well for you. Do not stop taking your medication for any reason without consulting your doctor. Beta-blocker dosages often need to be tapered gradually to avoid causing overactivity of the heart or increased blood pressure. Beta-blockers with some sympathetic activity (called intrinsic sympathomimetic activity, or ISA) will lower blood pressure and are used to treat hypertension, but are not effective for angina. Pindolol is an example.

Calcium Channel Blockers

As with nitrates, calcium channel blockers are vasodilators, but this newer class of drug dilates blood vessels by a different mechanism. As the name suggests, calcium channel blockers interfere with calcium transfer into cells. Because calcium plays an important role in muscle contraction, decreasing the flow of calcium into cells relaxes the layer of muscle within vessel walls. Vessel diameter increases, improving blood flow to the heart and reducing the force required to pump blood through the body. Individual calcium channel blockers may block calcium entry in slightly different ways. As a result, the drugs' positive—and sometimes negative—effects on the heart vary according to the particular drug used. The same holds true for noncardiac side effects.

Older (first- and second-generation) calcium channel blockers have the potential to weaken the heart's pumping action. The same mechanism that makes these drugs so helpful in controlling angina—discouraging muscle contraction within

Selected Oral Calcium Channel Blockers

Long-acting

Dihydropyridines
amlodipine (Norvasc)
felodipine, extended-release (Plendil)
isradipine, controlled-release (DynaCirc CR)
nicardipine, sustained-release (Cardene SR)
nifedipine, extended-release (Procardia XL, Adalat CC)
nisoldipine, extended-release (Sular)

Nondihydropyridines
bepridil (Vascor)
diltiazem, extended-release (Cardizem CD, Dilacor XR, Cardizem SR, Tiamate, Tiazac)
verapamil, extended-release (Isoptin SR, Calan SR, Verelan, Covera HS)

Short-acting

Dihydropyridines
isradipine, immediate-release (DynaCirc)
nicardipine, immediate-release (Cardene)
nifedipine, immediate-release (Adalat, Procardia)
nimodipine (Nimotop)

Nondihydropyridines
diltiazem, immediate-release (Cardizem)
verapamil, immediate-relase (Isoptin, Calan)

Capitalization indicates trade name.

vessel walls—also can affect the heart muscle's ability to contract properly. Newer calcium channel blockers, such as amlodipine (Norvasc) and felodipine (Plendil), have fewer adverse effects on the heart.

Some calcium channel blockers are used alone to control angina; others may be given in combination with nitrates or beta-blockers. Calcium channel blockers are also prescribed to treat hypertension. Another indication for certain agents (verapamil, diltiazem) is treatment of arrhythmias. The most common side effects associated with the various drugs are headache, low blood pressure, dizziness, edema (fluid retention), flushing, palpitations, and constipation.

Some questions have been raised about the safety of a particular type of calcium channel blocker, the so-called short-acting agents that raise heart rate. The issue is currently one of much debate. Physicians are awaiting results from large, long-term studies evaluating the safety of calcium channel blockers; meanwhile, they will do their best to answer any questions you might have about the particular drug you are taking.

Aspirin

Most patients with stable angina will be placed on daily (or every-other-day) low-dose aspirin. Aspirin decreases formation of blood clots and can reduce risk for heart attack and premature death in people with angina. In 1996 the U.S. Food and Drug Administration approved a new use for the old drug—prescribed administration at the onset of a heart attack. Costing only pennies a tablet, aspirin has properties that can help prevent clot formation. Such use was expected to save a significant percentage of people who now die prematurely of heart attack. The FDA's intent was that physicians add the drug to the arsenal of those at their command for combating heart attacks, not that patients treat their own heart attacks by taking aspirin.

Medications for Hypertension

Uncontrolled hypertension (high blood pressure) has potentially devastating effects on the body. This typically silent disease is a major contributor to heart attack, stroke, kidney damage, and heart failure. Careful monitoring and proper medication, however, can significantly reduce the risk of developing serious complications. Most people with hypertension will require lifelong medication, oftentimes with a combination of drugs.

The most commonly used blood pressure medications are diuretics, beta-blockers, calcium channel blockers, alpha-adrenergic agents, angiotensin-converting enzyme (ACE) inhibitors, and angiotensin-blocking agents.

Diuretics

Diuretics are a first-line treatment for hypertension. Sometimes referred to as "water pills," diuretics act on the kidneys, helping to remove excess water and salts from the body. Diuretics pull water from tissues, relieving fluid build-up (*edema*), and help convert the water to urine. This fluid removal reduces blood volume.

Selected Diuretics

Thiazide-type
bendroflumethiazide
   (Naturetin)
benzthiazide (Exna, Hydrex)
chlorothiazide (Diuril)
chlorthalidone (Hygroton,
   Thalitone)
cyclothiazide (Anhydron)
hydrochlorothiazide (Esidrix, Hydro-Chlor,
   Hydro-D, HydroDIURIL, Oretic)
hydroflumethiazide (Diucardin, Saluron)
indapamide (Lozol)
methyclothiazide (Aquatensen, Enduron)
metolazone (Diulo, Mykrox, Zaroxolyn)
polythiazide (Renese)
quinethazone (Hydromox)
trichlormethiazide (Metahydrin, Trichlorex)

Potassium-sparing Agents
amiloride (Midamor)
spironolactone (Aldactone)
triamterene (Dyrenium)

Loop Diuretics
bumetanide (Bumex)
ethacrynic acid (Edecrin)
furosemide (Lasix, Myrosemide)
torsemide (Demadex)

Capitalization indicates trade name.

Lower circulating blood volume allows blood pressure to drop, and less strain is put on the heart.

Several types of diuretics are available. These include thiazide, loop, and potassium-sparing agents. Your doctor may prescribe one or more medications. Side effects vary by class of drug. All diuretics have the potential to cause low blood pressure (hypotension). Hypotension, a particular concern for older people, can cause dizziness or a feeling of being faint, increasing the risk for falls.

Potassium loss is a concern with thiazide diuretics, which remove potassium along with other minerals. Excessive potassium loss can cause muscle cramps, weakness, and impotence and may trigger irregular heartbeats. A potassium supplement—or a potassium-sparing diuretic—typically is prescribed along with the thiazide diuretic. Thiazide medications can increase LDL-cholesterol and triglyceride levels. They have also been associated with elevations in blood sugar and uric acid in susceptible individuals, including some diabetics and people at risk for developing gout; these effects are dose dependent.

Loop diuretics are fast-acting agents that promote a high urine output over several hours. Like thiazide preparations, loop diuretics remove potassium. They also can deplete other electrolytes (minerals that help regulate fluid balance), and in fact are used to reduce high blood calcium levels (whereas thiazides can raise blood calcium). In high dosages, loop diuretics may affect hearing. Again, a potassium supplement or potassium-sparing diuretic may be given along with a loop-type diuretic. Loop diuretics can increase LDL-cholesterol.

Unlike thiazide diuretics, potassium-sparing diuretics, as the name suggests, preserve potassium and do not significantly alter lipid levels. Potassium-sparing agents typically are given with another type of diuretic. One drug—spironolactone—

can "spare" too much potassium, and it also can cause breast enlargement in some men and breast tenderness in some women.

Calcium Channel Blockers

Calcium channel blockers lower blood pressure through their vasodilating effects (discussed above). They are free of the adverse metabolic effects associated with diuretics. They do not significantly affect blood sugar, electrolytes, or blood lipid levels—and their beneficial effects on several other heart conditions may allow them to perform double duty in some patients. On the other hand, some of the first calcium channel blockers developed were known in patients at risk for heart failure to compromise the heart's pumping action further.

Beta-Blockers

Though the mechanism is not fully understood, beta-blockers lower blood pressure. Several actions probably are at work. These medications slow heart rate and decrease the force of the heart's pumping action (see pp. 437–438). Beta-blockers also control renin (an enzyme in the kidney that helps regulate fluid balance and blood vessel contraction through angiotensin formation), and they trigger release of prostaglandins (substances that have vasodilating effects). Side effects vary

according to the specific beta-blocker used. Fatigue, shortness of breath at low levels of exertion, depression, impotence, insomnia, cold hands and feet, and mental "fogginess" are some of the more common complaints. Because some beta-blockers can have negative effects on lipid levels, your doctor will monitor your cholesterol and triglyceride levels for significant changes.

Alpha-Blockers

Known formally as alpha-adrenergic antagonists, these drugs target another set of receptors found in blood vessels—alpha-receptors. By blocking these receptor sites, alpha-blockers disrupt nerve impulses that trigger muscle contraction, allowing vessels to relax. Alpha-blockers have beneficial effects on lipid levels as well. They decrease LDL-cholesterol levels, and some also decrease triglyceride levels and boost levels of HDL-cholesterol. They have recently proved useful in improving urine flow when there is blockage due to prostate obstruction.

The side effects associated with alpha-blockers typically are worse at the start of therapy and then dissipate with subsequent doses. These side effects include feeling faint or dizzy, orthostatic hypotension (an abrupt drop in blood pressure upon standing), drowsiness, headache, and, in women, stress incontinence.

Other Adrenergic Agents

Several other types of blood pressure medications target alpha-receptors. One medication, labetalol, blocks both alpha- and beta-receptors, at least initially. With continued use, labetalol's effects on alpha-receptors diminish and finally disappear. Among potential side effects are hypotension, tremors, and prickling or tingling sensations.

Drugs designated as "centrally acting agents" stimulate, rather than block, certain alpha-receptors in the central nervous system. Stimulating these receptors decreases vascular resistance, slows the heartbeat, and eases the heart's workload. Some of the side effects associated with centrally acting agents include dry mouth, orthostatic hypotension (a tendency to feel faint when rising to a standing position),

depressed heart rate, drowsiness, and sexual dysfunction. Abrupt discontinuation can lead to a dangerous rise in blood pressure and heartbeat irregularities.

ACE Inhibitors and Angiotensin Antagonists

Angiotensin-converting enzyme (ACE) is present in both blood vessel walls and the blood. ACE inhibitors constitute a relatively new class of blood pressure medications. They may improve insulin sensitivity and have beneficial effects on blood sugar and lipid levels. When given with a diuretic, ACE inhibitors counteract some of the diuretic's negative metabolic effects. Moreover, ACE inhibitors have beneficial effects on heart failure and on the nerve damage associated with diabetes. These drugs help dilate blood vessels by blocking an enzyme called angiotensin-converting enzyme. Under normal circumstances, ACE converts a chemical called angiotensin I to angiotensin II, a substance that induces blood vessels to constrict. By blocking ACE, these drugs shut down production of angiotensin II, allowing blood vessels to relax.

ACE inhibitors can cause hypotension, can elevate blood potassium levels, and have been known to worsen certain kidney conditions, but one of their most troubling side effects has been a dry cough. The cough is believed to be caused by high

Selected Combination Antihypertensive Drugs (Trade Names)

Diuretic + Diuretic
Aldactazide
Dyazide
Maxzide
Moduretic

Diuretic + Beta-Blocker
Corzide
Inderide
Inderide LA
Lopressor HCT
Tenoretic
Timolide
Ziac

Diuretic + ACE Inhibitor
Capozide
Lotensin HCT
Prinzide
Vaseretic
Zestoretic

Diuretic + Angiotensin II Antagonist
Hyzaar

Diuretic + Other
Aldoril
Apresazide
Esimil
Hydropres

levels of bradykinin, a natural chemical compound that dilates blood vessels and makes them more permeable. However, a newer drug class has been developed that is an angiotensin II receptor antagonist. These drugs do not block ACE, do not increase bradykinin levels, and generally are not associated with a cough. Approved angiotensin II antagonists are losartan and valsartan.

Fixed-dose Combination Agents

As noted above, combinations of antihypertensive drugs may be given. Antihypertensive drugs are prescribed in a *stepwise fashion*—for example, lower dosages and single agents are usually tried first. Finding the most effective and best-tolerated drug or drug combination for an individual patient may take several tries. Even when drugs are carefully chosen, individual responses may vary. Combination therapy may be given as separate drugs or may employ fixed-dose combination drugs, in which the drugs are already combined. These fixed-dose combinations are convenient for the patient, although some physicians prefer to adjust the dosage of each drug separately. The fixed-dose combination agents combine a thiazide diuretic with a potassium-sparing diuretic or another type of antihypertensive drug.

Selected Antiarrhythmia Medications

Beta-Blockers
(See list on p. 438)

Calcium Channel Blockers
diltiazem (Cardizem, Dilacor-XR)
verapamil (Calan, Isoptin, Verelan)

Digitalis Drugs
digitoxin (Crystodigin)
digoxin (Lanoxin, Lanoxicaps)

Other Medications
amiodarone (Cordarone)
disopyramide (Norpace)
flecainide (Tambocor)
lidocaine (LidoPen)
mexiletine (Mexitil)
moricizine (Ethmozine)
procainamide (Procan SR, Promine, Pronestyl)
propafenone (Rythmol)
quinidine (Cardioquin, Quinalan, and others)
tocainide (Tonocard)

Capitalization indicates trade name.

Medications for Arrhythmia

Drug treatment of irregular heartbeats depends on the type and severity of the arrhythmia. Some types of drugs commonly used to suppress rhythm disturbances are beta-blockers, calcium channel blockers, and digitalis medications. Several other antiarrhythmia medications have anesthetic and desensitizing effects.

Antiarrhythmia medications are given to restore normal heart rhythm. Their effects include suppressing or altering the electrical impulses that control heart rhythm and rate, or damping the heart muscle's response to these impulses. Some medications are given in intravenous form during an initial or life-threatening episode and then may be continued in oral form after heart rhythm has stabilized.

Cardiac arrhythmias are often simple and clinically insignificant, requiring minimal if any intervention. In other cases, they may be complex and require extensive diagnostic testing and trials with various medications to find the most effective agent or combination of agents. Here are some of the more commonly prescribed antiarrhythmia drugs and the general types of rhythm disturbance they are used to treat.

Beta-Blockers

Beta-blockers slow transmission of electrical impulses through the sinoatrial (SA) node—the heart's primary native pacemaker. Because these medications affect signals passing through the heart's central "switchboard," they are potentially beneficial in several types of arrhythmia. Beta-blockers frequently are prescribed after a heart attack, when the damaged heart is likely to develop abnormal rhythms. They also are used to treat atrial fibrillation, atrial flutter, and certain other supraventricular tachycardias.

On the downside, beta-blockers can drop the heart rate too low in some people and further compromise the heart's pumping action among patients with heart failure. Other potential side effects include respiratory problems, impotence, loss of mental clarity, cold hands and feet, depression, nightmares, and insomnia. Abruptly stopping a beta-blocker can also trigger arrhythmias.

Calcium Channel Blockers

Some calcium channel blockers help restore heart rhythm by damping the heart muscle's response to the erratic electrical impulses being transmitted. These select agents are often used to treat atrial fibrillation, atrial flutter, and supraventricular tachycardias. Most calcium channel blockers have no effect on cardiac arrhythmias. As with beta-blockers, certain calcium channel blockers may cause the heart rate to drop too low. Other potential side effects include headache, dizziness, fluid retention, and flushing.

Digitalis Drugs

Originally made from the dried leaves of foxglove plants, digitalis drugs slow transmission of electrical impulses within the heart. These medications restore normal rhythm by slowing and strengthening the heartbeat, enabling the heart to pump more efficiently.

Digitalis preparations are often used to treat atrial fibrillation and atrial flutter. These medications require close monitoring by your physician. Report fatigue or weakness, loss of appetite, nausea, vomiting, headache, confusion, visual disturbances, or heart palpitations to your doctor immediately.

Other Medications

Procainamide, quinidine, and disopyramide slow the conduction of electrical impulses through the heart and desensitize the heart muscle's response to these stimuli. Procainamide is often used to treat atrial fibrillation, atrial flutter, and ventricular tachycardia.

Quinidine can cause a rash or gastrointestinal complaints, such as loss of appetite, nausea, diarrhea, or abdominal pain. Procainamide can cause loss of appetite, diarrhea, lightheadedness, or the lupus syndrome. Drug-induced lupus is characterized by fever, arthritis, arthralgias, and rash, and is the most worrisome side effect of procainamide. Check with your doctor if you experience fever, chills, joint pain, or mental confusion, or if your breathing becomes painful or labored. Disopyramide may be associated with dry mouth, decreased urination, constipation, visual disturbances, or abdominal pain. Some of the other medications that may be prescribed for certain types of arrhythmia include lidocaine, mexiletine, moricizine, tocainide, flecainide, propafenone, and amiodarone.

These are all very powerful drugs, having significant and sometimes life-threatening side effects. Amiodarone, for example, is an ideal antiarrhythmia drug in many respects: it suppresses a variety of arrhythmias through several mechanisms and is one of the most effective medications available. It has been shown unequivocally to improve long-term survival. Its potential toxicity, however, requires careful consideration of the risk:benefit ratio before it is prescribed.

Antiarrhythmia medications can lead to *proarrhythmias*, the creation of a new rhythm disturbance or a worsening of an existing one. Antiarrhythmia drugs are paradoxical in that they can both suppress and cause arrhythmias. The induced arrhythmias can be quite serious because they may be harder to suppress or convert than the original arrhythmias. An individual's reaction to a particular medication often is unpredictable because of genetic differences or the coexistence of other heart problems.

Further complicating drug therapy for arrhythmias is that in some patients, successful suppression of the heartbeat abnormality does not always translate into improved survival. Several years ago, a large study found this to be the case with two medications in particular—encainide and flecainide. In the Cardiac Arrhythmia Suppression Trial (CAST), heart attack survivors given the drugs to control ventricular arrhythmias were more likely to experience sudden cardiac death than were patients who received no drug treatment at all. (Encainide is no longer available in the United States.)

Because of the potential problems with antiarrhythmia medications, the most powerful drugs are reserved for patients with life-threatening arrhythmias—patients whose risk for dying without treatment justifies taking a potentially dangerous medication. These drugs usually are first administered in the hospital under careful observation for as long as a week. Then they must be closely monitored for the duration of use.

Medications for Heart Failure

The ominous-sounding term *heart failure* is used to describe a loss of pumping efficiency in the heart. Less efficient pumping means that the heart must work harder to circulate blood throughout the body. The symptoms of heart failure include fatigue, weakness, shortness of breath, fluid build-up (edema), and lung congestion. The goal of medication is to reduce the heart's work load, eliminate excess fluid build-up, and, in severe cases, stimulate failing heart muscle. Vasodilators and diuretics are mainstays of treatment. Other types of medication may be added when necessary.

Vasodilators

Vasodilating drugs are important because of their ability to expand blood vessel diameter. Dilated blood vessels offer less resistance to blood flow—and that reduces the force required to circulate blood throughout the body. The principal vasodilators prescribed for heart failure are ACE inhibitors (especially captopril, enalapril, and lisinopril), nitrates, and hydralazine.

ACE inhibitors have proved to be particularly beneficial, especially in the aftermath of heart attack. Two studies—Survival of Patients with Left Ventricular Dysfunction (SOLVD) and Survival and Ventricular Enlargement (SAVE)—found that ACE inhibitor treatment lessens the structural changes and enlargement of the ventricles that may follow heart attack. (Such changes do not always follow heart attack and are very much a function of severity and extent of damage. The SOLVD and SAVE trials preselected patients who had severe impairment of ventricular function.)

Preserving ventricular structure and function, in turn, leads to improved survival. In the SAVE trial, for example, treatment with captopril reduced the risk for the development of congestive heart failure among heart attack survivors, and it reduced their risk for dying over the next four years by 19 percent. Research also suggests that captopril and enalapril lower the risk for death among patients already experiencing severe heart failure.

Diuretics

Diuretics help relieve the fluid build-up that typically accompanies heart failure. Mild heart failure often responds well to sodium and fluid restriction and diuretics. In more severe conditions, these drugs are used in combination with more powerful medications that act directly on heart muscle.

Digitalis Medications

Digitalis medications are particularly useful when arrhythmias accompany or contribute to heart failure. The benefits of treatment in cases without rhythm disturbances have been a matter of controversy. In one recent study, researchers found that patients with left ventricular heart failure who were treated with digoxin were no less likely to die than were those who took a placebo, but they were less likely to be hospitalized.

Studies indicate that 5 to 15 percent of patients experience digitalis toxicity at some point in their therapy. Digitalis has a narrow therapeutic range—meaning that a fine line exists between effectiveness and toxicity. Because effective doses can come precariously close to a dangerous level, close monitoring is essential, especially in patients without heart rhythm disturbances.

That makes it important to stay alert to the signs of toxicity—irregular heartbeats, loss of appetite, nausea, vomiting, diarrhea, mental confusion, agitation, lethargy, and visual disturbances.

Other Agents

Severe cases of heart failure may require treatment with drugs that stimulate muscle contraction in the heart. Some of the agents that can strengthen heart contraction include dopamine, dobutamine, amrinone, milrinone, and vesnarinone. Some block an enzyme called phosphodiesterase. These drugs can provide hemodynamic benefit for people whose heart's pumping ability is severely compromised. But as with most powerful cardiac medications, strength has a price—an increased risk for potentially serious side effects. These medications can overstimulate the heart and trigger arrhythmias, and they can worsen myocardial ischemia (reduced blood flow to the heart).

Carvedilol, a beta-blocker used to treat chronic heart failure, has been associated with reduced risks for death, hospitalization, and worsening disease in patients undergoing consistent concurrent therapy with diuretics, digoxin, and ACE inhibitors. In a study ended early because of the dramatic difference between the group treated with carvedilol and that taking a placebo, researchers found that while 7.8 percent of those taking the placebo died, only 3.2 percent of those on carvedilol did. Almost 1,100 patients participated in the study.

Again, treatment is a balancing act requiring your doctor to offset potential risks with benefits. He or she will select these medications carefully and closely monitor your heart's response.

Medications for Lipid Disorders

If you have an elevated cholesterol or triglyceride level that does not respond to lifestyle changes such as decreasing fat intake and increasing exercise and weight control efforts, your physician may prescribe a lipid-lowering drug. Such an agent may also be given to help increase your HDL-cholesterol level. These drugs are always given in addition to lifestyle modifications, never as a replacement for them. If your physician recommends that you begin lipid-lowering medication, you will need to continue your lifestyle efforts. There are excellent reasons to continue lifestyle modifications when drug therapy is prescribed: for example, changes in lifestyle may enable you to take a lower drug dosage, which reduces your risk for experiencing side effects from the drug. Also, lifestyle modifications improve your health in ways lipid-lowering drugs cannot, such as helping control blood pressure.

Unfortunately, in most cases in which lipid-lowering drugs are necessary, the drug therapy must be followed for a long time, perhaps even for the rest of your life. Abnormal blood lipid levels or blood pressure should be controlled with diet and exercise when at all possible. If drug treatment is necessary, your physician will consider factors such as your overall risk for coronary heart disease, your lipid goals, your age, and your medical history in deciding which drug or drugs are right for you. Many kinds of safe and effective drugs for controlling blood lipid levels are available, with differing effects on major blood lipids. Knowing how the various drugs affect lipids differently allows your doctor to tailor a drug therapy to your specific lipid problems.

The available lipid-lowering drugs fall into four classes: (1) nicotinic acid, (2) bile acid resins, (3) HMG-CoA reductase inhibitors, and (4) fibric acid derivatives. Lipid-lowering drugs may be given as single agents or in drug combinations. The major actions and side effects of the four classes of lipid-lowering drugs are described in this section.

Nicotinic Acid

Nicotinic acid, or niacin, is a B vitamin that is very effective for lowering low-density lipoprotein (LDL) cholesterol, sometimes called "bad" cholesterol. It also lowers triglyceride and raises beneficial HDL-cholesterol levels. Thus, it is useful in most lipid disorders, and it has the advantage of being fairly inexpensive. Do not confuse nicotinic acid with nicotinamide, which is also sometimes called niacin but does not lower cholesterol.

Many patients experience uncomfortable side effects with the use of nicotinic acid, including tingling sensations, warm feelings, headaches, nausea, gas, and heartburn. Nicotinic acid may also cause diarrhea, fatigue, itching, or a rash. Taking an aspirin 30 minutes before a dose of nicotinic acid, or taking the drug while you have food in your stomach, can lessen some of the side effects. Side effects are more likely to occur when you first begin taking nicotinic acid, or when the dosage is increased. Your physician will probably begin nicotinic acid at a low dosage and gradually increase it so that your body can get used to the drug.

Nicotinic acid is prepared in both immediate-release and slow-release formulas; however, the slow-release form entails increased risk for liver damage (the U.S. Food and Drug Administration has yet to approve slow-release preparations for treatment of cholesterol disorders). Nicotinic acid is not used in patients with chronic liver disease and not usually in patients with diabetes mellitus (it can worsen glucose intolerance). While taking nicotinic acid, be sure to discuss with your doctor the routine blood tests needed to make sure that other side effects are not occurring.

Another important consideration with nicotinic acid is its over-the-counter availability. The amounts of niacin found in multivitamin supplements are too small to affect cholesterol, and the dosages of niacin-only supplements needed to affect cholesterol are too high to be administered without safety monitoring. You should not attempt to self-medicate with niacin for the purposes of cholesterol lowering: the side effects can be serious, and proper medical supervision is required.

Bile Acid Resins

Bile acid resins are also called *bile acid sequestrants,* or simply *resins.* The resins available in the United States are cholestyramine and colestipol. The resins are chiefly active in lowering LDL-cholesterol. They may slightly increase HDL-cholesterol. They can also increase triglyceride level.

The resins are attractive solutions for lowering cholesterol because they do not seem to enter the bloodstream. The resins work by binding bile acids in the intestines and are eliminated in the stool. The body manufactures bile acids from cholesterol. When the bile acid level drops, the liver begins to produce more bile acid by drawing cholesterol out of the blood, thus reducing blood cholesterol. Some side effects associated with bile acid resins are constipation, bloating, gas, and heartburn. Increasing consumption of fluids and fiber can help relieve constipation if it occurs, and trying not to swallow air when taking the resin can help prevent gas. Mixing the scoops or packets of resin with noncarbonated rather than carbonated liquids may help prevent belching. Also, "light" and tablet preparations are available, and these may be more palatable. Side effects, if they occur, usually lessen over time.

Resins can interfere with the absorption in the intestine of other medications; therefore, it is important that you check with your physician about when to take other medications if you are taking a resin. Patients with a history of severe constipation or a triglyceride level higher than 500 mg/dl should not take bile acid resins because they may worsen these problems.

HMG-CoA Reductase Inhibitors

HMG-CoA reductase inhibitors, known more familiarly as *statins,* interfere with the body's ability to manufacture its own cholesterol, thus reducing blood cholesterol level. (*HMG-CoA* is an abbreviation for 3-hydroxy-3-methylglutaryl coenzyme A.) Approved in the United States are atorvastatin (Lipitor), fluvastatin (Lescol), lovastatin (Mevacor), pravastatin (Pravachol), and simvastatin (Zocor). The HMG-

CoA reductase inhibitors as a class are the most effective drugs for reducing LDL-cholesterol levels. All also may increase HDL-cholesterol moderately. Atorvastatin decreases triglyceride substantially; the other statins decrease it moderately. All the statins are easy to take and have good safety records.

Rare side effects have included inflammation and muscle ailments, so alert your physician if you experience any unexplained muscle weakness or pain while taking a statin. Statins are not used in patients with confirmed or suspected liver disease or in women who are pregnant, likely to become pregnant, or breast-feeding. As with any drug, your physician will consider other factors (such as other drugs you are taking) and potential side effects in deciding whether a statin is the best lipid-lowering drug for you. Your physician will order routine blood tests to measure your liver enzymes before you begin taking a statin and will monitor their levels periodically thereafter.

Fibric Acid Derivatives

Fibric acid derivatives, or fibrates, are well tolerated and are effective in lowering triglyceride and raising HDL-cholesterol levels. Their effect on LDL-cholesterol levels is variable: they can substantially lower them, but in some cases they may even raise them, depending on the triglyceride level. Fibrates available in the United States are gemfibrozil and clofibrate, but clofibrate is rarely used in this country. A third, fenofibrate, is approved for use, but currently unavailable.

Fibrates are not used in patients with liver or severe kidney disease, or in patients with gallbladder disease. As with statin treatment, your physician will need to use routine blood tests to monitor your liver enzyme levels during therapy with a fibrate. Such side effects as nausea, diarrhea, or gallstone development are rare.

Estrogen-replacement Therapy

In postmenopausal women, estrogen-replacement therapy has been shown to cause beneficial changes in blood lipid levels. However, the FDA does not classify estrogen therapy as a lipid-altering treatment. The issue of estrogen-replacement therapy is discussed in greater detail in Chapter 25.

Gene Therapy

Gene therapy is the process of introducing into a cell a functioning copy of a gene that is defective or missing. A gene is the biologic unit of heredity; it is located at a definite position on a particular chromosome. Because many disorders have been linked to mutated (irregular) or missing genes, introducing a replacement is one way scientists have attempted to resolve these diseases. If all goes well, the new gene will be incorporated into the cell's DNA (which carries genetic information) and will restore normal function. While the concept is simple, the execution is not. Genes can be delivered into cells in a special form called a vector. Two popular vectors are retroviruses and adenoviruses. A third method involves mixing the gene with special lipids to form a structure called a liposome for gene delivery.

Retroviral Vectors

Viruses, as we are all aware, can make us sick. They do this by taking over the genetic machinery of our cells to make copies of themselves. A retrovirus is a type of virus used in gene transfer therapy. Retroviruses used for this purpose are first changed so that they cannot make copies of themselves, thus neutralizing their danger as viral agents. The new gene that will be transferred is then inserted into the genes of the retrovirus, and the retroviral vector is delivered into the cell. Once inside the cell, the retrovirus cannot reproduce itself, but it can take over the cell's genetic machinery and insert its gene into the host cell's DNA. Once the cell's DNA has been altered, the cell will replicate and create copies of itself containing the new gene.

The main disadvantage of retroviral vectors is that they require a dividing cell in order to integrate the new gene into the cellular chromosome. Thus, all of this must be done in cells that have been taken out of the body. Once the cells have begun to express the retrovirus's gene, they are reinjected into the body. Retroviral vectors are often difficult and inefficient to make and to use, and it is hard to get enough of the modified cells back into the body to make a difference.

Adenoviral Vectors

Adenoviruses are another type of virus used for gene transfer therapy. For treating vascular diseases, adenoviral vectors are probably better than retroviral vectors. Adenoviral vectors can be applied directly to cells in the body and can affect cells that do not replicate, neither of which is possible with retroviral vectors. However, the effects of adenoviral vectors disappear quickly, because the body recognizes the cells that contain the adenovirus and destroys them.

Liposome–DNA Complexes

A liposome, which is a spherical particle, can be used to transport molecules and other particles into a cell. Liposome–DNA complexes are liposomes that contain DNA in which the desired gene has been inserted. Once the liposome has inserted its DNA complex into the cell, the DNA can work its gene into the host cell's DNA. Like adenoviral vectors, liposome–DNA complexes may be useful for vascular gene therapy.

Vascular Gene Therapy

Using the vectors described above, there are several potential applications that might improve cardiac health. Gene vectors might be useful to increase the cellular expression of molecules and compounds that improve or restore the normal function of diseased blood vessels. Also, gene therapy might be used to correct genetically caused lipid disorders such as familial hypercholesterolemia. Another possible application is to use gene therapy to encourage the body to develop collateral vessels, which are those vessels that bypass a severely blocked artery. This last application might be especially important, because it may reduce the need for bypass grafting and angioplasty. Another application may be the use of gene therapy to control the immune response to heart transplantation; such a treatment might reduce the chances of transplant rejection without the increased toxicity associated with some conventional immunosuppressive treatments. As the genetic mechanisms underlying left ventricular hypertrophy become better understood, possible gene therapies may present themselves.

Realistically, however, gene therapy is probably many years away from becoming a practical treatment option. Although studies of gene transfer in animals have provided encouraging results, results in humans have been more mixed. Gene vectors injected into humans often fail to produce the desired results, and changes prove to be temporary, disappearing within days or weeks after treatment. Given gene therapy's status as a relatively new technology, these setbacks seem a part of the expected process and do little to discourage optimism about gene therapy as a promising avenue of research for the twenty-first century.

CHAPTER TWENTY-EIGHT

Cardiac Rehabilitation: The Healing Heart

You've had a heart attack, had coronary bypass surgery, or undergone balloon angioplasty. What kind of life can you lead now? Can you return to the busy lifestyle your work and family demand? Is it safe to play tennis or swim? Will you need to hire someone to perform chores in the house and yard? Should you just take it easy to lessen the chance of doing additional damage to your heart? What kinds of foods should you eat? Should you try to avoid all stressful situations?

These questions and many more are familiar to every person who has undergone a major coronary event or surgical procedure. Heart attacks are scary experiences, and some find cardiac diagnostic and therapeutic procedures challenging as well. It is only natural to be concerned about what the future holds.

With modern technologic and medical advances, more people than ever before are surviving cardiac events. But survival is only the beginning. Healing the heart is a complex process that takes time, effort,

and the commitment of many people. An individual's rate of recovery will depend on his or her physical condition, cardiac risk factors, and emotional state. Numerous other factors are important, too. Thanks to the discoveries and efforts of modern rehabilitative medicine, thousands of patients with cardiovascular disease or damage eventually do return to living rich, satisfying lives with a new appreciation for the remarkable power of the human body to survive and recover.

Rehabilitation after stroke is discussed in Chapter 20. Remember that not every medical facility offers every rehabilitation service; options vary among facilities. This chapter describes general principles.

Recovery, Risk Reduction, and Renewal

The past 40 years have brought profound changes to the medical community's attitude toward patients with cardiovascular disease. In the early 1950s, patients who survived a serious heart attack, for example, typically were confined to bed for several weeks and faced a period of invalidism that could last for years and perhaps even for the remainder of their lives. Today, however, health care professionals work to restrict the progression of the disease, to return the patient to a full and productive life, and to reduce the risk for coronary death in the future. This process often is called *cardiac rehabilitation.*

In its earliest years, cardiac rehabilitation primarily focused on assisting the patient with uncomplicated heart attack (myocardial infarction). Today, advances in coronary artery disease treatment and the proven effectiveness of cardiac rehabilitation have drawn increased numbers of patients into rehabilitation activities. Some patients who have undergone coronary artery bypass surgery or coronary angioplasty receive rehabilitative care. Cardiac rehabilitation today also reaches more elderly patients, many of whom have severe, complicated coronary illnesses.

Cardiac rehabilitation includes education, risk factor modification, and exercise training activities designed to restore cardiac patients to physically, emotionally, socially, and economically satisfying lives. The short-term goals of cardiac rehabilitation are the following:

- To help patients regain physical conditioning so that they can return to their routine activities.

- To educate patients and family members about the disease.
- To offer emotional support.

The long-term goals are the following:

- To identify and modify the risk factors that were involved in the progression of the disease.
- To teach patients about healthy lifestyle behaviors.
- To improve physical conditioning.
- To help patients return to work and social activities.

Cardiac rehabilitation requires the efforts of a multidisciplinary team of experts, which may include, in addition to physicians and nurses, an exercise physiologist, a psychologist or psychiatrist, physical and occupational therapists, a registered dietitian, a social worker, and a chaplain. These team members work together to develop a comprehensive rehabilitative program that is tailored to the physical, intellectual, spiritual, and psychosocial needs of the individual patient.

The Cardiac Rehabilitation Program

Although cardiac rehabilitation programs can vary in their organization, they typically involve at least six months of time and are offered in a framework of four phases. Patients move through these phases at varying rates, depending on their age, their condition before they suffered the cardiac event, the severity of their illness, and their motivation. Other factors that may affect a patient's progression through the phases include insurance coverage and the availability of specific types of rehabilitation programs in the patient's geographic location.

Phase I: Inpatient Rehabilitation

Phase I of rehabilitation begins as soon as a patient who has suffered an acute coronary event or undergone cardiac surgery is stable; it lasts throughout the hospitalization period. While in the hospital, the cardiac patient may undergo a variety of diagnostic tests to help the physician determine the extent of the damage to the heart and plan the patient's recovery. Such tests may include electrocardiography (ECG or EKG), cardiac catheterization, an exercise stress test, and a thallium stress test. (See Chapters 5 and 6 for more information on diagnostic tests.)

An important component of phase I cardiac rehabilitation is early mobilization—helping the patient progressively resume physical activity. Mobilizing the cardiac patient is very important, since prolonged bed rest can lead to a variety of problems, including decreases in skeletal muscle mass and strength, orthopedic impairment, decreases in blood volume, and pulmonary abnormalities such as diminished lung volume and vital capacity. Early mobilization speeds the patient toward resuming normal daily activities and lessens the patient's feelings of anxiety and depression.

Therapists will begin the physical activity program by having the patient perform simple range-of-motion activities. At first, the therapist will move the patient's arms and legs, but the patient soon will progress to moving his or her own limbs. The patient then will perform such simple, nonstrenuous activities as sitting up in bed, brushing the teeth, and washing the face and hands. Since the length of the hospital stay after uncomplicated myocardial infarction or cardiac surgery is relatively brief, the amount of time that the rehabilitation team has with the patient during phase I often is limited. For this reason, the cardiac rehabilitation staff frequently will begin to work with cardiac patients on basic self-care activities very early in the hospital stay, sometimes even while the patients are still in the intensive care unit.

Once the patient is moved from the intensive care unit to a regular hospital room, the rehabilitation staff assists the patient in gradually resuming more physical and self-care activities. While the schedule will depend on the individual's condition, patients eventually progress from sitting up in a chair briefly to walking for increasingly longer time periods and to climbing stairs on a limited basis. Members of the rehabilitation team supervise the activities and monitor heart rate and blood pressure before, during, and after exertion.

The other important component of phase I cardiac rehabilitation is education and counseling for both the patient and the family. Initially, rehabilitation staff will talk with patients about their medical or surgical condition, answer any questions, and familiarize them with relevant hospital equipment, regulations, and procedures. As the time of discharge approaches, staff members will provide more detailed information about coronary disease management and teach patients how to take their pulse, how to recognize important symptoms, and how to obtain emergency medical care. In addition, team members will talk with patients about their cardiovascular risk factors.

Early intervention to control risk factors is advised. Patients should be instructed to follow a low-cholesterol, low-fat, diet (see pp. 422) before hospital discharge. For patients who have had a heart attack, many specialists recommend beginning cholesterol-lowering drugs called statins at the time of discharge if low-density lipoprotein (LDL) cholesterol is elevated (greater than 100 mg/dl). (The physician may base this decision on LDL-cholesterol levels before the heart attack,

because the LDL-cholesterol level may be artificially low after a heart attack and fail to stabilize completely for four to six weeks.) Other drugs, such as aspirin or beta-blockers, also may be given to reduce future risk.

During phase I, the patient's physician and the rest of the rehabilitation team will work together to develop a more formal program of rehabilitation activities for the future. They will tailor this program to the individual patient's needs, medical and surgical history, and functional capabilities and limitations. At the time of discharge from the hospital, each patient receives very specific advice about resuming familiar activities at home. The patient's spouse and other close family members should all be present when this information is given, if possible, so that everyone involved in the patient's care can ask questions and hear the same information at the same time. To get the most out of working with the rehabilitation team, patients must get the information they need to understand how to work toward full recovery (Figure 28.1).

Phase II: Therapeutic Exercise Training

Phase II begins the outpatient period of cardiac rehabilitation. It typically lasts for two to 12 weeks. Ideally, phase II should begin as soon as possible after a patient has been discharged from the hospital, and

A Patient's Guide to Working with the Cardiac Rehabilitation Team

- Do not be afraid to ask questions. No question should be considered foolish, trite, or inappropriate.
- Write down your questions in advance.
- Write down the answers from the rehabilitation team (or have a family member or friend write down the answers for you).
- Do not be embarrassed to ask for explanations and definitions of abbreviations and technical terms.
- Topics that you may wish to ask about include:
    - Your specific medical condition and prospects for recovery.
    - Exercise and physical activity.
    - Routine activities (such as housework and climbing stairs).
    - Self-care activities (such as bathing).
    - Sexual activity.
    - Diet.
    - Emotions.
    - Care of incisions.
    - Medications (names, purposes, dosages, desired effects, side effects).
    - Returning to work.
    - Symptoms to be concerned about.
    - Schedule for follow-up visits.
    - Coronary care support groups and other community resources for cardiac patients and family members.

Figure 28.1. Getting the most out of cardiac rehabilitation requires that the patient work with the rehabilitation team by asking questions and exploring options for all aspects of recovery and maintenance.

extend to the time when ordinary activities can be resumed. During phase II, patients gradually can resume additional self-care activities such as shaving, showering, and dressing, and can increase their level of supervised physical activity. They may be given exercises to do at home, such as walking at a moderate pace and stationary cycling. Patients with intermediate-risk and high-risk coronary disease will require medically supervised exercise training with ECG monitoring on either an intermittent or a continuous basis. The rehabilitation team will teach the patient about appropriate types of exercise, correct exercise techniques, how to check exercise intensity, and what symptoms to monitor. They also should give the patient detailed written instructions to refer to at home. All patients are encouraged to take part in medically supervised aerobic exercise programs when available at a local cardiac rehabilitation facility or hospital. If patients do not have access to such a facility, they may be able to resume exercising on their own if they are at low risk, but they must have their doctor's permission before they begin any type of exercise program.

Physical activity offers numerous benefits for the patient with cardiovascular disease. Not only does activity improve the patient's physical and emotional health, but also it maintains muscle tone and joint mobility and prevents physical deconditioning. The type of exercise plan that a rehabilitation team develops for a patient will be based on a number of factors, including age, medical condition, risk, current exercise capacity, and previous level of physical fitness. The individual's skills, likes and dislikes, and access to exercise facilities and equipment also are factors. Along with identifying the types of recommended physical activities, the exercise plan should specify the duration, frequency, and progression of practice.

Patient education and counseling are other important components of phase II cardiac rehabilitation, just as they are in phase I cardiac rehabilitation. Modifying risk factors and changing harmful health habits are not only important in preventing cardiovascular disease, but also is crucial in improving recovery. Quitting cigarette smoking, limiting dietary fat intake, losing weight if necessary, and controlling hypertension and diabetes can help limit progression of atherosclerosis and decrease risk for future adverse cardiovascular events. (See Chapter 7 for a discussion about risk factors and their role in the development and progression of atherosclerosis.)

Phases III and IV: Late Recovery and Maintenance

During phases III and IV of cardiac rehabilitation, patients should be able to maintain the benefits they have gained from phases I and II, while continuing to progress in their rehabilitation and recovery with less medical supervision. Once the patient has achieved the designated level of physical activity, maintenance becomes the primary goal of the exercise program. Patients usually remain in a phase III program for six to 12 months before moving to phase IV, which is primarily self-directed. However, participation in a phase III program may last indefinitely for some intermediate-risk or high-risk patients. Since the ultimate goal for almost every patient with cardiovascular disease is a physically active lifestyle, exercise programs in phases III and IV should include a variety of activities that the patient considers to be enjoyable, interesting, convenient, social, and appropriate.

Recovery from Specific Cardiac Events

Heart Attack

A heart attack can be a frightening experience, but the heart begins to heal soon after any nonfatal heart attack. Although part of the heart dies, the remainder continues to work. In some patients, within two to three weeks after the attack a system of new arterial branches forms, supplying the area previously served by the narrowed or blocked coronary artery.

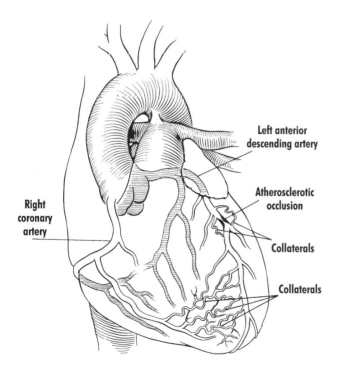

Figure 28.2. After a major cardiac event such as a heart attack, new arterial branches of collateral circulation, commonly called collaterals, develop.

This system is called *collateral circulation* (Figure 28.2; see also Figure 17.1).

When a major artery is narrowed or blocked by atherosclerosis or another problem, the blood may be able to detour around the blockage, reenter the artery beyond the damage, and continue on its way. To understand this process, imagine a highway that is blocked by damage from an earthquake. Drivers may be able to exit the highway and use small streets more or less parallel to the highway and then to reenter it at a point beyond the obstruction. Since the small streets will not easily accommodate the heavy traffic of the highway, engineers and their crews will try to widen them as quickly as possible. If their efforts are successful, widening the small streets may ultimately allow a nearly normal flow of traffic. In other words, the small streets may adequately replace the damaged section of highway.

These collateral vessels may have been present since birth. Blood flow redirected through these collateral vessels after major vessels are blocked makes the collateral vessels visible on angiograms (akin to spare tires or pinch hitters, they are usually not seen until they are put into service). Like the small roads described above, the collateral vessels need to be remodeled to handle their new duties. New cells are added to expand the vessels, including endothelial cells to pave the innermost lining of the vessel and smooth muscle cells to increase the strength of the vessel wall. Also, rather like alleyways, new microvessels, including arterioles and capillaries, form to direct the blood to its final destination.

Individuals who have good collateral circulation do better in terms of symptom relief and prognosis after an acute vascular event such as a heart attack. However, these individuals are not a majority, and the remodeling work is less than satisfactory in most people. The formation of collateral vessels is often too slow to maintain sufficient circulation, and the blood-deprived tissue (such as heart muscle) is damaged. Another way to go around the blockage in the artery is to transplant a vessel from another part of the body, as in coronary artery bypass grafting (see Chapters 15 and 18). Whereas collateral formation is like waiting for a local crew to expand small roads (which may or may not be present), bypass grafting is comparable to airlifting in a whole new section of highway.

What factors govern the growth of native collateral vessels is not entirely understood, although researchers have recently shown that both atherosclerosis and elevated blood cholesterol concentrations impair compensatory blood vessel growth. One reason is that the oxidized form of LDL inhibits the production of a very important growth factor called *basic fibroblast growth factor.*

Investigations are under way to promote collateral vessel growth, and it is very likely that in the future physicians will be able to give growth factors to patients to enlarge collateral vessels. This approach may someday allow a delay of, or eliminate the need for, surgical bypass in some patients.

The extent of a patient's collateral circulation is only one factor governing the rate of recovery from a heart attack. Rate of recovery also depends on a number of other factors, including the extent of the injury, the patient's general health, and the condition of the rest of the heart. Within six weeks, tough scar tissue forms to "strengthen" the damaged heart muscle. The healthy part of the heart muscle takes over the work of the damaged part and works to restore normal pumping action. While each person is different, healing of the heart muscle usually happens in four to six weeks.

A patient who has returned home after a heart attack may feel weak. The cause is probably loss of strength in muscles of the body due to physical inactivity. Once the patient begins the recommended program of gradually increased physical activity, the muscles will start to regain strength. The average interval between an uncomplicated heart attack and return to work is 70 to 90 days. This period may be substantially shortened, however, by carefully coordinating the rehabilitation program.

Most heart attack victims are able to resume their previous activities within a few weeks or months. Like all patients with heart disease or damage, those who have had a heart attack will need to make changes to move toward a more healthy lifestyle, including eating a low-fat diet and quitting smoking. Most heart attack victims survive their first attack and go on to recover and enjoy many more productive years of life.

Coronary Artery Bypass Surgery

Coronary artery bypass operations are designed to return patients with coronary artery disease to good health. Like heart attack or stroke survivors, patients who have undergone coronary artery bypass surgery should be strongly encouraged to make such lifestyle changes as reducing dietary fat and quitting smoking, and they may benefit from phase I rehabilitation.

A patient who has undergone a coronary bypass operation probably will feel weak upon returning home because of the period of extended bed rest in the hospital. In some cases, entry into a phase II rehabilitation program may be very beneficial. Strength should begin to return within a few weeks after the surgery, especially once the patient is able to begin such moderate physical activities as walking. The physician should be contacted if the patient experiences signs of infection at the incision, fever, increased fatigue, chills, shortness of breath, change in heart rate or rhythm, swelling of the ankles, or sudden weight gain.

After bypass surgery, patients who have sedentary jobs usually can return to work in about four to eight weeks. Those patients with jobs that require heavy physical activity probably will need to wait eight to 12 weeks before returning to their jobs. Bypass patients can begin driving whenever they feel physically able to operate a vehicle safely. Usually it is advisable to wait until at least a few weeks after leaving the hospital before starting to drive again.

Sexual activity may be resumed, on the average, about two months postoperatively; however, there may be considerable variability in the time of resumption of all the activities described above. Physician consultation is always advisable, and response to treadmill exercise testing is often helpful.

Special Concerns in Healing the Heart

Dealing with Emotions

An important, yet sometimes overlooked, factor in successful recovery after a cardiac event or procedure is confronting and dealing with the emotions faced by patients with cardiovascular disease. It is normal to feel apprehensive after suffering a heart attack, stroke, or other coronary event, or after undergoing cardiovascular surgery. After all, patients in rehabilitation have just been through a serious, life-threatening illness or procedure. Patients are in a strange setting, away from home and family, dealing with pain, and surrounded by unfamiliar equipment and instruments. They are unsure of the adjustments and lifestyle changes they are going to need to make in the future and do not know if they are going to be able to return to the routine activities of daily life. They probably also are worried about suffering another heart attack or having another type of cardiac problem. All these concerns naturally can lead to a variety of emotions: anxiety, depression, irritability, anger, fear, and a feeling of vulnerability. Family members may be feeling many of the same emotions.

Medical experts now realize that a patient's attitude can have a great impact on the outlook for his or her recovery. For this reason, many cardiac rehabilitation teams include experts who can help the patient and family members start to deal with their feelings and emotions before the patient even leaves the hospital. Community cardiac rehabilitation centers or hospitals often offer counseling and stress management classes that can be beneficial to both the patient and the family once the patient has returned home. Many patients find it helpful to become involved in organizations that allow patients and their families to share information and experi-

ences. Some of these are called *coronary clubs*.

Patients should be reassured by the fact that, by following the recommended physical activity plan, eating a healthy diet, not smoking, taking the appropriate medications, and adhering to the other recommendations made by the cardiac rehabilitation team, they are taking actions to decrease their chances of experiencing additional cardiac problems. It also may help patients improve their psychological well-being if they realize that there are many strategies for coping with illnesses and other serious situations, and that no one way is right or wrong. Some people tend to ask many *why* questions, and want to know all the details about *how* what has happened to them will affect them and *how* the rehabilitation plan that has been recommended for them will help. Other patients do not want to know *how* and *why*—all the technicalities—but just want to know *what* they need to do to improve their condition and future outlook. Whatever a patient's preferred coping strategy, he or she should feel free to ask the rehabilitation team about the medical condition, the recovery period, and any other concern. Education and understanding give most people a sense of control and make them feel more optimistic about the future.

For most patients, irritability, fear, and depression will fade with time, usually after two to six months. If the patient experiences warning signs of serious depression, the physician should be consulted. Such signs include sleep problems (either excessive sleeping or difficulty sleeping), appetite problems, extreme fatigue, emotional stress, loss of alertness, abnormal slowness of speaking, apathy, low self-esteem, and despair. While depression can be related to anxiety or feelings of loss of control, it also can be a side effect of medications used to treat cardiovascular problems. After evaluation, physicians can make a decision about the cause and recommend appropriate treatment.

Resuming Sexual Activity

Sexual activity is a major concern among patients in cardiac rehabilitation. Patients want to know when sexual activity can be resumed after the heart has been damaged. Sometimes, too, they are worried that sexual activity might lead to heart attack or even death. Recent research provides reassuring results that show that the risk of sexual activity's triggering a heart attack is low.

Giving a boost to rehabilitation efforts, researchers have concluded that regular exercise can reduce and perhaps eliminate the triggering of a heart attack. In contrast, a sedentary lifestyle has been linked with significantly higher risk of heart attack within two hours of sexual activity.

Physicians have generally recommended that a patient wait four to six weeks after a heart attack before resuming sexual activity, to allow sufficient time for healing. Because each individual's medical condition and personal situation are different, it is best for patients to discuss the subject with their own physician before leaving the hospital. If a person is enrolled in an outpatient rehabilitation program after suffering a heart attack or undergoing coronary artery bypass surgery, heart rate and blood pressure response to submaximal exercise will provide information useful in deciding when to resume sexual activity, as well as when to return to work.

Sexual activity is a topic that people often are embarrassed to discuss. Though initiating the topic may be difficult, patients should feel free to direct questions to their cardiac rehabilitation team. The patient's physician and other team members should be comfortable talking about sexual issues and be able to give individualized guidelines and advice for resuming sexual activity. Some medications can decrease sexual function, so any changes should be discussed with the physician. A patient should not quit taking any medications without the physician's approval.

Returning to Work

Not all patients in cardiac rehabilitation choose to return to work. Those who can return to work benefit psychologically, socially, and financially. The possibility of returning to work after hospitalization is influenced by a number of factors, including the patient's age, motivation, medical condition, satisfaction with his or her job, and the amount of physical activity that is involved in the job. Members of the cardiac rehabilitation team will look at such factors, as well as the results of exercise testing, to make recommendations for types of activities that a patient can safely pursue both at home and at work. Some cardiac patients decide to return to work on a part-time basis or to find a job that is less stressful or requires less physical exertion.

Summary

Cardiac rehabilitation reaches out to many patients with cardiac problems and works to ensure recovery through a phased phys-

ical rebuilding program, risk reduction through lifestyle changes and medication, and a psychological adjustment born of the cardiac event and a committed response. Like other health care relationships between professionals and patients, cardiac rehabilitation succeeds best when a partnership between professionals and patients forges forthright give-and-take and common understanding that encourage action. Like each patient, each specific cardiac condition, event, or surgery has characteristics of its own that need to be taken into consideration in rehabilitation. Also important to success are confronting and dealing with emotions, thereby freeing the patient to resume an active life that may extend for many years.

Glossary

ABDOMINAL ANGINA—A condition caused by occlusive disease of the celiac and superior mesenteric arteries, characterized by abdominal pain after eating and progressive loss of weight.

ABLATION—Removal of a part of the body by excision or amputation.

ACE INHIBITORS—A short name for angiotensin-converting enzyme inhibitors, which are blood pressure medicines that improve blood flow by dilating blood vessels, counteract some negative aspects of diuretic treatment, and ameliorate heart failure and diabetes-associated nerve damage.

ACIDOSIS—A metabolic condition characterized by a high acid content of the blood or body tissues. Acidosis may result from failure of the lungs to remove carbon dioxide (respiratory acidosis) or from overproduction of acid substances in the body's tissues (metabolic acidosis).

ADENOSINE TRIPHOSPHATE (ATP)—A chemical compound present in all cells representing a stored form of energy.

ADIPOSE TISSUE—Fat cells or fat tissue of the body.

ADRENAL CORTEX—The outer, firm, yellowish layer that comprises the larger part of the adrenal gland, where hormones of the cortisol family are produced.

ADRENALINE—A hormone secreted by the adrenal medulla that has profound effects on blood vessels, the heart, and the bronchioles in the lungs. It is synonymous with epinephrine. The hormone's actions on the heart, arterioles, and bronchioles have been classified as alpha and beta. At concentrations above those causing beta effects, the alpha actions predominate, especially the contraction of arterioles, which leads to a rise in blood pressure. The beta effects, which may be at relatively low levels, include relaxing the smooth muscle of the arterioles and bronchioles but stimulating the rate and contracting force of the heart.

ADRENAL MEDULLA—The innermost part of the adrenal gland; it secretes adrenaline and noradrenaline.

ADVENTITIA—The outermost layer of the arterial wall. Rich in connective tissue and nerve fibers, it contains a specialized group of blood vessels called the *vasa vasorum.*

AEROBIC CAPACITY—The maximum amount of oxygen uptake achievable during exercise.

ALBUMIN—A protein made by the liver and transported in the blood. It helps maintain the fluid level within the vascular tree and transports fatty acids.

ALDOSTERONE—The principal electrolyte-regulating steroid secreted by the cortex of the adrenal gland.

ALPHA-METHYLDOPA—An orally effective hyposensitive agent related to the catecholamines used in the treatment of essential hypertension.

ALVEOLI—Small air sacs in the lung from which blood receives oxygen and gives off carbon dioxide.

AMYLOID—A protein structure that may collect in tissues in certain diseases.

ANABOLISM—Those metabolic reactions in which cells or tissues and large molecules are synthesized or build up.

ANAEROBIC REACTION—A reaction that occurs in the absence of oxygen.

ANASTOMOSIS—A connection between vessels, grafts, or both.

ANEURYSM—Balloonlike sac formed by dilation of the walls of an artery damaged by arteriosclerosis.

ANGINA PECTORIS—Spasmodic chest pains, usually resulting from decreased blood flow to the heart caused by atherosclerotic disease of the coronary arteries.

ANGINA PECTORIS, STABLE—Angina pectoris that occurs in attacks of predictable frequency and duration after stimuli such as exercise or emotional stress.

ANGINA PECTORIS, UNSTABLE—Angina pectoris that is unpredictable or suddenly increasing in frequency or severity, often unprovoked, not responsive to nitroglycerin, and of unusually long duration.

ANGINA PECTORIS, VARIANT—Angina pectoris in which there is focal spasm of a coronary artery, often considered a form of unstable angina; also called *Prinzmetal's angina.*

ANGIOGRAM—X-ray visualization of blood vessels after injection of a radiopaque substance into a blood vessel.

ANGIOGRAPHY—Visualization by x-ray of arteries or veins after injection of a radiopaque substance.

ANGIOGRAPHY, RADIONUCLIDE—A noninvasive diagnostic technique for visualizing blood vessels and the heart that uses radionuclide-labeled substances and a scintillation camera.

ANGIOPLASTY—Surgical repair of a blood vessel.

ANGIOTENSIN II—A vasoconstrictor substance present in the blood and formed by the action of renin on a globulin of the blood plasma.

ANKLE/BRACHIAL INDEX—The ratio of systolic ankle blood pressure to systolic brachial (arm) blood pressure. The ratio, which should normally be 1.0 or greater, can help detect vascular disease in the lower extremities. Also called *systolic index.*

ANOXIA–The condition that results in the absence or lack of oxygen in the blood.

ANTAGONISTS, BETA-ADRENERGIC—*See* BETA-BLOCKERS.

ANTIBIOTIC—A chemical substance produced by microorganisms and capable of inhibiting or killing other microorganisms.

ANTICOAGULANT—A substance that suppresses, delays, or prevents clotting of blood.

ANTIPLATELET AGENTS—Drugs, such as aspirin, or other substances that prevent the aggregation of platelets to reduce the tendency to thrombosis (clot formation).

AORTA—The main artery carrying blood from the heart to the rest of the body. The ascending aorta is that part between the heart and the aortic arch where it turns to become the descending aorta. The aorta within the chest, or thorax, is known as the *thoracic aorta* and within the abdomen is called the *abdominal aorta.*

AORTIC ARCH—The place in the aorta at which it curves from an upward to a downward direction within the chest, or thoracic, cavity.

AORTOGRAPHY—The procedure of x-ray visualization of the aorta after injection of a radiopaque substance into the lumen of the aorta.

APHASIA—Loss of the ability of expression by speech.

APOPLEXY—An old term for stroke, mostly associated with intracranial hemorrhage.

APOPTOSIS—Programmed cell death.

ARRHYTHMIA—Any variation from the normal rhythm of the heartbeat.

ARRHYTHMIA, FOCAL—A type of abnormal heart rhythm caused when electrical impulses are fired independently from an abnormal focus, or area of tissue, upsetting normal patterns.

ARRHYTHMIA, REENTRY—An abnormal heart rhythm caused when a propagated impulse is blocked, slowing and redirecting the impulse on an alternate pathway from which it reenters the original path.

ARTERIOGRAM—X-ray picture of the lumen, or channel, of an artery made by injection of a radiopaque substance into the blood. *See* RADIOPAQUE.

ARTERIOGRAPHY—Method of x-ray visualization of the arteries after injection of a radiopaque substance into the lumen of the arteries.

ARTERIOLES—Small, muscular vessels that are formed from the small branches of the arteries. The arterioles then branch to form the capillaries.

ARTERIOSCLEROSIS—Disease of the arteries often referred to as hardening of the arteries. It includes and is often used synonymously with atherosclerosis. Whereas atherosclerosis refers primarily to disease of the intima (innermost layer of arterial wall), arteriosclerosis may also include disease of the arterial media (middle arterial wall layer).

ARTERITIS—Inflammation of the arteries.

ARTERY—A vessel that carries blood from the heart to the tissues of the body, ending in small branches called arterioles, which, in turn, branch to form the capillaries.

ASSIST DEVICES—Systems devised to support the functions of the heart that perform outside the body or within it after implantation.

ASYMPTOMATIC—Without symptoms.

ASYSTOLE—Complete cessation of contraction of the heart.

ATHEROMA—See ATHEROMATOUS PLAQUE.

ATHEROMATOUS PLAQUE—Focal deposition of lipid (fatty material) and other substances within the intimal layer of the artery, which may progress to narrow or block the lumen of an artery and is the most common cause of heart attacks and strokes. Sometimes called *atheroma*.

ATHEROSCLEROSIS—A form of arteriosclerosis in which lipids are deposited initially within the intimal layer of the artery and which causes most strokes and heart attacks. It is associated with growth of smooth muscle cells and other changes in the arterial wall.

ATHEROSCLEROTIC CORONARY ARTERY DISEASE—A form of hardening of the arteries in which cholesterol and other lipids accumulate within the arterial wall of the coronary arteries, at first affecting primarily the intimal layer of the artery, but eventually leading to narrowing or occlusion of the vessel.

ATP—Abbreviation for adenosine triphosphate, a chemical compound present in all cells, representing a stored form of energy.

ATRIA—The small antechambers of the heart that receive blood from the lungs and body.

ATRIAL FIBRILLATION—A type of heart irregularity in which the atrial contractions are poor, irregular, and not coordinated with those of the ventricle.

ATRIAL SEPTAL DEFECT—An opening in the septum between the right and left atrial (upper) chambers of the heart, permitting the mixing of blood between the chambers.

ATRIOVENTRICULAR BLOCK—See HEART BLOCK.

ATRIOVENTRICULAR DISSOCIATION—A condition in which no relation exists between atrial contractions and ventricular contractions.

ATRIOVENTRICULAR NODE—The specialized bundle of muscle and nerve tissue located in the wall of the right ventricle. It is stimulated by impulses from the sinoatrial node to discharge impulses that result in contraction of the heart muscle.

ATROPHY—The wasting away or diminution in size of a tissue or cell.

AURICLES—Upper chambers of the heart that receive blood from the veins.

AUSCULTATION—The diagnostic procedure of listening to sounds produced in the body.

AUTOREGULATION—In neurology, the automatic adjustment of blood flow to different areas of the brain according to need and despite blood pressure variance, ensuring a constant overall supply.

BACTERIAL ENDOCARDITIS—Inflammation of the endocardium (inner lining membrane of the heart) caused by bacteria, such as hemolytic streptococci or staphylococci, and often leading to deformity of the valves.

BALLOON ANGIOPLASTY—See PERCUTANEOUS TRANSLUMINAL ANGIOPLASTY.

BALL-VALVE PRINCIPLE—Involves a ball that fits in a cage over a cup-shaped opening in the seat. As the ball rises in the cage, fluid or air escapes through the opening in the seat; as the ball falls into the seat, the valve closes and thus prevents the escaped material from passing back through the opening.

BARORECEPTORS—Specialized sensory nerve endings sensitive to changes in blood pressure, located at certain sites in the walls of arteries, such as the aortic arch and carotid sinus, located at or above the bifurcation of the carotid arteries in the neck. They function to maintain the blood pressure within the normal range.

BASEMENT MEMBRANE—The delicate layer of extracellular condensation of the chemical substances, mucopolysaccharides, and proteins underlying the epithelium of mucous membranes and the outside endothelium of blood vessels. Diabetics develop a thickening of the basement membrane of blood vessels in smooth muscle cells and in the kidneys.

BETA-BLOCKERS—Another name for beta-adrenergic antagonists, the medicines that prevent beta-receptor activity, slowing the heart rate and decreasing the force of the heart's pumping action.

BIFURCATION—Division into two branches.

BLALOCK-TAUSSIG OPERATION—A surgical procedure developed by Dr. Alfred Blalock and Dr. Helen Taussig at The Johns Hopkins School of Medicine for the treatment of the congenital heart defect of tetralogy of Fallot. It consists in creating an artificial shunt from a nearby artery in order to bypass the narrowed pulmonary valve.

BLOOD GROUPS—A system of classification based on the presence of substances called *agglutinogens* on human red blood cells and antibodies to these substances in the serum. The major blood groups in man are A, B, AB, and O. Red blood cells contain agglutinogen A (group A), B (group B), A plus B (group AB), or none of these (group O). A person's serum contains antibodies to the agglutinogen(s) not present in his red blood cells. There are other subgroups and additional markers besides these major ones.

BLOODLETTING—A procedure consisting in removal of blood from a vein, once used as a form of treatment for many types of disease.

BLOOD PRESSURE—Pressure of the blood as it moves through the arteries, divided into systolic and diastolic. Systolic blood pressure is the top number in the blood pressure fraction and is the measure of pressure when the heart is contracting, or pumping. Diastolic blood pressure is the bottom number in the blood pressure

fraction and is the measure of pressure when the heart is relaxed and filling with blood.

BLOOD TRANSFUSION—The removal of blood from a vein of one person (donor) and its intravenous administration into the vein of another person (recipient).

BRACHIAL—Pertaining to the arm.

BRADYCARDIA—A heart rate of less than 50 beats a minute.

BRADYCARDIA, SINUS—Bradycardia as a normal response to everyday demands.

BRADYCARDIA-TACHYCARDIA SYNDROME—A type of sick sinus syndrome, in which periods without a heartbeat (asystole) alternate with periods of rapid heartbeat (atrial flutter or fibrillation).

BRAIN DEATH—Irreversible brain damage causing complete cessation of cerebral cortex function and brain stem activity.

BRUIT—A swishing noise produced by blood as it rushes through an artery narrowed by an obstructive lesion.

BUNDLE OF HIS—These specialized muscle fibers originate in the atrioventricular node, connect to the atrioventricular junction, and pass under the endocardium into the ventricles, transmitting the contraction rhythm from the atria to the ventricles through the Purkinje fibers.

BYPASS OPERATION—A surgical procedure in which a graft is attached to an artery above and below the site of obstruction to provide normal blood flow distal to the diseased vessel.

CABG—*See* BYPASS OPERATION.

CALCIFICATION—The process by which tissues, including those of the arterial wall, become hardened by a deposit of calcium.

CALCIUM DEPOSITION—*See* CALCIFICATION.

CANNULA—A tube used for insertion into a blood vessel or the heart.

CAPILLARIES—Small vessels, only one cell in thickness, from which blood supplies oxygen and nutrients to tissues. Formed by the branchings of arterioles, they combine into larger vessels called venules.

CARDIAC ARREST—Cessation of heart function.

CARDIAC ASTHMA—*See* PAROXYSMAL NOCTURNAL DYSPNEA.

CARDIAC CATHETERIZATION—Passage of a catheter through a peripheral artery or vein to the heart to measure flow or pressure in the heart chambers, and to inject a radiopaque substance to observe by x-ray the function of the heart and the coronary arteries.

CARDIAC OUTPUT—The total volume of blood ejected by the heart each minute.

CARDIAC REHABILITATION—A formal program consisting in a dietary regimen, medication, and progressive exercise, directed toward improving cardiac function.

CARDIAC TAMPONADE—A condition, usually caused by bleeding from the heart or a major vessel near the heart, in which the pericardial sac around the heart rapidly fills with blood. This causes compression of the heart, which usually is fatal in a very short time unless corrected by removal of the blood or fluid.

CARDIAC TRANSPLANTATION—Replacing a severely diseased heart with a functional one from a donor.

CARDIOMYOPATHY—A group of diseases, often of undetermined cause, characterized by dysfunction of heart muscle and heart failure due to weakness and dysfunction of the heart muscles per se. Other causes of heart failure must be excluded.

CARDIOMYOPLASTY—An operation for heart failure in which muscle from the patient's latissimus dorsi muscle is wrapped around the heart, and pacing is used to synchronize muscle stimulation with heart contraction, theoretically improving contraction.

CARDIOPLEGIA—Stopping contraction of heart muscle, usually by a chemical substance such as potassium.

CARDIOPLEGIC DRUG—A drug used to produce paralysis, or arrest, of the heart.

CARDIOPULMONARY BYPASS—Used synonymously with the heart-lung machine. Venous blood is diverted to the artificial lung of the machine, where it is oxygenated and carbon dioxide is removed. The oxygenated blood is then pumped back into the patient's arterial system.

CARDIOVASCULAR SYPHILIS—An infection caused by the spirochete *Treponema pallidum* involving the heart and major arteries.

CARDIOVERSION—Restoration of a normal heartbeat by administration of an electrical shock or drug.

CARDIOVERTER/DEFIBRILLATOR, IMPLANTABLE—A battery-driven device implanted within the chest that is capable not only of pacing the heart when abnormal rhythms occur but also of delivering a shock to it to convert chaotic (abnormal) rhythms to normal ones.

CAROTID ARTERIES—The principal arteries that supply blood to the brain. They arise from the innominate artery on the right and the aortic arch on the left.

CAROTID SINUS—A bulbar structure at or above the bifurcation of the common carotid artery into the external and internal carotid arteries in the neck. The sinus, which is in the wall of the artery, contains specialized nerve endings that respond to distension of the wall produced by a rise in blood pressure. These receptors function to maintain normal blood pressure.

CATABOLISM—Those metabolic reactions in which cells or tissues and large molecules are broken down.

CATECHOLAMINES—A group of compounds that contain the structure catechol to which a portion containing an amine is attached. Adrenaline (epinephrine), noradrenaline (norepinephrine), and dopamine are examples. They exert actions on the cardiovascular system associated with the sympathetic nervous system.

CATHETER—A long, extremely narrow tube used in cardiac diagnostic and therapeutic procedures to introduce fluids or devices into the blood vessels.

CATHETER ABLATION—Nonsurgical removal or elimination of cardiac tissue through a catheter using radiofrequency energy. Sites responsible for arrhythmias identified by electrophysiologic mapping studies may be removed by special catheters whose tips transmit the radiofrequency energy to the tissue.

CAT SCANNING—*See* COMPUTED TOMOGRAPHY.

CELIAC ARTERY—An artery that arises from the abdominal aorta and divides into arteries supplying blood to the liver, spleen, and stomach.

CELLULITIS—An inflammation under the skin of connective tissue.

CEREBELLUM—One of the divisions of the brain, concerned with the coordination of movements.

CEREBROVASCULAR—Pertaining to the blood vessels of the cerebrum (the principal portion of the brain).

CHEYNE-STOKES RESPIRATIONS—An alternating pattern of fast, deep breathing and slow, shallow breathing.

CHOLESTEROL—Type of animal fat called a sterol. The body gets cholesterol both by making it and from the diet.

CHOLESTEROL RATIO—Usually refers to the ratio of total cholesterol to HDL-cholesterol. A high ratio of total cholesterol to HDL-cholesterol (more than 5 for individuals without atherosclerotic disease and more than 4 for individuals with atherosclerotic disease) indicates increased risk for coronary artery disease.

CHORDAE TENDINEAE—Stringlike attachments that connect the edges of the mitral and tricuspid valves to the papillary muscles in the ventricles of the heart. They resemble ropes attached to the edges of a parachute.

CHOREA—Disorder of the central nervous system characterized by spastic twitchings of the muscles.

CHYLOMICRON—A large lipoprotein in the blood that is manufactured in the intestine by using fats and cholesterol obtained in the diet. Chylomicrons deliver triglycerides to cells.

CIRCLE OF WILLIS—A network of arteries resembling a circle, formed by the main arteries supplying the brain and located at the base of the brain.

CIRCULATION—The movement of blood through the circuit of blood vessels (the vascular tree). *See also* EXTRACORPOREAL CIRCULATION.

CIRCUMFLEX CORONARY ARTERY—One of the two main branches that normally originate from the left coronary artery. These branches supply blood to the left lateral and posterior aspects of the heart.

CLOT BUSTERS—*See* THROMBOLYTIC THERAPY.

COARCTATION OF THE AORTA—A congenital heart defect characterized by a severe narrowing of the aorta, usually in the distal part of the arch.

COLLAGEN TISSUE—A type of fibrous connective protein tissue that supports the skin, tendons, arterial wall, and similar structures.

COLLATERAL CIRCULATION—The development of connections around an obstruction to blood flow by growth of small arteries above and below the obstruction. This is nature's method of compensating for obstruction in blood flow.

COMPUTED TOMOGRAPHY—A study by radiography of the body's internal structures in which three-dimensional images are created by computer from plane images taken along an axis. Also called *CT* or *CAT scanning.*

CONGENITAL CORONARY ARTERY DISEASE—A form of inherited abnormality in the coronary arteries.

CONGESTIVE HEART FAILURE—A form of heart failure characterized by venous congestion producing prominent neck veins, fluid retention in the lungs, hepatic enlargement, and edema of the legs.

CONTRACTILITY OF THE HEART—The ability of the heart muscle to contract and pump blood.

CONTRAINDICATION—Something, such as a preexisting condition, that makes a particular therapy or procedure inadvisable.

CONTRAST AGENT—A substance introduced into the body to enhance differentiation during diagnostic radiology visualization.

CORONARY ARTERIES—Two main arteries and their associated branches that supply the heart with the oxygen and nutrients it needs to function.

CORONARY ARTERIOGRAPHY—Radiographic visualization of the coronary arteries, performed by introducing a catheter through which radiopaque dye is injected into these vessels.

CORONARY ARTERY BYPASS GRAFTING—*See* BYPASS OPERATION.

CORONARY ARTERY DISEASE—Atherosclerotic plaque within the coronary arteries.

CORONARY-PRONE BEHAVIOR PATTERN—*See* TYPE A PERSONALITY.

CT SCANNING—*See* COMPUTED TOMOGRAPHY.

CULPRIT LESION—The type of atherosclerotic lesion that researchers now believe may be responsible for most heart attacks. The culprit lesion has a lipid-rich core and usually a thin rather than thick cap, so is prone to rupturing. The degree of vessel narrowing may be only 30 to 50 percent. Also called *unstable* or *vulnerable atherosclerotic lesion*.

CYANOSIS—A clinical condition characterized by a bluish appearance caused by lack of oxygen in the blood.

CYSTIC MEDIAL NECROSIS—Death of cells in the media of the arterial wall, with formation of a cyst or open space at the site of tissue destruction. This condition may lead to dissection of the layers of the artery's wall, a catastrophic cardiovascular situation.

CYSTOSCOPE—A lighted tubular instrument that can be inserted through the urethra into the urinary bladder for visualization.

DEFIBRILLATION—Termination of an extremely rapid, irregular, and ineffective heartbeat, usually by electric shock.

DEPOLARIZATION—The process from the endocardium to the epicardium of changing the resting (polarized) state to an activated (positively charged) state in myocardial cells, resulting in activation of ordinary ventricular muscle.

DIASTOLE—The phase of the heart's cycle during which it relaxes and fills its chambers with blood.

DIASTOLIC BLOOD PRESSURE—The minimal blood pressure observed during ventricular diastole.

DIGITALIS—A drug that, when administered in the proper dosage, stimulates contractility and slows the failing heart. Excess digitalis can result in poisoning and produce severe toxicity.

DISSECTION—Separation, or division, of the tissues of the body.

DISTAL—Remote, farther from any point of reference; the opposite of *proximal*.

DIURETIC—A pharmacologic agent that promotes excretion of urine.

DOPPLER ULTRASONOGRAPHY—A noninvasive diagnostic technique that employs high-pitched sound waves to calculate the speed and direction of flowing red blood cells. These measures are reported both audibly and visually by echocardiography. A special type of Doppler study reports its findings on blood flow in color, with each color indicating a speed and a direction in a two-dimensional image. These studies are especially valuable in evaluating blood flow through valves or any abnormal blood flow.

DROP ATTACK—Sudden loss of consciousness because of arrhythmia or complete heart block, also called *Stokes-Adams attack* or *Stokes-Adams syndrome*.

DROPSY—In cardiac dysfunction, the abnormal accumulation of fluid in bodily tissues.

DUCTUS ARTERIOSUS—The fetal blood vessel that connects the pulmonary artery with the aorta. It may fail to close at birth—a malfunction that causes the congenital abnormality called *patent ductus arteriosus*.

DUCTUS VENOSUS—A vessel that brings oxygenated blood from the mother's placenta to the fetus. This vessel bypasses the liver of the fetus and goes directly to the right atrium.

DYSARTHRIA—Speech difficulty or imperfect articulation.

DYSPNEA—Labored or difficult breathing. When shortness of breath is detectable during activity but disappears when exertion stops, the condition is termed *exertional dyspnea*.

ECHOCARDIOGRAPHY—A method of imaging and recording the motion of the wall and internal structures of the heart by echo from beams of ultrasound waves directed through the chest wall.

ECTOPIC FOCUS—A heartbeat caused by an impulse generated somewhere in the heart other than in the normal sinoatrial node.

EDEMA—The presence of abnormally large amounts of fluid in the intracellular tissue spaces of the body. When swelling does not rebound quickly when pressed, it is called *pitting edema*.

When the fluid accumulates in the lungs, it is called *pulmonary edema.*

EDEMA, PITTING—Edema in which indentation caused by external pressure remains after the pressure is removed. Pitting helps distinguish fluid edema from myxedema, which is a dry, waxy swelling of the skin associated with hypothyroidism.

EDRF—*See* NITRIC OXIDE.

EJECTION FRACTION—That part, or fraction, of all blood in the ventricle that is actually ejected at each heartbeat. A normal ejection fraction is 50 percent or more.

ELASTIN—A type of elastic tissue that occurs in the wall of the arteries and other tissues of the body.

ELECTROCARDIOGRAM—A recording of a tracing of the heart's electrical activities, usually measured in a standard way.

ELECTROCARDIOGRAPHY—Recording of the electrical impulses of the heart, usually in the form of the electrocardiogram.

ELECTROPHYSIOLOGIC STUDY—The diagnostic procedure of mapping the conduction pathways of the electric impulses and any abnormalities.

EMBOLECTOMY—An operation in which an embolus (*see* EMBOLUS) is removed from a blood vessel.

EMBOLIC STROKE—A stroke caused by the blockage of an artery to the brain by a clot or other form of obstruction brought there by the blood current.

EMBOLISM—The sudden blocking of a blood vessel by an EMBOLUS. *See also* THROMBOEMBOLISM.

EMBOLIZATION, PERIPHERAL—Obstruction or occlusion of a distal artery in the arms, legs, brain, or kidney, usually by a clot, but sometimes by a mass of bacteria or other matter transported in the blood stream from some proximal or central source.

EMBOLUS—A clot or other matter that travels through the blood stream to lodge in a small vessel and obstruct the circulation. *See also* PULMONARY EMBOLUS.

EMPHYSEMA—The loss of elasticity of the bronchi in the lungs, resulting in chronic overexpansion in the lungs and leading to shortness of breath.

ENCEPHALOPATHY—Any degenerative disease of the brain.

ENDARTERECTOMY—A surgical procedure in which the artery is opened and the atherosclerotic plaque is peeled away from the arterial wall and removed. The incision may be closed by suturing the remaining normal walls or by using a patch graft that provides a widely patent lumen in the previously diseased vessel.

ENDOCARDIAL FIBROELASTOSIS—A condition characterized by overgrowth of the endocardium, or lining, of the left ventricle, resulting in a thickening that decreases the volume capacity of the left ventricle.

ENDOCARDIUM—The inner lining of the heart that is in contact with the blood.

ENDOGENOUS—Caused by or related to factors *within* the body or a given system.

ENDOTHELIUM—The innermost layer of cells lining a blood vessel.

EPICARDIUM—The outer layer of the heart in contact with the pericardial sac that contains the heart.

ERYTHROCYTES—The red blood cells containing hemoglobin. Their main function is to transport oxygen.

ESTERS—Chemical compounds that are formed from an alcohol and an acid by the removal of water.

ETIOLOGY—The study of the cause of any disease.

EXCISION—The surgical removal of a diseased segment of tissue or vessel.

EXCITOTOXICITY—The result of a process that occurs during ischemia, in which excitatory influences tend to predominate, stimulating neurons to fire, further consuming scarce energy and oxygen and resulting in the faltering of neuronal function.

EXERCISE STRESS TEST—A type of stress test in which patients usually walk on a treadmill or pedal a stationary cycle while physicians use electrocardiography, echocardiography, and scanning techniques to study heart function and coronary artery blood supply.

EXOGENOUS—Caused by or related to factors *outside* the body or a given system.

EXSANGUINATION—Forceful expulsion of blood from the body.

EXTRACELLULAR—Outside of a cell or cells.

EXTRACORPOREAL CIRCULATION—Circulation of the blood through a mechanical device, usually a heart-lung machine, outside the patient's body.

EXTRACRANIAL ARTERIES—Arteries supplying blood to the brain before they enter the skull.

FATTY STREAK—A small, flat, yellowish patch in the artery wall that appears to be the earliest lesion in the development of atherosclerosis. Fatty streaks are found even in very young children.

FEMORAL ARTERY—An artery in the upper part of the leg.

FIBRILLATION—Contraction or twitching of individual muscle fibers.

FIBRIN—An elastic filament protein that is formed by the action of thrombin to produce the clotting of blood.

FIBRINOGEN—A long fibrillar protein found in the blood. It is transformed into a smaller protein called fibrin during the formation of a blood clot.

FIBROELASTIC—Tissue composed of fibrous and elastic elements.

FIBROMUSCULAR HYPERPLASIA—The abnormal increase in the number of normal muscle cells in an artery, causing thickening of the wall and narrowing or occlusion of the vessel. It usually occurs in the renal arteries, where it may cause hypertension.

FIBROSIS—The formation of fibrous tissue.

FIBROUS PLAQUE—A type of atherosclerotic lesion that is covered by a cap of fibrous tissue containing collagen, elastic fibers, and smooth muscle cells filled with fat. Most of the total fat in the plaque, however, is found outside the cells.

FLUTTER, ATRIAL—A heartbeat irregularity in which atrial contractions exceed ventricular contractions in number.

FORAMEN OVALE—An oval opening in the septum of the fetal heart between the right and left atria that normally closes after birth.

FUSIFORM—Spindle-shaped.

GALLOP RHYTHM—An abnormal heart rhythm in which there are three or four heart sounds (rather than the normal two) in each heartbeat, like the sound of a galloping horse.

GANGLIA—Knotlike masses of a group of nerve cell bodies located outside the central nervous system.

GLOBULINS—A group of blood proteins, some of which function as antibodies.

GLYCOGEN—Chemically, a polysaccharide that is formed and stored in the liver, muscles, and, to a lesser extent, other tissues. The chief carbohydrate storage material in the body, it is readily converted into glucose when needed.

GRAFT—As a verb, to implant (living tissue) surgically; to join by grafting.

GROIN—The region between the abdomen and thigh.

HDL-CHOLESTEROL—The cholesterol contained in high-density lipoproteins, which are lipoproteins in the blood that are believed to return excess cholesterol to the liver for excretion. HDL-cholesterol is known as "good" cholesterol because high levels correlate with reduced risk for coronary artery disease in population studies.

HEART BLOCK—A condition in which conduction of the heart's electrical impulses is blocked or slowed by an impedance, or barrier, along the conduction pathway.

HEART BLOCK, COMPLETE—Complete cessation of electrical communication between the atria and the ventricles. *See* HEART BLOCK, THIRD-DEGREE.

HEART BLOCK, FIRST-DEGREE—An irregular heart rhythm in which atrial and ventricular contractions are matched, but the electrical impulse slows during conduction through the atrioventricular node and causes a change in the P–R interval on the electrocardiogram.

HEART BLOCK, SECOND-DEGREE—An irregular heart rhythm in which multiple atrial contractions occur to each single ventricular contraction because of the failure of the sinus node impulse to proceed properly through the atrioventricular node.

HEART BLOCK, THIRD-DEGREE—An irregular heart rhythm in which electrical impulses from the sinus node to the ventricle cease to pass through the atrioventricular node, and ventricle pacing becomes controlled by a pacing mechanism within the ventricle and unrelated to sinoatrial node impulses. Severe bradycardia results.

HEART FAILURE—Generally, a clinical syndrome in which cardiac output is inadequate to meet the body's needs, associated with reduced exercise tolerance and a high incidence of ventricular arrhythmias.

HEART–LUNG MACHINE—A mechanical pump used during heart surgery to shunt blood away from the heart, oxygenate it, and return it to the body, thereby maintaining blood circulation. *See also* CARDIOPULMONARY BYPASS.

HEMOGLOBIN—A conjugated protein within the red blood cells (erythrocytes) that is capable of transporting oxygen and carbon dioxide.

HEMORRHAGE—Bleeding or the escape of blood from the blood vessels.

HEPARIN—A mucopolysaccharide acid occurring in various tissues but most abundantly in the liver. When injected into the circulation, it blocks blood coagulation and promotes the clearing of triglyceride fat.

HETEROGRAFT—The graft of donor tissue transplanted from one animal species to another animal species.

HIGH-DENSITY LIPOPROTEIN CHOLESTEROL—*See* HDL-CHOLESTEROL.

HOLTER MONITOR—A portable electrocardiography device for tracking heart function that is worn by patients outside the hospital during daily activities.

HOMEOSTASIS—A state of equilibrium in which the chemical substances and various components of the body are in balance with each other.

HOMOCYSTEINE—An amino acid, elevations of which can predispose blood factors to form clots and which are linked to increased risk for heart attack and stroke.

HOMOGRAFT—Human tissue used to replace a diseased blood vessel or organ, usually obtained from a cadaver.

HYDROLYZE—To cleave (or break) a chemical bond with water. For example, a triglyceride is hydrolyzed, or broken down, into glycerol and free fatty acid components.

HYPERCHOLESTEROLEMIA—Elevation of the plasma or serum cholesterol concentration.

HYPERLIPIDEMIA—An abnormally high concentration of lipids (fats) in the blood.

HYPERLIPIDEMIC SERUM—Serum that contains an elevated concentration of the blood lipids. This term is used most often to refer to serum in which the triglyceride blood fats are elevated.

HYPERTENSION—The condition in which the blood pressure within the arteries is elevated.

HYPERTHYROIDISM—Excessive thyroid activity.

HYPERTRIGLYCERIDEMIA—Elevation of the concentration of the plasma or serum triglycerides.

HYPERTROPHIED MUSCLE—Muscle that is enlarged because of increased activity.

HYPERTROPHY—Enlargement or overgrowth of an organ or body part.

HYPONATREMIA—Deficiency of sodium in the blood.

HYPOPLASIA—Incomplete or underdevelopment of a tissue or organ.

HYPOTENSION—Abnormally low blood pressure.

HYPOTHERMIA—The use of low body temperature to reduce cardiac output, pulse rate, blood pressure, and oxygen consumption, since cells survive longer when chilled.

HYPOTHYROIDISM—Deficiency of thyroid activity.

HYPOXIA—The condition in which the oxygen level of the body or a tissue is too low.

IDIOPATHIC—Any pathologic condition of unknown cause.

ILIAC ARTERIES—The terminal branches of the abdominal aorta; the principal arteries supplying blood to the pelvic or hip region and legs.

ILIOFEMORAL ARTERIES—Pertaining to the iliac and femoral arteries.

INFARCTION—An area of dead tissue resulting from obstruction of the artery supplying that area.

INFERIOR MESENTERIC ARTERY—The artery from the abdominal aorta that supplies the lower part of the large intestine.

INFERIOR VENA CAVA—The main vein returning blood to the heart from the lower part of the body. *See also* SUPERIOR VENA CAVA.

INNERVATION—The supply of nerves to a part of the body.

INNOMINATE ARTERY—The first of three major arteries that arise from the aortic arch. It divides into the right subclavian and right common carotid arteries.

INOTROPIC AGENTS—Those substances favorably affecting the force of muscular contraction, particularly of the heart.

INTERMITTENT CLAUDICATION—Excessive fatigue or pain in the buttocks, thighs, or calves of the legs, produced by exertion on walking a short distance and relieved by a brief period of rest.

INTERSTITIAL FLUID—The fluid in which the individual cells of the body are bathed.

INTIMA—The innermost layer of the arterial wall that is in contact with the blood.

INTRACRANIAL ARTERIES—Arteries within the skull.

IRRITABLE FOCUS—An area in the heart other than the normal sinoatrial node that is generating impulses to cause contraction of the heart muscle.

ISCHEMIA—Tissue anemia (as of heart muscle) resulting from lack of flow of arterial blood.

ISCHEMIC—The state in which a cell or tissue has an insufficient supply of blood.

LACUNE—A type of stroke resulting from atherosclerotic occlusive disease, typically occurring in major arteries supplying blood to the brain.

LDL-CHOLESTEROL—The cholesterol contained in low-density lipoproteins, which are lipoproteins in the blood that carry most of the cholesterol. Even though LDL is a necessary component of the body, LDL-cholesterol is known as "bad" cholesterol because increased levels correlate with increased risk for coronary artery disease in population studies.

LEFT ANTERIOR DESCENDING CORONARY ARTERY—One of the two main branches that normally originate from the left coronary artery. It supplies blood to the anterior wall of the heart.

LERICHE'S SYNDROME—Described by René Leriche in 1926, the condition, occurring more often in men, is characterized by intermittent claudication (excessive fatigue and pain in the legs after walking a short distance, with relief on resting) and impotence, caused by atherosclerotic occlusive disease in the aorto-iliac arteries.

LESION—An abnormality in any structure of the body.

LEUKOCYTES—The white blood cells whose main function is to protect the body against infection. The major types are polymorphonuclear leukocytes, lymphocytes, and monocytes.

LIPID PROFILE—A full, fasting lipid profile (also called a *lipoprotein profile*) consists of determinations of total cholesterol, HDL-cholesterol, triglyceride, and LDL-cholesterol. The lipid profile requires a 10- to 12-hour fast because of the variability of triglyceride level according to whether the individual has recently eaten.

LIPIDS—Fatty substances, including cholesterol, triglyceride, and phospholipid, that are present in the blood and tissues.

LIPOPROTEIN[a]—A lipoprotein identical to LDL except for the addition of a special protein called apolipoprotein[a], or apo[a]. Elevation of lipoprotein[a] in the blood has been correlated with increased risk for coronary artery disease in many population studies. Lipoprotein[a] is often referred to as "Lp little a."

LIPOPROTEINS, PLASMA—Macromolecular complexes of lipid and protein that transport all the plasma lipids or fats, including cholesterol, triglyceride, and phospholipid.

LOW-DENSITY LIPOPROTEIN CHOLESTEROL—*See* LDL-CHOLESTEROL.

LUMEN—The inner, open cavity of a tubular structure, such as an artery or vein.

LUNG EMBOLISM—Blockage of the pulmonary arteries in the lung resulting usually from thrombus or clots that break off a thrombus in the peripheral veins, usually in the legs.

LYMPHOCYTE—A type of white blood cell involved in antibody reactions. Lymphocytes are produced in lymphoid tissue and constitute 20 to 30 percent of the white blood cells (leukocytes) of normal human blood.

MAGNETIC RESONANCE IMAGING—A noninvasive diagnostic technique that relies on the magnetic resonance of the body's atoms in response to radio waves within a magnetic field to produce computerized images of internal structures. This method is used to study structural malformations (congenital defects, tumors) and to evaluate diseases of the myocardium, pericardium, and heart valves. Also called MRI.

MARFAN'S SYNDROME—A group of multiple congenital abnormalities involving connective tissue and often occurring in conjunction with cystic medial necrosis of the aorta. Patients with this syndrome generally are tall, with unusually long bones of the arms, legs, feet, and hands.

MEDIA—The middle, muscular layer of the arterial wall. The media contains smooth muscle cells, elastic tissue, and collagen.

MEMBRANE OXYGENATOR—A device made of flat bags of cellophane or Teflon used to oxygenate blood. It is a component of the heart–lung machine.

MESENTERIC ARTERIES—The major arteries that supply blood to the gastrointestinal tract.

METABOLISM—The body's chemical processes. Metabolic processes are divided into anabolic and catabolic.

MI—*See* MYOCARDIAL INFARCTION.

MITOCHONDRIA—Specialized structures within the cell that function for the oxidation of food substances and the production of energy.

MITRAL REGURGITATION—Dysfunction of the mitral valve produced if the valve is incompetent or "leaky" and allows blood to flow back into the left atrium during systole, the phase in which the heart contracts.

MITRAL STENOSIS—Narrowing or constriction of the mitral valve.

MITRAL VALVE—The valve separating the left atrium from the left ventricle of the heart. It is also called the *bicuspid valve* because it is composed of two cusps. *See also* TRICUSPID VALVE.

MOBITZ TYPE I HEART BLOCK—A type of second-degree heart block in which electrical impulses from the sinoatrial node become progressively slower and are eventually blocked at the atrioventricular junction. This pattern is followed by a pause and then resumption of the same cycle, or by transmission of an impulse through the atrioventricular node or a separately arising ventricular beat.

MOBITZ TYPE II HEART BLOCK—A type of second-degree heart block in which electrical impulses from the sinoatrial node remain normal but ventricular impulse conduction is blocked below the atrioventricular node and perhaps even below the bundle of His.

MONOCYTE—A type of white blood cell that is believed to interact with lymphocytes in immune reactions.

MONOGLYCERIDE—A glycerol molecule to which only one fatty acid molecule is attached.

MONOUNSATURATED FAT—A fat (or fatty acid) containing one double bond. Monounsaturated fat helps lower total cholesterol and LDL-cholesterol levels when it is substituted for foods high in saturated fat. The most concentrated dietary sources are olive oil, canola oil, peanut oil, and high-oleic safflower oil. Other sources are avocados and nuts (hazelnuts, pecans, macadamia nuts), as well as beef fat and pork fat (which also contain saturated fat).

MORPHOLOGIC—Pertaining to the science of forms and structure of organized beings.

MR—*See* MAGNETIC RESONANCE IMAGING.

MRI—*See* MAGNETIC RESONANCE IMAGING.

MURMUR—A sound heard on auscultation (listening through a stethoscope) of the heart, lungs, and blood vessels.

MYCOTIC ANEURYSM—An aneurysm produced by the lodging of an infected embolus in the vessel's wall.

MYOCARDIAL INFARCTION—Used synonymously with *heart attack* or *coronary thrombosis* but refers specifically to the death of part of the heart muscle (myocardium). The diagnosis is established by clinical manifestations, changes in the electrocardiogram, and measurement of blood enzymes released from the damaged heart muscle.

MYOCARDITIS—Inflammation of the heart wall's muscular layer.

MYOCARDIUM—The muscular tissue of the heart.

MYOCYTE—A muscle cell.

NEPHRITIS—Inflammation of the kidneys.

NERVE—A structure in the form of a fiber that transmits impulses between the central nervous system and parts of the body.

NEURON—A nerve cell.

NEUROPATHY—A general term describing dysfunction, with or without pathologic changes, in the peripheral nervous system.

NEUROTRANSMITTER—A substance, such as acetylcholine or norepinephrine, that transmits the nerve impulse across the synapse.

NITRIC OXIDE—A simple chemical substance, synthesized in diverse human tissues, that plays many biologic roles. In the vasculature, it is a principal determinant of resting vascular tone. Endothelium-derived relaxing factor (EDRF) is now known to be nitric oxide.

NITROGLYCERIN—A drug used to treat angina pectoris. It usually provides rapid relief of chest pain (within one to three minutes) in a patient suffering an attack of angina pectoris.

NORADRENALINE—Synonymous with norepinephrine. This hormone, secreted by the adrenal medulla, has profound effects on blood vessels, the heart, and the entire cardiovascular system, and causes the arterioles to contract and the heart rate to increase.

OCCLUSION—Closure or obstruction of a passageway or blood vessel.

OFFICE HIGH BLOOD PRESSURE—*See* WHITE COAT HIGH BLOOD PRESSURE.

ORTHOPNEA—Breathing difficulty evident when patient is lying flat.

ORTHOTOPIC—The grafting of tissue in a normal position.

OSTIUM—An opening, for example, the opening into a blood vessel (as at the tip of a straw).

PACEMAKER—The sinoatrial node. A small bundle of muscle fibers and nerves within the right atrium, the sinoatrial node sends out electrical impulses at regular intervals to cause contraction of the heart.

PACEMAKER, ARTIFICIAL—A mechanical device that can be used to control the heart rate and take the place of the patient's own natural pacemaker, the sinoatrial node.

PALLIATIVE—Treatment that provides relief for a condition but not a cure.

PALPATION—Examination with the hands and fingers to feel body structures.

PALPITATION—A subjective feeling of an irregular or unduly rapid heartbeat.

PAPILLARY MUSCLES—The muscles inside the ventricles of the heart that are attached to the mitral and tricuspid valves by means of the chordae tendineae.

PARAPARESIS—Weakness or paralysis of the lower extremities.

PARAPLEGIA—Paralysis of the legs.

PARASYMPATHETIC—Pertaining to one of the two divisions of the autonomic nervous system. Parasympathetic activity tends to slow the heart rate and cause widening or dilation of arterioles.

PARASYMPATHETIC NERVES—A subdivision of the anatomic nervous system with cranio-cerebral fibers that are, in general, functionally antagonistic to the sympathetic division and cause vasodilation in the abdominal viscera and slowing of the heart.

PARESIS—Partial or incomplete paralysis.

PAROXYSMAL NOCTURNAL DYSPNEA—Nighttime attack of breathing difficulty.

PATCH-GRAFT ANGIOPLASTY—A surgical procedure that consists in suturing a patch into an incision in the wall of an artery in order to widen the lumen of the vessel.

PATENT—Open and unobstructed, as in an unobstructed blood vessel.

PATENT DUCTUS ARTERIOSUS—A congenital anomaly consisting in a persistently open lumen of the fetal vessel (ductus arteriosus) between the aorta and pulmonary artery after birth.

PENETRATING ARTERIES—Extremely small blood vessels that branch off main arterial trunks of the basilar and middle cerebral arteries.

PENUMBRA, ISCHEMIC—A "shadow" zone around a core zone of cardiac ischemia in which blood flow is decreased but not completely lost in a stroke.

PEPTIDE—One of a class of compounds of low molecular weight that contains two or more amino acids. It may be formed by the breakdown of proteins or by linking together two or more amino acids. When a peptide reaches a certain arbitrary size, it becomes known as a protein.

PERCUSSION—A diagnostic method to determine by response the condition of an internal organ by tapping on the surface of the chest and abdomen.

PERCUTANEOUS TRANSLUMINAL ANGIO-PLASTY—An angiographic procedure in which a balloon is inflated to flatten atherosclerotic plaque against an artery wall; also known more casually as "balloon angioplasty." The balloon catheter is inserted through the skin ("percutaneous") and through blood vessel lumens ("transluminal") to reach the site of vessel narrowing. When the procedure is applied to the arteries of the heart, it is known as *percutaneous transluminal coronary angioplasty,* or *PTCA.*

PERFUSION—The flow (or spread) of blood to an area.

PERICARDIAL—Pertaining to the fibroserous sac that contains the heart.

PERICARDIECTOMY—Surgical procedure that consists in stripping off a section of the pericardium (the sac that contains the heart).

PERICARDITIS—Inflammation of the pericardial sac.

PERICARDIUM—The saclike covering that contains the heart.

PET SCANNING—*See* TOMOGRAPHY, POSITRON EMISSION.

PHEOCHROMOCYTOMA—A tumor, derived from cells in the medulla of the adrenal gland or from similar tissue growing outside the gland, that secretes the adrenal hormones adrenaline and noradrenaline, resulting in high blood pressure.

PHLEBITIS—Inflammation of a vein, often associated with thrombus (clot) formation.

PHOSPHOLIPID—A lipid or fatty constituent of the blood and of cell membranes containing glycerol, two fatty acids, and a phosphorus-containing component. It is essential for the structure of the cell membrane. In the blood it probably functions to keep the cholesterol and triglyceride in solution.

PLAQUE—A well-demarcated, raised patch or swelling on a body surface. Atheromatous plaques occur on the inner surface of an artery and are of a yellowish color produced by fatty deposits.

PLASMA—The fluid part of the blood.

PLATELET—A disk-shaped structure in the blood that plays an important role in coagulation.

PLETHYSMOGRAPHY—A method that records changes in the volume of organs, used most often to measure blood flow in the limbs or fingers.

PNEUMATIC CUFF—A cuff inflated with air used to constrict the artery in the arm to measure blood pressure.

POLYARTHRITIS—Inflammation of more than one joint.

POLYMORPHONUCLEAR LEUKOCYTE—A type of white blood cell involved in the protection of the body against infection through ingestion of bacteria.

POLYUNSATURATED FAT—A fat (or fatty acid) containing more than one double bond. Polyunsaturated fat helps lower total cholesterol and LDL-cholesterol levels when it is substituted for foods high in saturated fat. The two major types of polyunsaturated fat in the diet are omega-6 fatty acids (vegetable oils such as corn, safflower, sunflower, and soybean) and omega-3 fatty acids (fish oils). High-fat fish (mackerel and salmon) are higher in polyunsaturated fat than low-fat fish (flounder and redfish).

POPLITEAL ARTERY—An artery behind the knee that carries blood from the femoral artery to the lower portion of the leg.

POSTPHLEBITIC SYNDROME—A chronic condition, usually after occurrence of thrombophlebitis in the legs, characterized by swelling, dermatitis, pigmentation, and ulceration.

PREMATURE VENTRICULAR COMPLEXES—A type of tachycardia characterized by heartbeats that occur too soon, which are caused by premature contraction of the ventricle. These are also called *premature contractions.*

PRINZMETAL'S ANGINA—*See* ANGINA PECTORIS, VARIANT.

PROARRHYTHMIA—A rhythm disturbance or worsening of an existing rhythm irregularity induced by medication.

PROFILE, FULL LIPID—*See* LIPID PROFILE.

PROGRESSION—In reference to atherosclerotic disease, a decrease in the diameter of an artery narrowed by atherosclerosis, that is, an increase (or worsening) of the disease. Progression of atherosclerosis has been slowed or stopped in many patients by using lipid-lowering therapies.

PROPRANOLOL—A drug called a beta-blocking agent that blocks certain actions of the adrenal hormones and is used to treat angina pectoris and cardiac arrhythmias.

PROSTACYCLIN—An oxygenated unsaturated animal fatty acid that, acting like a hormone, dilates blood vessels and inhibits platelets from clustering in a mass.

PROSTHETIC DEVICE—An artificial material or device used to replace a normal structure that has been removed. In the cardiovascular system, a prosthesis may replace a defective heart valve or a diseased blood vessel.

PROXIMAL—Nearest (closer to any point of reference); the opposite of *distal*.

P/S RATIO—The ratio of the polyunsaturated to saturated fats in the diet.

PULMONARY ANGIOGRAPHY—X-ray visualization of the pulmonary arteries in the lung after injection of a radiopaque substance.

PULMONARY ARTERY—The vessel transporting blood from the right ventricle to the lungs. The pulmonary artery contains relatively deoxygenated blood that is replenished with oxygen in the lungs.

PULMONARY EDEMA—A condition associated with heart failure in which the left ventricle of the heart does not pump adequately, so that fluid accumulates within the lungs.

PULMONARY EMBOLUS—A substance that is carried from a distal part of the vascular tree to the lungs, where it is too large to pass through the pulmonary vessels. Usually, an embolus arises from a blood clot in a vein.

PULMONARY HYPERTENSION—The condition in which the pressure in the pulmonary arteries is increased, which may lead to thickening and damaging of the walls of the vessels, with back pressure exerted on blood flow from the right ventricle.

PULMONARY VALVE—The valve between the right ventricle and the pulmonary artery.

PULMONARY VEIN—The vessel carrying blood from the lungs back to the left atrium. The pulmonary veins contain blood that has been oxygenated in the lungs.

PULSE RATE—The number of beats per unit of time (per number of the radial or other superficial arterial pulse), which is usually the same as the heart rate.

PULSUS ALTERNANS—A pulse that alternates between weak and strong beats.

PURKINJE FIBERS—Fibers within the endocardium that are the terminal ends of the heart's conduction system.

PYELOGRAM—A radiograph of the kidney and ureter, usually obtained after intravenous injection of a radiopaque material.

PYROPHOSPHATE TECHNETIUM-99m SCANNING—A noninvasive nuclear scanning technique that uses the radioactive tracer pyrophosphate technetium-99m to evaluate blood flow. This tracer is used after a heart attack to identify areas of the heart affected by inadequate blood supply and to evaluate the risk of embolism after a heart attack.

RADIOPAQUE—The property of blocking x-rays, resulting in a light or white appearance on the exposed x-ray film.

RADIOPHARMACEUTICAL—A radioactive chemical or drug used in diagnosis or therapy.

RAUWOLFIA—A group of drugs used to treat hypertension. Their name comes from their origin, a genus of tropical trees and shrubs, many species of which have been used in South America, Africa, and Asia as sources of arrow poisons.

REDUCTION (REMODELING) SURGERY—An operation for heart failure in which portions of a severely dilated heart are removed, with the intention of improving function by relieving wall stress, reducing valve leakage, and remodeling the pumping chamber.

REGRESSION—In reference to atherosclerotic disease, an increase in the diameter of an artery narrowed by atherosclerosis, that is, a decrease (or improvement) in the disease. Regression of atherosclerosis has been achieved in some patients by using lipid-lowering therapies.

REGRESSION TRIAL—In reference to lipid lowering and atherosclerotic disease, a clinical trial that examines (usually by angiography or ultrasonography) whether lowering blood lipids results in improvement in atherosclerosis in the arteries. Many large regression trials have shown slowed progression and even regression of atherosclerotic disease with lipid lowering.

REJECTION—An immune response that amounts to a refusal by the body to accept a transplanted organ, resulting in the organ's failure to survive.

RENAL ARTERIES—Major arteries from the abdominal aorta to the kidneys.

RENIN—An enzyme liberated by the kidney when the blood flow to it is reduced. Renin acts on a blood globulin to cause the formation of angiotensin II, a vasoconstrictor peptide.

RESTENOSIS—Recurrent stenosis.

RHEUMATIC FEVER—An inflammatory disease that usually follows an infection by a group A beta-streptococcal organism. It is not an infection itself, but a response to previous infection, probably on an allergic basis. The heart valves and heart tissue are inflamed, as are the large joints, and the nervous system may be involved.

ROENTGENOGRAM—X-ray.

SACCIFORM—Shaped like a sac, bag, or pouch.

SAPHENOUS VEINS—The two large superficial veins of the leg.

SARCOPLASM—The cytoplasm of a muscle cell in which are embedded the fibrillae of the muscle fiber.

SATURATED FAT—A fat (or fatty acid) containing no double bonds. Saturated fat is the primary dietary factor that raises total cholesterol and LDL-cholesterol levels. It occurs in all foods of animal origin, for example, butterfat and meat fat. Tropical plant oils such as palm, coconut, and palm kernel oils are high in saturated fat.

SCINTIGRAPHY—A diagnostic technique in which a scintillation camera records the distribution of radioactivity after a radionuclide is introduced into tissues of the body.

SCLEROSING—The process of obliterating by the formation of extensive scarring.

SEDENTARY—Doing much sitting; used to refer to a physically inactive lifestyle.

SEPTICEMIA—Severe bacterial infection of the blood stream.

SEPTUM—A dividing wall or partition.

SERUM—The fluid part of the blood that remains after a blood clot is formed and removed.

SERUM CHOLESTEROL—The cholesterol contained in the serum (see SERUM and CHOLESTEROL).

SICK SINUS SYNDROME—A set of abnormalities related to failure of the sinus node to perform its pacemaker duties satisfactorily. Characteristics include producing impulses too slowly or too quickly, producing impulses that fail to cause the atria to contract, or failing to produce any impulse.

SINOATRIAL NODE—Called the *pacemaker;* a small bundle of muscle fibers and nerves within the wall of the right atrium that sends out electrical impulses at regular intervals to cause contraction of the heart. May also be called *sinus node.*

SINUS BRADYCARDIA—Slowness of the heart rate with regular rhythm, usually less than 50 beats a minute, originating in the normal sinus pacemaker.

SINUS NODE—*See* SINOATRIAL NODE.

SINUS OF VALSALVA—Pouchlike enlargements in the aorta just above the aortic valve.

SINUS RHYTHM—Heart rhythm produced by impulses of the sinoatrial node.

SINUS TACHYCARDIA—Rapid but regular heart rate, usually more than 100 beats a minute, originating in the normal sinus pacemaker.

SMALL, DENSE LDL—LDL particles with a higher proportion of protein than normal LDL particles. Having a preponderance of small, dense LDL particles (LDL pattern B) has been linked to increased risk for heart attack.

SPHYGMOMANOMETER—An instrument for measuring blood pressure in arteries.

SPLANCHNIC—Pertaining to the viscera. (*See* VISCERAL.)

STASIS DERMATITIS—Inflammation of the skin due to obstruction of blood to the area.

STATINS—Short name for HMG-CoA reductase inhibitors, a class of lipid-lowering drugs (currently including atorvastatin, fluvastatin, lovastatin, pravastatin, and simvastatin). *HMG-CoA* is an abbreviation for 3-hydroxy-3-methylglutaryl coenzyme A.

STENOSIS—Narrowing (constriction) of an orifice or the lumen of a hollow or tubular organ.

STENT—In the treatment of vascular diseases, a rodlike device used to induce or maintain the patency of blood vessels or to support anastomosed blood vessels.

STERNOTOMY—A vertical incision made in the sternum (breastbone) by a surgical saw to open the chest and expose the heart.

STEROIDS—A group of organic compounds that contain the cyclopentanoperhydrophenanthrene ring system, exemplified by sex hormones, adrenal gland hormones, and bile acids.

STETHOSCOPE—An instrument originally used to conduct sound from the chest wall to the ear, but now used to conduct sound from other areas of the body as well.

STOKES-ADAMS ATTACK or SYNDROME—A condition resulting from heart block causing unconsciousness. *See* DROP ATTACK.

STREPTOCOCCAL INFECTION—An inflammation or infection caused by streptococcal bacteria.

STRING GALVANOMETER—Designed by Willem Ëinthoven in Leyden in 1901, it consisted in a fine platinum or silvered quartz thread that was held taut in a powerful magnetic field, for recording electrical potential generated by the heart, and was the forerunner of the modern electrocardiograph. Also known as *einthoven galvanometer* or *thread galvanometer.*

STROKE—A sudden and dramatic decrease or loss of consciousness caused by rupture, blocking of a vessel with a clot, or hemorrhage in the brain.

STROKE VOLUME—The amount of blood pumped by the ventricle with each heartbeat.

SUBCLAVIAN ARTERIES—Arteries that supply blood to the upper part of the chest, shoulders, and arms. The left subclavian arises from the aorta, and the right subclavian from the innominate artery.

SUBCUTANEOUS—Beneath the skin.

SUPERIOR MESENTERIC ARTERY—The artery from the abdominal aorta that supplies the small intestine.

SUPERIOR VENA CAVA—The main vein returning blood to the heart from the upper parts of the body. *See also* INFERIOR VENA CAVA.

SUPRAVENTRICULAR—Above the ventricles.

SYMPATHECTOMY, LUMBAR—Surgical procedure consisting in excision of a small segment of the lumbar sympathetic nerve ganglia to interrupt the nerve impulses to the muscles in the walls of the arteries of the legs. Its purpose is to permit dilation of the smaller arteries and thus to increase the blood flow and to allow a greater degree of collateral circulation in the lower portion of the legs.

SYMPATHETIC—Pertaining to one of the two divisions of the autonomic nervous system. Sympathetic activity tends to speed up the heart rate and cause narrowing of the arterioles.

SYNAPSE—The area of contact where a nerve impulse is transmitted from one neuron to another.

SYNCOPE—Fainting; loss of consciousness.

SYNDROME X, CARDIOLOGIC—The finding of angina pectoris or anginalike chest pain in the presence of normal coronary angiography.

SYNDROME X, METABOLIC—A described syndrome characterized by insulin resistance or hyperinsulinemia, elevated blood triglyceride, low HDL-cholesterol, and elevated blood pressure, among other findings. It may account for a significant number of cases of atherosclerosis in which LDL-cholesterol levels are relatively normal. This syndrome, also called *insulin-resistance syndrome,* is under investigation.

SYNTHETIC GRAFT—An artificial artery of synthetic material that is used to replace a segment of a diseased artery.

SYPHILIS, CARDIOVASCULAR—Syphilis affects the cardiovascular system many years after the primary infection occurred. The aortic valve ring may become dilated with resultant aortic insufficiency, and pathologic changes may develop in the wall of the aorta that may lead to development of an aneurysm.

SYSTOLE—The phase of the heart's cycle during which the heart muscle contracts to pump blood to the body.

SYSTOLIC BLOOD PRESSURE—The maximum blood pressure occurring at the time of ventricular systole.

SYSTOLIC INDEX—*See* ANKLE/BRACHIAL INDEX.

TACHYCARDIA—A heart rate of more than 100 beats a minute.

TACHYCARDIA, SINUS—Tachycardia as a normal response to everyday demands.

TACHYCARDIA, SUPRAVENTRICULAR—A sustained, rapid heartbeat that originates in the atria or the atrioventricular node.

TACHYCARDIA, VENTRICULAR—A sustained, rapid, and regular heartbeat that arises in the ventricle.

THALLIUM SCANNING—A noninvasive method for visualizing blood flow with radioactive thallium labeling, often used in exercise stress testing to evaluate infusion of blood to the heart's muscular layer. This term is sometimes used interchangeably with *perfusion scanning*.

THORACIC—Pertaining to the chest.

THROMBIN—A protein involved in blood clotting. By causing the conversion of fibrinogen to fibrin, it promotes formation of a clot.

THROMBOEMBOLISM—Obstruction of a blood vessel by a thrombus, or clot, swept by the blood stream from its site of origin.

THROMBOENDARTERECTOMY—A surgical procedure that consists in removing a blood clot associated with an atheromatous lesion by dissecting or separating it from the arterial wall. The opening in the artery is repaired by suturing the two edges together or by inserting a patch to widen the arterial lumen.

THROMBOLYTIC AGENTS—Drugs such as streptokinase or other substances that dissolve clots.

THROMBOLYTIC THERAPY—Therapy that uses drugs to dissolve a blood clot, for example, when a blood clot has obstructed blood flow to the heart and caused a heart attack. Thrombolytic agents are also known as "clot busters." Well-known examples are tissue plasminogen activator (t-PA) and streptokinase.

THROMBOPHLEBITIS—Inflammation of a vein with thrombus, or clot, formation.

THROMBOSIS—The development or presence of a thrombus (*see* THROMBUS).

THROMBOSIS, ARTERIAL—Formation of a blood clot within the arterial system. This is the type of thrombosis that can cause heart attacks and strokes. It is rich in blood platelets and is sometimes called a *white thrombosis* because of its appearance.

THROMBOTIC STROKE—A stroke caused by thrombosis, or clot formation, in the arteries supplying blood to the brain.

THROMBUS—A clot in a blood vessel or one of the cavities of the heart, formed by coagulation of the blood. A *mural thrombus* is a blood clot attached to a diseased part of the inner lining of the heart wall.

TISSUE HYPOXIA—Low oxygen content in a tissue.

TOLERANCE—Absence or reduced response to a drug, other agents, or test substances, or immunologic unresponsiveness to an antigen that is ordinarily capable of producing a response.

TOMOGRAPHY, ELECTRON-BEAM—*See* TOMOGRAPHY, ULTRAFAST COMPUTED.

TOMOGRAPHY, POSITRON EMISSION—A tomographic scanning method whose ability to evaluate myocardial metabolism noninvasively enhances physiologic and pathophysiologic study. This technique provides a cross-sectional image of local metabolism by measuring the gamma radiation emitted when electrons in cells collide with positrons linked to radiotracers. Also called PET scanning.

TOMOGRAPHY, ULTRAFAST COMPUTED—A very fast tomographic scanning method used to assess the amount of calcification in blood vessels. Also called *electron-beam scanning* or *ultrafast CT* or *CAT scanning*.

TOTAL CHOLESTEROL—The concentration of all of the cholesterol in the blood stream, adding up the cholesterol packaged in LDL particles, HDL particles, and other lipoproteins.

TRANSESOPHAGEAL ECHOCARDIOGRAPHY—A method in which the transducer is placed in the esophagus, and thus closer to the heart, in order to obtain a more accurate echocardiogram.

TRANS FATTY ACID—A type of fatty acid (fat) created when polyunsaturated fat is converted to monounsaturated fat during the process of hydrogenation (the addition of hydrogen atoms, used to convert vegetable oils to a more solid fat). *Trans* fatty acids may increase blood cholesterol levels as much as cholesterol-raising saturated fatty acids.

TRANSIENT ISCHEMIC ATTACK—Often referred to as TIA, it is characterized by brief periods of headache, weakness, or partial paralysis of the legs or arms, and difficulty in speech.

TRANSPOSITION OF THE GREAT ARTERIES or VESSELS—A severe form of congenital heart disease. Although the basic abnormality is transposition of the aorta and pulmonary artery, there are a number of variations.

TRANSVENOUS—Through a vein.

TRICUSPID ATRESIA—A congenital heart defect in which the tricuspid valve is absent, associated with a small right ventricle and an atrial septal defect.

TRICUSPID VALVE—The valve between the right atrium and the right ventricle, so called because it has three cusps. *See also* MITRAL VALVE.

TRIGLYCERIDE—A fat containing a backbone of glycerol to which fatty acids are attached. It may be of animal or vegetable origin, and it is also manufactured by the body.

TRUNCUS ARTERIOSUS—A form of congenital heart defect in which the pulmonary artery arises from the aorta.

TYPE A PERSONALITY—The hard-driving, time-conscious person who is thought by some physicians to have an increased risk of getting premature coronary artery disease.

TYPE B PERSONALITY—The relaxed, less compulsive person who is thought by some physicians to have a lower risk of getting coronary artery disease than does the person with the hard-driving Type A personality.

ULTRASONOGRAPHY—A diagnostic imaging modality that enables visualization of deep structures in the body by recording reflections of ultrasonic waves directed into the tissues. Also called simply *ultrasound*.

ULTRASOUND—Vibrations the same in nature as sound by outside the range of human hearing. Also used to mean *ultrasonography*.

UNSATURATED FAT—A fat (or fatty acid) containing one or more double bonds; includes *monounsaturated fat* and *polyunsaturated fat*.

UREMIA—An increase in the concentration of urea and other constituents in the blood normally excreted through the kidney. It is caused by failure of kidney function and is used synonymously with kidney failure.

URIC ACID—A compound excreted in the urine of man that represents the end product from the breakdown of nucleic acids and a group of substances known as purines. Elevations of blood uric acid are often found in patients with gout.

VAGAL MANEUVERS—An attempt to terminate tachycardia or induce bradycardia and decrease myocardial contractility by stimulation of the vagus nerve.

VAGAL TONE—Inhibition of the heart, primarily the atria and sinoatrial and atrioventricular nodes, by impulses of the vagus nerve.

VALVES—Tissues in the passageways between the atria and ventricles that control passage of blood and prevent regurgitation.

VALVULAR DISEASE—Dysfunction or abnormality of the heart valves.

VALVULOPLASTY—A surgical operation on a heart valve to restore its normal function.

VASA VASORUM—The network of small vessels within the outer portion of the arterial wall. Its function is to supply oxygen to the outer wall of medium and large arteries and veins.

VASCULAR—Pertaining to the blood vessels of the body.

VASCULAR RING—A congenital abnormality of the aortic arch in which a part of the developing arch fails to disappear and may obstruct the esophagus, trachea, or both.

VASCULAR TREE—The network of blood vessels that carries blood from the heart to the tissues and back again. It comprises arteries, arterioles, capillaries, venules, and veins.

VASOVAGAL ATTACK—A transient neurovascular reaction characterized by nausea, sweating, pallor, and rapid drop in blood pressure.

VEIN—A vessel that transports blood from the capillaries in the tissues back to the heart.

VENESECTION—Incision of a vein to remove blood; once used as a form of treatment for many types of disease. *See also* BLOOD-LETTING.

VENOGRAPHY—Radiographic visualization of veins after injection of a radiopaque substance.

VENTRICLES—The large chambers of the heart from which the blood is propelled out to the lungs and the rest of the body.

VENTRICULAR FIBRILLATION—A heart irregularity or arrhythmia in which the heart beats very fast but ineffectively, so that blood is not pumped out to supply the body. This condition results in death if not corrected quickly.

VENTRICULAR SEPTAL DEFECT—An opening in the septum (wall) between the right and left ventricles (lower chambers) of the heart that permits the mixing of venous and oxygenated blood.

VENTRICULOGRAPHY, RADIONUCLIDE—A method of nuclear scanning that calculates the size and shape of the ventricles at systole and diastole, indicates the functioning of all areas of the ventricular wall, and shows ischemia from heart attack or coronary artery blockage.

VENULES—Small vessels that carry blood back toward the heart from the capillaries. They combine to form larger vessels called veins.

VERTEBRAL ARTERIES—Two arteries that arise from the right and left subclavian arteries and supply blood to the posterior and basal aspects of the brain.

VERY LOW DENSITY LIPOPROTEIN—*See* VLDL.

VISCERAL—Relating to a *viscus* (internal organ; plural *viscera*), especially the heart, liver, or intestine.

VLDL—Very low density lipoprotein. A lipoprotein, manufactured in the liver, that delivers triglyceride to cells. Some VLDL particles eventually become LDL particles (LDL particles derive from VLDL particles). In a fasting measure of blood triglyceride, the triglyceride in VLDL particles usually accounts for most of the triglyceride value.

WENCKEBACH PHENOMENON—A form of heart block characterized by longer conduction with each heartbeat until conduction is completely blocked, after which conduction is restored and the cycle is repeated.

WHITE COAT HIGH BLOOD PRESSURE—High blood pressure caused by the stress of being evaluated by a physician. May also be called *office high blood pressure*.

XENO—A prefix that denotes relation to foreign material.

XENOGRAFT—The grafting of tissue from an animal of one species to that of another species. Same as *heterograft*.

Index

QRS wave, 29-31, 60, 118, 157
Quinidine, 138, 145, 446

R wave, 29-31, 60
Radiation, affect on heart, 330, 332
Radionuclide test. *see* Angiography;
    Ventriculography
Radiopaque injection, 221-222
Rehn, Ludwig, 223, 376
Renaissance, 3, 5, 7, 8-9
Renal arteries
    blood flow to, 43
    disease in, 193
    occlusive disease affecting, 294-295
    see also Kidneys
Renal artery stenosis, 172-173
    see also Hypertension; Kidneys
Renin, 295
Resnick, W.H., 16
Respiration. *see* Breathing problems
Restenosis
    in atherosclerosis, 196-197
    in coronary artery disease, 279
Rheumatic fever, and heart disease, 15, 325,
    335-336, 343
Rheumatic heart disease
    effects of, 300
    see also Coronary artery disease; Heart disease
Richards, Dickinson W., 223
Risk factors
    in aging, 80, 83-85, 96, 138, 408
    of alcohol, 52, 98, 105-106, 133, 137, 425
    for atherosclerosis, 79, 80-85, 96-100
    for caffeine, 52, 121-123, 419
    for cholesterol, 52, 79-80, 83-84, 86, 92-100,
        92-93, 95, 192, 196, 300, 408-411,
        421-428
    for coronary artery surgery, 195, 196, 197-198,
        407
    for coronary heart disease, 79-112
    definition, 79
    emotional, 107-112, 431-432
    for hypertension, 84, 89-90, 172, 173-177,
        188, 407, 412, 419-421
    for oral contraceptives, 87, 176-177, 408, 409,
        410, 421
    of physical inactivity, 80, 95-96, 103-105, 174,
        410, 428-431
    risk reduction factors, 107-108, 111-112
    for smoking, 52, 79, 84, 86-89, 101-102, 107,
        189, 409, 410, 416-419
    for stroke, 83, 84-85, 87, 299-300
Riva-Rocci, Scipione, 45-46
Robb, G.P., 223
Roentgen, Wilhelm Konrad, 221
Roth, C., 222

S wave, 31, 60, 118, 261
Sabiston, David, 269
St. Jude prostheses, 341-342
St. Vitus Dance, 335
Salt. *see* Sodium
Santos, J. Cid dos, 217
Santos, R. dos, 222
Saphenous vein autograft, 203, 269-272, 275-276,
    294
    see also Bypass surgery
Sarcoidosis, 329
Sauerbruch, Ernst Ferdinand, 223
Scarpa, Antonio, 211
Schmieden, V., 224

Scintigraphy. *see* Angiography
Sclerotheraphy, for varicose veins, 182
Septicemia, 336
Septum, defects of, 242-245, 281-282
Servetus, Michael, 6
Seven Countries Study, 92
Sex
    after heart attack, 465
    after sympathectomy, 292
    effect on heart rate, 23
    impotence, 416, 438, 442, 446
    relation to heart failure, 130
Shock
    cardiogenic, 374
    evaluation of, 77
    in occlusive disease, 298
    symptoms of, 54
Shumway, Norman, 378-379
Siccard, J.A., 221
Sick sinus syndrome, 141
Simvastatin Survival Study (4S Study), risk factors
    evaluation, 83-84, 99-100
Sinoatrial node
    dysfunction, 139, 141
    function, 19, 28, 29, 133, 134, 153, 445
Sinus of Valsalva, aneurysm of, 247-248, 356
Sinus venosus, 243
Skin, examination of, 53-54
Skoda, Joseph, 21-22
Smoking
    and atherosclerosis, 195
    effect on heart rate, 32, 123, 133, 136, 137, 142
    and hypertension, 176-177
    risk associated with, 52, 79-80, 84, 86-89,
        101-102, 107, 189, 409, 410, 416-419
    and stroke, 300
Sodium
    relation to heart failure, 121, 122, 373
    risk associated with, 80, 438
    role in hypertension, 175, 420, 427
    see also Diet; Hypertension
Sokoloff, Louis, 66
Sones, F.M., 223
Souttar, Henry S., 224
Speech, affected by stroke, 301-302, 310, 316
Sphygmomanometer, 45-46, 170
    see also Blood pressure
Spironolactone, 441-442
Spleen
    blood flow to, 43
    occlusive disease affecting, 294-298
Statin. *see* HMG-CoA reductase inhibitor
Steinberg, I., 223
Stenosis
    aortic, 249-251
    arterial, 273
Stent implantation, 203-205, 367-368
Stethoscope, 21-23, 170
Stimulants
    affect on heart rate, 32, 33, 133, 136
    see also Alcohol; Caffeine
Stokes-Adams attack, 36, 155, 157, 158
Stomach
    blood flow to, 40
    occlusive disease affecting, 294-298
    ulcer in, 109
    see also Abdominal aorta
Streptokinase, 207
Stress
    and angina, 259
    and heart rate, 133

and hypertension, 176
    medication affecting, 442
    risk associated with, 107-112, 431-432
    see also Emotions
Strieder, John, 224
String galvanometer, 29
Stroke
    biochemical events of, 311-313
    breathing problems in, 51
    causes, 40, 75, 110, 138, 169, 186, 300-301,
        339, 397, 408, 416
    embolic, 301
    evaluation and treatment, 306-307
    from embolus, 34
    ischemic, 308-309, 311-313, 314
    lacune, 301
    medical aspects of, 299
    physiology of, 303-306
    rehabilitation for, 310-311
    risk factors for, 83, 84-85, 87, 299-300
    surgical treatment of, 313-322
    symptoms of, 301-303
    thrombolytic therapy for, 307-310
    thrombotic, 301
Stroke volume, evaluation of, 70
Subclavian arteries
    function, 40
    occlusive lesions in, 317
Subvalvular aortic stenosis, 249
Superior vena cava, 17
Support network, 130, 149, 464
    see also Cardiac rehabilitation
Surgery
    cardiovascular, 211-228
    development of, 8-9, 13-14
    endovascular, 367-368
    open heart surgery development, 15
    see also Bypass surgery
Survival of Patients with Left Ventricular
    Dysfunction (SOLVD), 448
Survival and Ventricular Enlargement (SAVE), 448
Suture
    of blood vessels, 9, 211-212, 233
    of heart, 223
Swallowing difficulties, in stroke, 302, 309, 310
Swelling. *see* Edema
Swick, M., 222
Sylvius, 7-8
Sympathectomy
    for angina pectoris, 267
    for occlusive disease, 292-294
Sympathetic nerves, affect on heart, 26-28
Symptoms diary, 50
Synapse, 311
Syncope. *see* Fainting
Syphilis
    aneurysm from, 350
    and heart disease, 343
    treatment of, 6, 15
Systolic phase. *see* Circulatory system

T wave, 31, 32, 60, 118, 261
t-PA. *see* Tissue plasminogen activator
Tachycardia, 55-56, 135, 141, 446
    pacemaker for, 163-165
    paroxysmal atrial (PATs), 137
    sinus, 31-32, 136
    supraventricular, 136-138, 163, 166, 445
    treatment for, 145, 166-167
    ventricular, 34, 138-139, 145
    see also Arrhythmia

Order form for related books by Drs. DeBakey and Gotto

The New Living Heart Diet provides easy-to-follow information on the role of diet in losing weight, preventing and treating high blood cholesterol and triglyceride, decreasing high blood pressure, and managing diabetes. The book also has chapters on vegetarian eating and vitamins and minerals. It includes 311 recipes, 72 menus, and nutrient analysis for 1,000 foods. Softcover, 414 pages, 1996.

The Living Heart Guide to Eating Out is a guide to heart-healthy eating away from home. It includes 160 tips on selecting foods lower in fat and sodium in American and ethnic restaurants, as well as fast food establishments. The book lists the amount of calories, fat, saturated fat, and cholesterol in 1,630 restaurant foods. Softcover, pocket size with 170 pages, 1993.

The Living Heart Brand Name Shopper's Guide—Third Edition, lists more than 5,000 supermarket foods low in saturated fat; values are given for calories, fat, saturated fat, carbohydrate, fiber, and sodium. It is designed to aid in the selection of foods to help you (1) lose weight, (2) lower blood cholesterol and triglyceride levels, (3) lower high blood pressure, and (4) reduce cancer risk by eating fiber. Softcover, 286 pages, 1995.

Print Name _____

Address _____

City _____ State _____ Zip _____

Please send the book(s) indicated below:

_____ copy(s) of *The New Living Heart Diet* @ $16.00 each . . . . $ _____

_____ copy(s) of *The Living Heart Guide to Eating Out* @ $9.95 each . . . . $ _____

_____ copy(s) of *The Living Heart Brand Name Shopper's Guide* @ $14.95 each . . . . $ _____

Add $3.00 for postage and handling for the first book $ _____

and $1.50 for each additional book $ _____

TOTAL $ _____

Make check or money order payable to Diet Modification Clinic.
Please return to: Diet Modification Clinic, 6565 Fannin, F770, Houston, TX 77030
Phone: (713) 798-4150

━━━━━━━━━ **To order additional copies of *The New Living Heart* . . .** ━━━━━━━━━

Copies of *The New Living Heart* are available wherever books are sold. If you cannot find *The New Living Heart* at your favorite retail outlet, you may order it directly from the publisher for $17.95 plus $4.50 shipping and handling. **BY PHONE:** Call 1-800-872-5627 (in Massachusetts 781-767-8100). We accept Visa, Mastercard, and American Express. **BY MAIL:** Write out the full title of the book you'd like to order and send payment, including $4.50 for shipping and handling, to: Adams Media Corporation, 260 Center Street, Holbrook, MA 02343. 30-day money-back guarantee.